Peter Shalit

Living Well

Living Well

The Gay Man's ESSENTIAL Health Guide

by **Peter Shalit, M.D., Ph.D.**

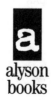

alyson books

LOS ANGELES • NEW YORK

NOTICE TO READERS

THIS BOOK IS INTENDED AS A REFERENCE VOLUME ONLY. IT IS NOT A MEDICAL MANUAL. THE INFORMATION CONTAINED IN THIS MANUAL WAS WRITTEN TO HELP READERS MAKE INFORMED DECISIONS ABOUT HEALTH ISSUES ASSOCIATED WITH THEIR SEXUALITY. IT WAS NOT DESIGNED AS A SUBSTITUTE FOR ANY TREATMENT THAT MAY HAVE BEEN PRESCRIBED BY YOUR PERSONAL PHYSICIAN. IF YOU SUSPECT THAT YOU HAVE A MEDICAL PROBLEM, SEE A COMPETENT PHYSICIAN TO DISCUSS YOUR CONCERNS.

A PORTION OF THE PROCEEDS FROM THIS BOOK WILL BE DONATED TO THE PRIDE FOUNDATION IN SEATTLE.

MANUFACTURED IN THE UNITED STATES OF AMERICA.
PRINTED ON ACID-FREE PAPER.

THIS TRADE PAPERBACK ORIGINAL IS PUBLISHED BY ALYSON PUBLICATIONS INC.,
P.O. BOX 4371, LOS ANGELES, CA 90078-4371.
DISTRIBUTION IN THE UNITED KINGDOM BY TURNAROUND PUBLISHER SERVICES LTD.,
UNIT 3 OLYMPIA TRADING ESTATE, COBURG ROAD, WOOD GREEN, LONDON N22 6TZ ENGLAND.

FIRST EDITION: NOVEMBER 1998

02 01 00 99 98   10 9 8 7 6 5 4 3 2 1

ISBN 1-55583-444-2

LIBRARY OF CONGRESS CATALOGING-IN-PUBLICATION DATA
SHALIT, PETER.
    LIVING WELL : THE GAY MAN'S ESSENTIAL HEALTH GUIDE / BY PETER SHALIT.
    INCLUDES BIBLIOGRAPHICAL REFERENCES AND INDEX.
    ISBN 1-55583-444-2
    1. GAY MEN—HEALTH AND HYGIENE—POPULAR WORKS. I. TITLE.
RA777.8.S52 1998
613'.0423'08664—DC21   98-39946 CIP

CREDITS
FRONT COVER PHOTOGRAPH BY BRIAN TO. BACK COVER PHOTOGRAPHY BY CHRISTOPHER HARRITY.

For Andy

Contents

Acknowledgments

First I want to thank my patients for being so supportive and for teaching me so much about the beauty and diversity of gay men. I am also grateful to my coworkers, Jeff, Pam, Bea, Mark, Anne, Marshon, James, Edie, and Steve. They have graciously and unselfishly made it possible for me to take chunks of time out from my busy practice to write during the past 18 months.

I am indebted to my brother Andrew, who read an early version of the manuscript and gave me his frank and helpful comments when I was between editors. I thank my other family members, Gene, Willa, Emily, Amanda, and Nevin, for a lifetime of unconditional love and support.

Friends and hugs are an essential of life. I am grateful to my friends Jim, Ralph, Rick, Bill, Frank, Audie, and Douglas, and most especially my partner of 18 years, Andy. They all have helped me keep things in perspective when I felt overwhelmed by work, and they reminded me about what is really important about being a human being and a gay man.

I am grateful to the city of Victoria, Canada. This beautiful spot, just a two-hour jetfoil trip from my home in Seattle, is where I found the peace and solitude that enabled me to write much of this book.

I feel blessed to have lived in Seattle for the past 21 years. The Emerald City is a wonderful place to be a gay man. In gratitude, a percentage of the profits from this book will be donated to the Pride Foundation, a community foundation working to strengthen the lesbian, gay, transgendered, and bisexual community in the Pacific Northwest.

Last I want again to thank my patients, who have taught me most of what I know about gay men's health.

The Origins of This Book

Since 1990 I have provided general medical care for a large number of gay men. In fact, gay men are the vast majority of patients in my practice. As a gay man myself, I find this situation particularly wonderful and rewarding. It is a privilege to work with my own tribe in this way. In the process I have come to learn that gay men have their own particular spectrum of health care needs.

Much of my time as a doctor is spent teaching my patients about their health. Writing a book about health for gay men is therefore a natural outgrowth of what I do in the office all day. There are many reasons why gay men need a book of health advice written by a gay physician specifically for them.

Most general health books ignore our existence. They do not speak to us as gay men. Even books and magazines specifically about men's health seem to be unaware that many men are gay. I believe there is a reason for this, and it is not because of malice or homophobia on the part of authors and editors. Rather, it is because many straight men would be made uncomfortable or turned off if gay men's needs were addressed in discussions of male health. Instead of alienating these potential readers, the authors pretend that gay men—and homosexuality—do not exist.

Society in general tends to do the same. We gay men live in a society that assumes everyone is heterosexual unless stated otherwise. This is frustrating for many gay men. It doesn't feel good to feel invisible. So we create our own gay spaces—social settings where we are the majority, where being gay is the norm. This book is a gay space. It is populated with stories of gay men, and it is written with the assumption that you, the reader, are gay.

Gay Men's Health Issues

What health issues specifically pertain to gay men? The typical public images of gay men's health tend either to be buffed models who obviously never have to worry about a medical problem or people who have AIDS. But of course we gay men have the usual spectrum of health concerns that all human beings have. The more serious a condition is, the more important that it be seen in the setting of the person's whole life.

Gay men have earaches, sprained ankles, heart attacks, and cancer. We may smoke, drink, or use other drugs, and we may or may not want to stop. We exercise or want to start. We want to lose weight or gain weight. We complain about growing older, though we also want to live to a ripe old age. We love, lose, and grieve. But we are not the same as straight people. We deal with medical challenges in the context of our lives as gay men.

There certainly are a number of specific medical problems more common among gay men than in the general population. In my heavily gay medical practice I see many men dealing with HIV and AIDS, hepatitis, and various other sexually transmitted diseases. My patients also sometimes develop "male diseases" that are a concern for all men, such as prostate cancer, testicular cancer, and male sexual dysfunction. These disorders can bring up special concerns for a gay man, concerns that are often inadequately addressed by a medical profession that tends to assume all men are straight.

As gay men, we have our own spectrum of psychosocial stresses and life issues. Every day I see in my patients the mental and physical impact of life challenges particular to gay men in our society. Such issues include repeated losses from AIDS, discrimination by society, low self-esteem, coming-out issues, depression, growing older, and same-sex domestic violence.

Education Is Needed

I wrote this book because I believe that as gay men we need to be better educated about our health. Many gay men will not get this type of information from the general self-help medical guides, which ignore us, or from their doctors. It should come as no surprise that doctors don't know everything, and many doctors know next to nothing about gay men. Believe me. Gay and lesbian physicians are working from within the profession to try to change the situation, but change takes time.

I try to do my part. Every year I give a one-hour lecture to the class of second-year medical students at the University of Washington to try to expose them to what they should know about gay men's particular health care needs. Only one hour, but it's a start. Similar lectures are given at many other medical schools across the United States. Each year students in the class seems more and more receptive to what I have to say.

So, the next generation of physicians should be more respectful of our lives and a little more knowledgeable about our needs. But that's the next generation. Most doctors currently practicing have had no training in the special needs of gay men. Given that, if you take the responsibility to learn about your health by reading this book, it will benefit you, your health care practitioner, and the overall health care system.

Knowledge=Power

If you are an informed medical consumer, you will be better able to make decisions about your health and your use of the health care system. You will be able to have more confidence in your health care provider if you start from a position of knowledge rather than ignorance. You will become a more active participant in the treatment process and be more proactive about your health. In addition, the results of any treatment will be better the more actively you participate and the better educated you are about your health.

If you read this book, you may well become better informed than your doctor about your particular health care needs as a gay man. By bringing this knowledge into the doctor-patient relationship, not only will you improve the quality of the care you receive, but you will improve the situation for other gay men who see that doctor in the future.

What You'll Find Here

In writing this book I have tried to include all the aspects of health care that are particularly important to gay men. My intention is not that this be a complete encyclopedia of health. I have tried to limit the coverage to those medical situations that are more common among gay men and to medical issues that, while they may affect anyone, may be experienced differently by a gay man.

I have tried to write this book the same way I would talk to a patient or advise a friend. I encourage you to read it from start to finish as a discussion of what you and I, as gay men, need to know about our health. The table of contents and the index will certainly allow you to locate a topic of interest, and there are some resources listed at the end if you want to explore a given area further.

In this book I discuss how to go about finding the right doctor for you and how to deal with that weird subculture known as the health care system. You'll learn what to expect from your relationship with your doctor and how to make the most out of your medical visits.

A significant portion of the book will be devoted to aspects of sexuality, which is an area where we gay men have our own unique concerns. We will discuss the varieties of sexual expression among gay men and how to enjoy sex as safely as possible. A separate section describes the various sexually transmitted diseases that gay men can get. I also talk about general male health: the anatomy and physiology of the male parts of your body, how to keep them in good working order, the kinds of things that may go wrong with them, and what can be done to fix them.

Incidentally, remember that there are two sets of vocabularies that can be used when talking about body parts and sex: short, Anglo-Saxon terms, such as *fuck* and *cock,* and their clinical, Latin-derived counterparts, such as *intercourse* and *penis.* When chatting with a patient, I use any term that the patient is comfortable with, and frequently the Anglo-Saxon terms are more direct and meaningful. I'll use both sets of terms in this book, as appropriate to the particular situation under discussion. I hope you don't mind.

Because HIV is such an important concern for gay men, it is given special attention in this book. There are many books written for the general public entirely on the topic of HIV. What I have tried to include here is HIV 101—the basic things that any gay man, HIV-negative or HIV-positive, should know about HIV infection. If you happen to be HIV-positive or if someone important in your life is positive, then the material in this section can serve as a starting point in your learning process about this virus, what it does, and how to deal with it.

Not all medical care has to do with treating illnesses. Far from it. Preventive care is extremely important. Much of this book deals with preventive care: how to stay healthy and how to improve your overall level of health. I talk about exercise, fitness, nutrition, and prevention of cancer and heart disease. You'll also learn how to protect your health when you travel. All, of course, from a gay man's perspective.

Many men see their doctors because they are unhappy with their physical appearance and they want to change their body in some way. There are sections on cosmetic surgery and on the medical aspects of grooming as well as tattooing and piercing, popular activities that could be considered a form of cosmetic surgery practiced by nonphysicians.

Lifestyle and psychological issues are very important to one's health also. They come up repeatedly in my interactions with patients, and so they have been given their full share of space in this book. Gay men don't have a monopoly on alcohol, tobacco, and other types of substance abuse, but these problems are very, very common in our community. Drug abuse, addiction, and recovery in our community must be seen as gay issues if they are to be dealt with successfully. Gay-specific information on substance abuse and treatment is therefore included in detail. Depression and lack of self-esteem are found frequently among gay men, so they have been given attention as well.

Finally, my patients often ask my advice about their lives: medical-legal issues, domestic violence, parenting, aging, grief, loss. Although these issues are not obviously medical concerns, they are important aspects of gay men's lives and well being, and they can have a great impact on one's physical and emotional health. I have included my two cents on them as well.

Some Disclaimers

Knowledge doesn't sit still. It is changing all the time. What is true today might well not be considered true in a few years. In addition, it's important to keep in mind that much of the advice in this book represents my own opinions, based on my professional experience and judgment. A given piece of advice certainly might not be right for you. So read with a critical eye. Take the information as a starting point as you strive to be healthy.

I have attempted to make this book as accurate and up-to-date as possible. There are bound to be errors, and inevitably some facts will be out-of-date as time goes on. So feel free to contact me if you find errors or disagree with what I say, and if it makes sense to me, I'll change it in the next edition. I can be reached through the publisher or via E-mail at ps83@cornell.edu.

Many of the medical situations in this book are illustrated with anecdotes inspired by situations from my practice or experiences of friends or acquaintances or even my own. It's fun to read about people's experiences, and the anecdotes help drive home the concepts and make them seem more real. In every case I have changed the names and some of the details to protect the privacy of the men involved. Many of the anecdotes are composites of two or more true events. No individual can be recognized from the stories I have included. If you think you recognize someone, it is probably because the situation is a common one.

One last thing: Please keep in mind that this book is not a substitute for having a real, live health care professional working for you. Rather, the information here should help you stay well and enhance your ability to get the proper health care when you need it. So, if you don't already have a doctor, my first piece of advice to you is to go out and get one. Nothing can replace a face-to-face encounter with your personal physician when you have concerns about your health.

What Is a Gay Man?

Gay men, like any other group of people, have a right to culturally sensitive, medically appropriate health care. The next section of this book deals with finding the right health care provider, one who will meet your needs as a gay man. In this section I will discuss who we gay men really are in an attempt to describe our tribe, our "ethnic group." Many people do not understand that gay men need to be viewed this way. But I think it's essential to our receiving proper medical care.

Now, we know that gay men are not all alike. We are everywhere, and we are a very diverse group of people. But it's helpful to try to describe what we have in common in order to understand why we have particular concerns when we seek health care. So who exactly are we?

There are several ways a man can be described as gay: by his sexual orientation, by his sexual behavior, and by his gay socialization, or culture. Some gay men are gay in all of these aspects, although many of us possess only one or two out of these three aspects of gayness.

Sexual Orientation

Being gay certainly has to do with our sexuality. All people are sexual beings. We begin to have romantic and sexual fantasies and desires starting in childhood, and they develop as we grow. In some people sexual desire focuses on other members of the same sex; in some, desire focuses on members of the opposite sex; and some are attracted to members of both sexes. This is known as sexual orientation: homosexual, heterosexual, or bisexual.

Those of us with a predominantly homosexual orientation nowadays generally call our-selves gay men.

Humans seem to have a need to know why, and there has been much debate about what factors influence sexual orientation. The biological reason for sex is procreation. So why are some people programmed for same-sex attraction, which does not facilitate procreation? No one knows.

Certainly for most men, sexual orientation is not a conscious choice. It's easy to know that by simply looking within oneself and asking, "Did I make a choice to be attracted to mem-bers of the same—or opposite—sex?" Usually the answer is no. Just as one does not choose to be right-handed, left-handed, or ambidextrous, so a man does not choose his sexual orienta-tion. Rather, it is something within each one of us that makes itself known through feelings of attraction.

Sexual orientation often seems to be "set" at an early age; many gay men remember feel-ing different as children, though not understanding what that difference was until entering puberty. We may have had crushes on a male teacher or classmate. Some of us may have liked sewing or playing with dolls rather than football. Others may have had none of these feelings but, on entering puberty, simply began to realize that it was a man's body, not a woman's, that aroused us sexually. For many gay adolescents this can cause a great deal of emotional turmoil, as we'll discuss later.

There is debate over whether sexual orientation is genetically influenced or whether it is solely environmentally determined—by early upbringing, for example. Certainly homosexuali-ty seems to run in some families with sets of gay brothers and uncles being more common than should occur by chance. Some researchers claim to have found a genetic link to homosexuali-ty in certain families with more than one gay man in the family, although a specific gene that influences sexual orientation has not been identified. Even if such a gene exists, its effect must not be absolute. The proof comes from pairs of identical twins. By definition, a pair of identical twin brothers are genetically identical. Often, perhaps a majority of the time, if one twin is gay, the other is too. Yet sometimes a pair of identical twins includes one individual who is gay and one who is not. So genes do not completely determine sexual orientation.

Why is it important to know where our homosexuality comes from? Because even though we know that our sexual orientation is a deeply personal issue that comes from within, our society has made it a religious, legal, and political issue with a huge impact on our lives. We are various-ly viewed as deviant, evil, or felonious because of our homosexuality. This stems from the mistaken belief that people choose to be gay, and that that is an immoral, unhealthy, or illegal choice.

Some gay pundits feel that if it were proved that sexual orientation is biologically or genetically determined, then that would help others see that homosexuality is morally neutral and not a choice, and that this would help end antigay discrimination. Others are not so sure. They say that if sexual orientation were proved to have a biological basis, this would not stop discrimination. Instead it would lead to a view of homosexuality as a birth defect and might even lead to genocidal efforts to prevent the conception and birth of any baby who might turn out to be gay.

In any case, whatever leads to one's sexual orientation, in most gay men it is a state of being that cannot be changed. Our gayness seems to be an integral part of the fabric of our being, our identity, our soul. The current accepted medical view is that an individual's sexual orientation is a stable and healthy personal characteristic rather than a disease state.

Some gay men feel social or religious pressure to somehow become heterosexual. However, all medical or psychological efforts to change men's sexual orientation—whether through conditioning, aversion therapy, psychotherapy, or prayer—have ultimately led to failure, not to mention severe emotional damage for the men involved. A man's behavior might be changed but not his innate sexual orientation. Organizations such as the American Medical Association and the American Psychiatric Association have condemned such efforts to turn gay men straight. Instead, these organizations point out that a gay man's happiness is to be found by accepting and learning to be proud of his sexual orientation, which is an integral part of his being.

Certainly sexual behavior can be modified by the pressure of circumstances. We know that heterosexually oriented men can have sex with another man if they are in prison or on board ship where there is no other choice or if they are rewarded highly enough, as with some gay-for-pay porno actors or male prostitutes. Similarly, a gay man can be persuaded to have sex with a woman if he feels enough pressure or reward to do so—for example, if his culture expects him to marry and father children. This does not mean he is straight or even bisexual in orientation. His sexual orientation has not changed; he has just changed his behavior.

Of course, some men are truly bisexual and are attracted relatively equally to members of each gender. Bisexual men may relate sexually to both men and women. But by acting on their attraction, they too are being true to their innate sexual orientation, so they are not an exception to the rule that sexual orientation cannot be changed.

What proportion of men are gay? The frequently quoted 10% figure is almost certainly an overestimate. The best surveys of sexual behavior indicate that something like 2 to 4% of men are exclusively homosexual, and perhaps an equal number are bisexual to some degree. There is a tendency to focus on the number of gay men, as if the more of us there are, the more important we are. But the actual numbers are trivial. There are plenty of gay men around, whatever our percentage of the total population. As far as I am concerned, we contribute far more than our proportionate share to society.

Having a stigmatized sexual orientation can have a strong influence on a person's emotional development. Men who grow up knowing they are gay realize that they are different from the accepted model of the way a man should be. This sometimes leads to self-esteem problems and other psychological difficulties. But it can also lead to great insight, creativity, and compassion, with which many gay men are especially gifted.

Sexual Behavior

Separate from sexual orientation, there is sexual behavior. As mentioned above, although a man may feel attracted primarily toward men, his actual behavior may not reflect this. Although many homosexually oriented men identify themselves as gay and have all of their sexual and affectional relationships with other men, not all do. Some gay men marry women for various reasons, including the pressures of family, religion, or society at large. And some gay men—some clergy for example—are celibate. Their orientation but not their sexual behavior is homosexual.

Many men have some degree of attraction to members of both sexes, and they may choose to have relationships primarily with men, with women, or both. They may label themselves as bisexual, or they may prefer to call themselves gay or heterosexual if they feel that that is a better term for their predominant orientation and/or behavior.

The information in this book is intended for any man who is emotionally and/or sexually attracted to other men, and/or at times has sex with other men. If a man is also attracted to women and considers himself to be bisexual or heterosexual, so be it; but if ever he relates sexually to men, he has a gay side, and that is the side I am speaking to.

For simplicity's sake I will use *gay* rather than a more cumbersome term such as *gay or bisexual* or *men who have sex with men*. I mean to be inclusive of bisexual men and of heterosexual men who choose to relate sexually to other men at times. I use the terms *gay* and *gay man* to include both those who are gay-identified and those with a gay aspect to their lives.

As gay men, our capacity for affection and sexual expression with other men is an important factor that sets us apart from the rest of society. In addition to the psychological stress involved with activities that for many are taboo, our sexual behavior remains illegal in many places, and nowhere are our relationships given the same legal recognition as opposite-sex couplings. As a by-product of our sexual intimacy, we have the potential to spread various infections to each other, and it is our responsibility to deal with these as effectively as possible.

Gay Culture

This capacity for same-sex affection has led to the development of our rich gay culture. Gay men tend to form social groups. In a small town it may be the "tea circle" that meets one evening a month, at the home of the "bachelor" high school teacher who serves as the social director or queen bee. In a big city there may be a population of hundreds of thousands of gay men who congregate in neighborhoods and form their own gay communities with their own particular social structures, institutions, and norms.

Like members of other social groups, gay men are more at risk for particular medical conditions because of sexual and social behavior patterns within our subculture. Like other social or ethnic groups, our gay society forms a support network that is often more important to the individual gay man than is the family he was born into. Doctors are beginning to realize that each patient must be viewed in the context of his personal support network. So these networks become highly relevant to the doctor-patient relationship.

As part of our gay culture, we often create "families of choice" that may be more significant in our lives than the biological families we came from. The larger society does not recognize these families of choice, and they have no legal standing. In particular, our marital relationships are not legally recognized. There are ways to legally define these relationships so that in case of major life events—such as parenthood, illness, or death—our relationships are properly recognized by the powers that be.

Working With a Health Care Provider

In the following sections we begin with advice on how to access the health care system, what to look for in a primary care doctor, and how to find the right one. Then we'll discuss how best to communicate with your doctor once you have found that person. If you don't already have a personal physician who knows you and whom you can trust, I highly recommend you start looking for one now.

If you have a medical condition that requires ongoing care, such as HIV or diabetes or high blood pressure, you will certainly need to have a doctor. But even if you currently have no particular medical problems, there are many benefits to having a relationship with a primary health care provider. You can work with your doctor on preventive care to help maintain your health. If you do develop a medical problem, you will already have a professional to go to. In an emergency it's reassuring to know there is someone you can call on for guidance and help. Your primary care doctor can be your advocate in dealing with the rather daunting maze of health care bureaucracy.

For many people, their relationship with their doctor is one of the deepest, most significant relationships in their life. It can be uniquely intimate in that the doctor may be privy to delicate details about a person's fears, secrets, and intimate bodily functions that the patient may not share with anyone else, not even his lover or family. A doctor-patient relationship can last for many years, often far longer than many other intimate relationships.

Having taken care of many gay men for several years, I have often known a patient longer than he has known many other important people in his life. Often I know more about certain details of his life than his current lover does. It's a privilege to have that kind of intimate helping relationship.

I have accompanied many of my patients through innumerable major life events, both happy and sad: bonding with new partners, losing friends or loved ones to illness, personally facing serious or even life-threatening illnesses, dissolution of loving relationships. It is an honor to be part of these men's lives. The experience is very enriching. For many men I expect that I will be their doctor for the rest of their lives. More than once a patient has told me, "Peter, I'm glad I'm older than you. I'm counting on you to outlive me so I won't ever need to find another doctor."

This is all just a long way of saying that it is important to find the right doctor because your relationship with that person may be one of the longest and most intimate relationships you will ever have. So put some energy into getting started with one you'll want to stay with. It's worth the effort.

The next sections describe how to deal with the health care system, how to look for the right primary care doctor for you, and how best to communicate with that person. A concluding section discusses alternative or "natural" approaches to health care. These have great appeal to many people, and they have value—but in my opinion they do not eliminate the need for a personal, Western-type physician.

Finding Your Primary Care Provider

How to Obtain Health Care

The health care system is a strange subculture with its own bizarre rules, hierarchies, and etiquette. Some people like to pretend it is like any other business with consumers (patients) and providers (doctors, nurses, clinics, hospitals). But obtaining health care is much more complicated than buying a quart of milk at the supermarket. I don't think it's good to approach your health care the same way you would purchase other things you consume. Besides, the days are gone when a doctor visit cost $5, everybody paid cash (or bartered), and what tests and treatments there were were simple and inexpensive. Health care is no longer a simple transaction.

Nowadays most health care is "delivered" by large entities such as health maintenance organizations, multispecialty clinics, and physician-hospital organizations. The cost of care is financed by third parties (you and your doctor being parties number 1 and number 2). In the United States these third parties include private health insurance companies (sometimes working with employers) and also the government (providing Medicare and Medicaid for the elderly, poor, and disabled, as well as certain medical benefits for some veterans of the armed forces).

Elsewhere (Canada and Great Britain for example) most health care is financed by the government through taxes. In the United States, health care is not a right of citizenship. Instead it is up to each individual to find a way to pay for his or her health care, usually by getting insurance that pays for some or all of the cost.

It is easiest to get health care if you work for a large corporation that provides medical benefits as part of the employment package. If you are self-employed or work for a small business, you are likely to be responsible for your own health care insurance, which can be difficult and/or expensive to arrange. If you are poor, you may be eligible for Medicaid, the State-run health care program for low-income people. It's a patchwork system, and many people unfairly lack the health care coverage they need, but so far it's what we've got, and legislative efforts to improve access to health care have not gotten anywhere.

Your first step in entering the wondrous world of the health care system is to make sure you have coverage, if possible, to help pay for your care. It's possible to pay for health care as you go, but this can be risky, especially if you come up with an expensive medical problem. Besides, you'll pay more because insurance companies usually have contracts with doctors that give them a deep discount on the doctor's cash rates. These contracts also forbid the doctor from giving a discount to cash-paying patients.

Primary Care: Your Personal Health Care Provider

After obtaining medical coverage, the next step is to find yourself a good doctor who will be your entry point into the system. This doctor will need to have a relationship with the insurance plan you have chosen, whether it is an HMO or a private insurer with a list of "preferred" physicians.

Ideally you should have a relationship with a doctor who not only will be your counselor about your health but also will serve as your advocate in the health care system. The word *doctor* comes from the Latin for "teacher." Your doctor's job is not only to teach you how to stay as healthy as possible but also to help you manage medical problems as they arise and, additionally, to guide you through the intimidating maze of the health care delivery system when you need it.

The best way to get good overall health care is to have a close relationship with your own personal primary care physician. Without one it's very hard to get decent care. *Primary care* is a term referring to general medical care. Usually men get their primary care from a type of doctor known as a family practitioner or one called a general internist or (becoming old-fashioned in the United States) general practitioner. All of these sorts of doctors provide general, or primary, medical care.

In addition, much primary health care is provided by medical workers other than doctors: physician's assistants and nurse practitioners. These well-trained professionals have not gone through medical school, but rather they have studied to become "physician extenders," to provide the same basic care that many primary care docs provide. They are licensed similarly to doctors; the extent of their medical privileges varies from one jurisdiction to the next.

Depending on your situation, a physician's assistant or a nurse practitioner may well be an excellent primary care provider for you. Although they are commonly found on the staffs of HMOs, they are employed more and more frequently in private medical offices as well, and in some places they are licensed to set up their own clinics. When I say *doctor* in this book, I really mean "health care provider," who may be a physician's assistant, a nurse practitioner, or a physician.

To illustrate: In my office, we have three health care providers, all of whom provide the same sort of primary care, though each of us comes from a different educational background. I am trained as a general internist, or internal medicine specialist. This is a rather archaic and confusing term. It does not mean that I am an intern (a doctor in his first year of training after medical school), nor does it mean that I only take care of people's internal organs. Rather, the fact that I am an internist means that in my medical training I focused on the general health care of adults. I am not trained to deliver babies, take care of infants, or perform surgery.

Jeff, the doctor who is my office partner, trained as a family practitioner, which means that, unlike myself, he is also qualified to take care of infants and children and has had experience in obstetrics and minor surgery during his training.

Pam is our physician's assistant. She trained originally as a nurse, then went back to school for a two-year physician's assistant program in which she learned to provide direct patient care. She provides medical care to patients semi-independently under Jeff's and my supervision.

Because our practice focuses on the needs of gay men, lesbians, transgendered people, and people with HIV, we all have developed special expertise in working with these populations.

Every patient who comes to our office has someone (Pam, Jeff, or me) whom he or she identifies as their primary care provider. That means that when the patient becomes ill or has a health question or when it is time for preventive care or screening, there is someone to call or visit. That someone is a health care provider who is familiar with the individual's medical history, his or her health habits, and (hopefully) something about the other important parts of the person's life.

Specialist Health Care Providers

Where do medical specialists fit in? They have a very valuable role in the system but not on the front lines. Specialists are the troops we primary care providers call in when we need more help. If a patient comes to me with a problem I don't have the expertise to handle or if we don't seem to be getting anywhere in treating a problem, then I need to be able to say "I don't know," and then refer that person to a specialist. But I like to be asked first. I can handle a lot of medical situations that some people might think they need a specialist for.

Besides, if a patient of mine sees a specialist, I want to make sure they see the right one. I am very protective of my patients. Any specialist that a patient of mine sees has got to be intelligent enough to help us with the problem at hand and also needs to respect my patient for who he is. I don't want my patient going to the surgeon whose homophobic diatribe on AIDS being God's punishment just appeared on the op-ed page of the local paper. Or to the gastroenterologist who misdiagnosed my last patient's colon cancer. I want my patient to go to the best—and most respectful—specialist I can find for his particular problem.

So, for many reasons, it makes much more sense to see your own personal doctor, who knows you, before going to a specialist. But in the United States, for years there has been a strange tendency for people to bypass primary care and go straight to medical specialists with their problems. Curious about a mole? Find a good dermatologist. Cough been bothering you? Go to a lung specialist. Earache? See the ear-nose-throat person. This leads to a type of fragmented medical care where each doctor may view the patient as an isolated body part—an ear or a set of lungs or a layer of skin.

Fortunately, there now is pressure to move away from that approach. For one thing, it is too expensive. The services of a specialist cost more than those of a generalist, and specialists tend to order more expensive tests and more of them. Insurance companies realize this, and now many plans will not let you see a specialist without first consulting your primary care doc. In Canada and Britain, the system just plain does not permit it, and primary care docs are the only way to access medical care. This is more and more the case in the United States

Besides, it is very inefficient to get all of your medical care from specialists. Why run around and see three different doctors, none of whom knows your entire medical history or has the time to find out? Your primary care doc, who already knows you, may well be able to take care of the mole, the cough, and the earache—all in the same visit. And when you see your doctor and start talking about how these three problems have been on your mind, you may discover that the real agenda is that you had unsafe sex a few months ago, and you're worried that the symptoms might be signs of HIV infection, and what you are really looking for is reassurance and an HIV test.

The Medical Profession's Attitudes Toward Gay Men

So, you need someone to provide you with primary care, someone who can be there for you when you need help or advice with just about any health problem. Just like Marcus Welby on TV—if you're old enough to remember him—the ideal, kindly doctor who could fix anything. You'll be looking for a gay-friendly version of Marcus Welby. What are your chances of success?

It's a jungle out there, so be careful. Things are changing for the better, but the medical profession has a long, unfortunate history of homophobia. Even though there have always been doctors who were gay or gay-friendly, the profession's official attitude has not been so accepting. Society's prejudices about homosexuality have influenced medical attitudes, and the former medical view of homosexuality as a mental illness has influenced society's acceptance.

In the past decades as we gay people have asserted our right to be who we are, changes in society and changes in medical attitudes have run parallel to each other. Of course we gay people know that our gayness is not an illness; society's homophobia is the real illness. Beginning with the American Psychiatric Association's removal of homosexuality from its list of mental disorders in 1980, organized medicine has steadily demedicalized and destigmatized homosexuality.

Finally in 1995, after years of behind-the-scenes wrangling, the American Medical Association adopted an official policy of nondiscrimination toward gay and lesbian physicians. The following year, this historically rather conservative organization came out with a position paper on the health care needs of gay and lesbian patients. In it the AMA reversed its previous stance condoning aversion therapy as a means of "curing" homosexuality. Instead it advised doctors to help unhappy gay people become comfortable with their sexual orientation. These changes in official AMA policy were the result of much hard work by many gay and lesbian physicians and other supportive members of the organization.

Still, homophobia remains common among individual members of the medical profession. Surveys of doctors performed within the last ten years indicate that many are still uncomfortable in dealing with gay men and lesbians, and a significant percentage continue to believe that homosexuality is an illness.

Nor do medical schools teach students much about the health care needs of gay men or about our lives. Medical students, like the public in general, often harbor prejudices and misconceptions about gay men, and an hour or two of lectures in medical school does little to change that. But because more of us are open about our sexual orientation, many medical students now have gay or lesbian family members, friends, or colleagues, or are openly gay or lesbian themselves. These future doctors are much more likely to respect and honor the gay identity of their gay male patients.

As a patient, you may have occasion to deal with a medical student or a resident (doctor in training). You can help educate and desensitize that future doctor—and benefit that doctor's future patients—by being open about the fact that you are a gay man.

Coming Out to Your Doctor

Many doctors will not know that you are gay unless you tell them. Fewer than half of physicians even bother to obtain a sexual history from their patients. Maybe they are too busy, or maybe they are uncomfortable with the issue; they're only human. In fact, in surveys of physicians many claim to have no gay or lesbian patients! Of course they have gay and lesbian patients—they just don't know they do because they haven't asked. But if they think they don't, then they can pretend they don't need to know about our particular medical needs.

For many reasons, it's important that your doctor know you're gay. There are a number of conditions that are more common among gay men, and all aspects of a gay man's health need to be seen in the context of his life as a gay man. If your doctor doesn't know you're gay, it will be that much harder for you to get the best medical care. Knowing about this important aspect of your life, your doctor will be better able to diagnose and treat medical conditions as they occur and will be able to offer you preventive care specific to your needs. You should be able to share this important aspect of your life with your doctor. As you go through this book, you'll see numerous specific examples of why it is important for your doctor to know you are gay.

As stated in the AMA position paper on the health care needs of gay men and lesbians, "All patients, regardless of their sexual orientation, have a right to respect and concern for their lives and values." So in looking for a gay-friendly M.D., you will want a doctor who not only isn't prejudiced against you but also can actively honor and respect your identity as a gay man. You'll feel better about a doctor who supports you in this way. If you come out to your doctor, and the reaction is less than warm, then maybe another doctor would be better for you.

What to Look for in a Doctor

Your prospective doctor should be aware that as a gay man your health care needs are somewhat different from those of other people—not only with regard to the obvious issues around HIV but also regarding other infections that gay men are more often exposed to and other health risks, such as substance abuse and the psychosocial stresses that can go along with being gay. Your prospective doctor should be able to understand who the important people are in your life—your partner, friends, family—and involve them in your care when appropriate. If you are HIV-negative, you don't want a doctor who equates being gay with having HIV or assumes that any new medical problem you have must be related to an HIV infection that has not been found yet.

If you are HIV-positive, you need to be even more careful in choosing a doctor. Obviously, your doctor should have all of the nonhomophobic attributes described above. But in addition, it has been shown that people with HIV do better and live longer when they are under the care of doctors who are experienced in dealing with HIV infection. This is becoming more important every day as the treatment of HIV becomes more sophisticated, delicate, and complex. The wrong doctor, however well-intentioned, could cause you a lot of problems—even permanently damage your health. So it is very important that you seek a doctor who has taken care of a number of HIV-positive people and whose knowledge keeps current in the area. Let the inexperienced, well-meaning doctor who wants you to be his first HIV patient learn on someone else, not on you.

There are many primary care docs who are pro-gay and understand the special medical needs of gay men. And there are many more who may not be highly knowledgeable about general gay men's health, but are willing to learn from you. In some situations it may not be possible to find a doctor who knows that much about the non-HIV health concerns of a gay man, even if you find a one who is sympathetic and nonjudgmental. In that case it is important to educate yourself, and then let the doctor know what your needs are. There are sections of this book that discuss the basic health care issues that are unique to gay men. Read them, and make sure they are addressed by your doctor. You can even give a copy to your doctor if you like.

Your prospective doctor need not be a gay man himself. There are many wonderful female and straight male health care providers who offer excellent care to gay men. And don't assume that if you do find a gay male physician, that he would be a good doctor for you. In fact, a few of the most homophobic doctors I know are closeted gay men. Their own internalized homophobia gets in the way of their providing sensitive care to other gay men. They bend over backwards to be ignorant of the needs of gay men. Thankfully, this breed is disappearing as the closet gets smaller and less appealing every day. Seldom do I hear stories like Pedro's any more, who after his first visit to me expressed relief at seeing an openly gay M.D.

Pedro: *Peter, I feel so much more comfortable going to a gay doc. My last doctor was straight, and he never understood where I was coming from. He didn't understand me as a gay man. In fact, he was one of the most homophobic people I have run into in a long time. You should hear what he had to say about anal intercourse.*

I didn't tell Pedro that his last doc was actually a gay man who was pathologically afraid of being outed and losing his position in a prestigious practice. This man did everything he could not to attract a gay male clientele. He purposefully projected a homophobic attitude that drove gay men away from his practice.

But as a gay male doctor myself, I must say that there are many wonderful, openly gay male physicians in many places, who practice primary care, and welcome gay men into their practice. I feel I have a special bond with my gay male patients. My office is a safe place for gay men, where the gay aspect of our lives is a given, not a secret to be revealed and coped with.

As a gay man, I am motivated to provide the best possible care for all of my patients but especially my gay male patients because they're my species. I am their advocate in a system that many still see as homophobic. I make sure that they are treated respectfully by my specialist colleagues and by hospital personnel. My straight physician colleagues even send me gay men who are looking for a gay primary care doc.

But again, it's not at all necessary or even feasible for every gay man to have a gay physician. In most places, there are few openly gay primary care docs, and the demand often exceeds their capacity to take new patients. And besides, some gay male patients prefer to see a female physician because they feel sexual tension being examined by a man. That's fine. What's most important is one's rapport with his physician, the physician's medical and interpersonal skills, and the physician's knowledge and support of gay men's lives.

The Search Is On

So now you know what qualifications to look for in a doctor. How do you go about finding your own personal Doctor Welby? There is no single, simple way. You might start out by asking friends—ideally gay male friends—to see if any of them have a doctor that might be good for you. Depending on where you live, that may or may not be feasible. For instance, if you live in a rural area and don't know any gay people locally, you may not have this option or even much choice in a doctor.

Many hospitals, clinics, and HMOs have phone numbers you can call to request a referral to a primary care doc. Unfortunately, most of these services will not be able to help you find a gay-friendly doc because they just don't have that kind of information. It doesn't hurt to ask, but you probably won't get far. But by asking for or demanding a gay-knowledgeable physician, you may help change the system for the future.

Many larger cities have gay and lesbian business associations with listings of gay, lesbian, or friendly businesses that often include doctors. But remember, you are looking for a primary care physician. A gay pathologist or radiologist may belong to the business association, but they aren't qualified to be your personal physician, so look at the specialty of the doctors listed. Many of my patients have found me this way, by cross-referencing the doctor listings provided by our local gay and lesbian business association with the list of "preferred" or "participating" primary care docs issued by their insurance company. Recently some of my straight-but-not-narrow colleagues have expressed an interest in advertising themselves as gay-friendly. Change is occurring.

Also, the Gay and Lesbian Medical Association and the National Lesbian and Gay Health Association offer referrals to gay or gay-friendly health care providers nationwide. Their phone numbers are listed in the back of this book.

The Internet is another place to find leads on gay-friendly doctors. People talk about their doctors in gay chat rooms all the time. A patient recently brought me a sheaf of papers containing a printout of such chat, with strong opinions on many local doctors (myself included) by the gay male participants.

In some places, doctors advertise, and you can find display ads in the local gay newspaper. Los Angeles must be the capitol of the doctor-advertising industry, for reasons I don't understand. I am sure that some excellent physicians promote their practices this way, but on a recent trip to LA, I must say I was amazed at the full-page ads in the gay papers and the enormous billboards advertising physician services. Certainly I do not recommend deciding on a doctor solely on the basis of an ad. And if a doctor is advertising heavily, I would wonder why, and I would question where the money for the ads is coming from.

If you belong to an HMO, your choice of docs may be more limited. If you have any friends who belong to the same HMO, you may want to get advice from them. Gay people have always been good at networking. Within some HMOs there is a gay or gay-friendly physician who can advise you on choosing a primary care doc. It may take some detective work to find such a person, though. In some large HMOs you may find advocacy groups of gay HMO members, and this is a great way for you to find an appropriate doctor for yourself.

The Doctor-Patient Relationship

Once you have the name of a prospective doctor, you should make an appointment to meet this person. But it's important to remind yourself that you don't have to stick with the first one you try. Remember, this is going to be an intimate and unique relationship. I don't just mean that your doctor is going to see you naked. That part is trivial. Your doctor will be involved with some of the most important aspects of your life: health, illness, issues of life and death and sex.

You will want to be able to be completely open and honest with your health care provider, to give him or her your total trust with this intimate business of your health. You will want someone who is smart enough to be a good diagnostician, but who, more importantly, is also a caring, gentle human being who you can respect and on whom you can depend to be there for you.

So consider your first appointment a trial run. See if you are going to get along with this person. Give yourself permission to look for someone else if you don't hit it off with the first doctor you interview.

Even if you have no immediate medical concerns, you should take the time to establish a relationship with your new doctor. Bring a list of questions to the interview. See if you will be comfortable with this person. Once you choose someone, you will feel confident in knowing you now have a doctor to help you with your medical needs as they arise. And if a medical crisis should occur, you'll be working with a doctor with whom you already have a relationship, rather than with a new doctor you've just met and who is just getting to know you.

Now suppose you already have a doctor that you work well with, and then your health insurance changes. You may well have to start fresh with a new doctor. It is an unfortunate reality of the current U.S. health care system that not all doctors are covered by all plans. You may be forced to change doctors if your employer contracts with a new insurance company that does not include your current doctor. Or you may change jobs and find that your new job provides health insurance exclusively through a closed HMO with a limited list of primary care providers.

In such a situation, the first thing you should do is protest to your employer and explain the importance of your ongoing relationship with your primary care doctor. That probably won't change your situation, but at least it will let your employer know that you are being impacted by having to change doctors and pressure the employer to offer a more flexible plan.

Other situations may precipitate the need to change doctors. Your physician may retire or move away, and the practice may be turned over to someone you don't like. Or maybe you have moved to another city.

In any case, when the need arises for you to seek a new doctor, use the advice in this section. Remember that you have a right to obtain, free of charge, a copy of your medical record from your previous doctor, within a reasonable period of time. Especially if you are moving to another city, it's a good idea to take advantage of this and bring a copy of your records with you. That way, your new doctor can review your past records right away, making for a smoother transition. Alternatively, if you are interviewing several prospective doctors, you may want to wait until you have chosen one. At that point you can sign a release and have your records copied and sent to the new doctor. Again, there should be no charge for this service.

What to Expect at the Doctor's Office

So now you have your first appointment with your new doctor. What should you expect? There are various types of medical visits. Maybe you just want to meet with your prospective new doctor for a chat to see if you two are going to get along and if so, to set up a more complete visit later. Perhaps your visit was precipitated by a particular problem, like a swollen knee or diarrhea or insomnia. Or perhaps you are interested in a general checkup, or "physical," to check out your current state of health and discuss how to optimize it.

Whatever your expectations are, it is important to state them when you first call for your appointment so that the proper time can be allotted for your visit and then to repeat the reason for your visit when you show up. But don't worry. If you don't volunteer this information, you will be asked. If you have a complicated medical situation and have been under another doctor's care, it really helps if your prospective new doctor has had a chance to review your medical records before your first appointment.

Once you report for your appointment, different offices have different ways of doing things. In general, you can expect to have to do some paperwork the first time you go to a new doctor, to register as a patient in the clinic. After that, you will usually be "checked in" (have your blood pressure, temperature, etc. taken) by a nurse or medical assistant. Ultimately you will see the doctor.

But you may well have to wait. Many jokes have been made about doctors running late. The thing is, it's true. Many doctors habitually run late. If you have been given an appointment at a particular time, try to understand that medical appointment times are approximations. There are so many uncertainties in a doctor's work schedule. Medicine is unpredictable. For example, the doctor may have just had to deal with an unanticipated emergency. Or the last patient may have turned out to have had a very complicated problem that took extra time to address.

Just don't imagine that the doctor was sitting there on the phone with a stock broker while you were fuming in the waiting room. I'm often running behind at work, and all day I feel like I'm dancing as fast as I can. It's not because I think that my time is more valuable than the time of the patient who is waiting. It's because I feel that the concerns of the patient I am dealing with right at the moment are no less important than the concerns of the next patient who is waiting, and I need to make sure they are adequately addressed before I move on to the next person.

Meeting Your Doctor

So anyway, finally you find yourself in the consultation room with the doctor, and the visit is beginning. Doctors are accustomed to starting every encounter with "the history," which means that they talk to you and ask you how you are doing and what the purpose of the visit is. For an overall checkup, that means a complete medical history. Otherwise, the history focuses on the problem(s) that led you to come to the doctor that day. We docs like to do this part first because it helps us know what to look for when we do the exam and (possibly) order other tests.

If you have questions for the doctor, or if there are things you don't want to forget to mention, it really helps to make a list and bring it with you to the appointment. Don't be embarrassed. Patients apologize to me when they pull out a list of 12 questions. I tell my patients I love lists. Really. Answering questions about your health is the doctor's job. If it's your first visit, or you're simply interviewing a prospective doctor, it's very important to bring a list of questions that you would like answered about the doctor: qualifications, background, philosophy of treatment, for example.

How do you talk to your doctor? In plain English! Doctor or patient, we're all human beings, and just because we doctors have a certain educational background does not mean we need to be put on a pedestal or shielded from certain words. Use words that you are comfortable with. These might be clinical words or more crude terms. When a patient comes to me and says he's been suffering from lots of gas, for example, I'm not sure what that means. The best way to find out is to ask: "Are you belching or farting or both?" So don't be afraid to tell your doctor that you are farting a lot if that is what the problem is. Another common scenario is the person who comes to me and shyly tells me, "I'm having a problem down there," and expects me to know what he means. Down where? Penis? Balls? Anus? Toe?

And never be afraid to ask questions. There is no such thing as a stupid question, so you should never have to apologize for anything you may ask your physician. No doctor is all-knowing, but we docs sure spent a lot of time in medical training, and so we should know a little more about people's bodies and how they work than the average person.

I love it when I can answer a question that's been bugging one of my patients. All those years of medical training actually help sometimes! Even if it's a simple question like "What side is my liver on?" And sometimes I can't answer the question because I don't know the answer. A good doctor will say "I don't know" rather than bluff or will look up the answer if there is one. Sometimes no one knows the answer. I think my patients are surprised sometimes when I say "I don't know," but there is a whole lot I don't know. Any doctor who purports to know the answer to everything is doing a lot of bluffing.

What should you call your doctor? Traditionally, medical decorum has dictated that you as a patient should call me "Dr. Shalit" and I call you "Mr. Smith." Many people—myself included—now feel that that is more formal than they are comfortable with. I address nearly all of my patients by their first names, and I ask that in return they call me Peter. A few feel more comfortable with "Dr. Shalit," or even "Dr. Peter," and that's OK if it's what they prefer. I try to establish this at the first visit. If your doctor does not ask you what you would like to be called, then bring the subject up, and find out what the doctor would like to be called.

As part of your first visit, in general I think it's a good idea to come out to your doctor. There are a few exceptions to this—for example, if you live in a small town and you feel it would be dangerous if people found out you were gay, or if you are in the military and using their health care system. But otherwise, it is almost always the best thing for your doctor to know you are gay.

The American Medical Association Council on Scientific Affairs, in their recent position paper on the health care needs of gay men and lesbians, made this statement: "The AMA believes that the physician's nonjudgmental recognition of sexual orientation and behavior enhances his or her ability to render optimal patient care in health as well as in illness. In the case of the homosexual patient, this is especially true, since the physician's failure to recognize homosexuality or the patient's reluctance to report his or her sexual orientation and behavior can lead to failure to screen, diagnose, or treat important medical problems." So, when you come out to your doctor, the AMA, a fairly stuffy and conservative group, is on your side!

Sometimes it's easy to come out. When you fill out the registration paperwork at a doctor's office, there is usually a question regarding marital status. If you are in a relationship, that is the opportunity to for you to come out, even before you meet the doctor, by listing your partner as your spouse. Otherwise, try to bring up the subject during the first visit. You can do this even if it is not relevant to the earache or knee pain that brought you in. It is especially important if you are there for a complete checkup or a "get acquainted" visit because the fact that you are gay is a very important piece of information that the doctor should know from the start.

Confidentiality

When you discuss your sexual orientation with you doctor, you may also want to discuss confidentiality. The doctor records information about you in a medical record, or "chart." Theoretically, this information is confidential and cannot be released to anyone else without your permission. However, when you enroll in a health insurance plan, you are automatically giving the insurance company access to your medical records. They have a right to know what it is they are paying for. And if you decide to apply for life or disability insurance, the company has a right to review your medical records or refuse to insure you. In many cases, being gay may be no big deal for any of this. But in some cases, having that information in your chart could get you in trouble.

Sam: *I have been in the U.S. Navy for 20 years, and I have kept my gay life to myself. Under the military's current "don't ask, don't tell" policy, that is just fine. But my health care is through the military as well, and if I tell my doctor I am gay, it becomes part of my military record. It's a catch-22 situation. When I went to the baths and came down with VD, the doctor wanted to know how I got it. I had to make something up about a female prostitute because I didn't want it in my record that I got it from a guy. I know it's not honest, but my job and my pension depend on this.*

Despite stories like Sam's, I hope most gay men can trust their doctor enough to reveal their sexual orientation. If asked, many doctors will honor your request to keep sensitive information out of the written record.

Fred: *I tested HIV-positive at a free clinic, anonymously. They said I needed follow-up care and referred me to a doctor. I was uncomfortable at first because my health insurance is through a group policy at work. My boss is pretty homophobic and AIDS-phobic, and I thought he might find out somehow. So when I went to the doctor, I didn't want him to write anything about HIV or my being gay in my chart, and I didn't want him to do any blood testing that might be a clue about my HIV infection. The doctor explained that it would be hard to take care of me under these circumstances and, besides, my insurance was supposed to pay for my medical care whatever my medical problems were. He also told me that there was no way for my boss to have access to my medical records and that even though the insurance company would know I was being treated for HIV, they do not report that information back to my employer. So I agreed to let the doctor write about my HIV status in the chart and do the proper HIV-related blood work so that the insurance would cover the cost of my medical care. After all, it's their job.*

Ethics and Boundaries

The doctor-patient relationship is a very intimate one. I continue to be surprised at how frankly patients talk to me about the most intimate details of their bodies and their psyches. In the exam room I can ask people questions about their bodily functions, their sexuality, their moods—questions that would seem intrusive or rude in most any other setting. And people usually answer these questions.

Despite this intimacy, there is nothing sexual about a doctor-patient encounter. (I can see you smiling. "You mean, I am naked except for this paper gown, and this man is touching my body, and that is not sexual?") Sure, there can be some sexual tension during a medical visit. Especially if you are not used to going to the doctor.

But remember, it is the doctor's job to examine people's bodies. For most doctors, fortunately, their work is not charged with sexuality nor is it particularly embarrassing to them. After all, this is what they do all day. When I was just starting practice, I remember one evening after work thinking about how many penises I had seen that day and how nonerotic it was for me.

Occasionally, a patient will get an erection during an exam, particularly a genital exam. Again, this is nothing the doctor hasn't seen before. If this happens to you, it doesn't necessarily mean that you're just so attracted to the doctor that your body is giving you away. Usually the erection is nothing more than an involuntary response to the embarrassment of the situation. The doctor will generally ignore it or reassure you to try to keep you from being too embarrassed, or (hopefully) at least not make some rude comment like "looks like you're glad to see me."

So anyway, it is OK if you feel a bit of sexual tension or discomfort during your exam. You are even allowed to have sexual fantasies, later, about the experience. We all fantasize about sexual situations that are inappropriate to act on. And after all, there are many porno stories and films that use a doctor-patient encounter as their starting premise.

But in real life such activities are a huge no-no. Ethical principles prohibit any sort of sexual relationship between doctor and patient because the power situation is just too unequal. It's very similar to the situation between a teacher and pupil or a military drill instructor and recruit— all situations best kept in the fantasy realm. So don't try to make it any more than a fantasy. Don't ask your doctor out for a date, and don't expect that hunky doc to ask you out either. And if he does, don't say yes if you expect to continue being his patient. If your doctor propositions you, that is a major ethical violation. My advice in that case would be to end your doctor-patient relationship with that individual and to report the incident to the local medical society.

Second Opinions and Frank Communication

All human relationships have their ups and downs, and doctor-patient relationships are no exception. If your doctor does something you don't like, let the doctor know. If your doctor tells you something that doesn't make sense to you, then say so. If you don't like the options a doctor is offering you, it is your right to have a second opinion. This shouldn't have to hurt anyone's feelings. Medicine is not an exact science, and we have all been wrong more than once.

If I feel I'm right, but a patient is not accepting of my opinion, I am happy for him to have a second opinion so that he'll be more comfortable. And if I'm not so sure about what is wrong with my patient, I may even suggest a second opinion so that we are both more comfortable. You should never accept a diagnosis or a treatment plan that you are uncomfortable with. It's your body and your life.

Personally I feel it is very important that I be able to be honest with my patients. If I have a concern about their health, I need to be able to let them know and not shield them from it. If I discover a serious problem, such as HIV infection or cancer, I need to be able to tell them frankly about what is wrong. No one likes to be the bearer of bad news, but it must be done.

Sometimes people become angry at the doctor who discovers their serious problem. They are confusing the messenger with the message. More often my patients will tell me, "Peter, I never want you to hide anything from me. If it's bad news, I want to know right away." That works well for me, and that is the way I would want my own doctor to relate to me as a patient.

Switching Doctors

Sometimes things just aren't working out, and there comes a time when you feel the need to find a new doctor. Occasionally I see a new patient who has the following kind of story to tell:

Gene: *Dr. Merman was my family doctor. He has taken care of me since I was a baby, and he even helped me come out to my parents when I was fifteen. But lately it doesn't seem like he listens to me. I get whisked into the room for a minute, he runs in, runs out, and barely sits down. The last time I had a bout of tonsillitis, he prescribed an antibiotic he should have known I was allergic to, and when I told him, he yelled at me. I don't know if he's getting overworked or burned out or using drugs or what, but I'm not going back to him.*

This kind of situation happens. Doctors are human beings. I don't know what Dr. Merman's problem was, but Gene had no obligation to continue going to him under the circumstances. I did suggest to Gene that he write a short note to Dr. Merman explaining why he was leaving his practice. I also suggested he might want to write a note to the local medical society if he felt that Dr. Merman's judgment was impaired.

Alternative Health Care

C hicken soup helps a cold, eating fish makes you smarter, carrots help you see better at night—folk remedies are part of our lives. We were often first exposed to these by our mothers. My mother wasn't very good at it, though. She did the chicken soup thing all right, but that was about it. I remember her saying one day, "Now is it 'feed a cold and starve a fever' or the other way around?"

Many cultures have a variety of folk remedies that have been handed down for generations. In recent years, a variety of alternative health care practices have become popular. Practitioners of alternative therapies, usually not M.D.s, use a range of techniques, some traditional and some of more recent origin. A significant percentage of Americans take advantage of alternative therapies, and the annual number of visits to alternative practitioners exceeds the number of visits to primary care medical providers. Some health insurance plans are even starting to provide coverage for some of these therapies. In addition, many people self-treat with herbs, vitamins, or other "natural" remedies.

Overview of Alternative Approaches

Millions of Americans visit alternative healers, often with a high degree of satisfaction in the services they receive. There is no such thing as an average or typical alternative healer. Alternative providers are a very diverse group of people, practicing such arts as herbal medicine, acupuncture, acupressure, reflexology, Reiki, or nutritional therapy—to name just a few. It is beyond the scope of this book to describe in detail all the different modalities of alternative healing that are available.

Alternative healers often follow models of health and disease that are different from the model followed by Western, or allopathic, medicine. For example, acupuncture addresses energy channels and flows in the body, called meridians, that are not recognized by Western doctors. Acupuncture needles are placed in order to influence these flows and restore balance. Traditional Chinese medicine relies on pulses and "warmth/cold" and "wet/dry" states to diagnose and treat illness. The system of reflexology teaches that the entire body is represented in the sole of the foot, and by manipulating the foot, the health of other parts of the body can be affected. Herbalists base their treatments on folk wisdom that has been handed down for generations. An herb is known to be useful for a specific situation, without necessarily understanding why it might be so.

Western medicine employs a different model, one that may be called *scientific medicine*. Health and disease are defined in terms of physical and biological processes, and treatments are aimed at intervening in those processes or correcting abnormal physiology. Treatments (including many medications that originated from herbal sources, incidentally) are studied for their effect on numbers of patients. Western physicians claim to require evidence of efficacy, although in truth many of the treatments we accept as efficacious have never been studied rigorously. There is a recent movement toward evidence-based medicine, meaning the acceptance of treatments only if they have been rigorously proven to be effective.

Naturopathic physicians, trained and licensed in parts of the United States, usually have expertise in a variety of alternative methods. Chiropractors are licensed in all fifty states. Acupuncturists and massage therapists are also licensed and certified in the majority of states. For many other alternative practitioners, however, there is no licensing or certifying process to ensure that a given healer has the expertise claimed. The prospective client must trust that the healer is competent, sometimes guided by the recommendation of satisfied clients.

Some alternative treatments are not so "alternative" anymore and are accepted by Western medicine as having proven efficacy in certain situations. Chiropractic manipulation and acupuncture are examples. At the other extreme, some methods of diagnosis and/or treatment—such as astrology, crystal healing, or hydrogen peroxide enemas—are not widely accepted even by many practitioners of alternative healing.

One thing that many alternative healers have in common is the belief that the human body possesses the intrinsic ability to heal itself. They generally see themselves and their therapies as gentle guides that help nudge the body systems in the right direction or remove obstacles to health. The body's innate healing processes do the rest.

Any Treatment May Have Risks

Not all "natural," "herbal," or "alternative" therapies are benign. For example, spinal manipulation done by an incompetent person can be dangerous. Some people assume that just because a substance is sold as an herbal supplement, it is completely safe to take in any situation and in any quantity. Many herbs certainly are quite safe, especially when taken in moderation. But this is not always the case. Toxicities or adverse interactions are possible.

If you take significant quantities of herbal remedies, vitamins, or other supplements, you may want to seek the guidance of an herbalist or naturopathic physician. At the very least, if you are taking such substances, do let your primary care provider know what you are taking, to make sure that no potentially harmful drug interactions occur.

A naturopathic physician colleague of mine says that his new patients often bring him a shopping bag full of self-prescribed herbs and supplements. He goes through the bottles and points out the ones that conflict with each other and the ones that may be more harmful than helpful. Usually the patient leaves with a much smaller sack of pill bottles.

Complementary Health Care: A Collaboration

Alternative therapies are best seen as complementary to the type of medicine I practice. We each have abilities the other does not. We each have our uses.

If you have a chronic illness, such as diabetes, HIV, or cancer, you should have a relationship with with a Western-type physician at a minimum. Most people agree that it would be unwise to expect an alternative practitioner to "heal" any of these disorders. But alternative medical approaches may be a good complement to mainstream therapy. For example, the alternative practitioner may help a diabetic patient lower his blood sugar with diet and/or herbal remedies. A man with HIV may combat the side effects of antiviral medications through the use of acupuncture and acupressure for neuropathy and nausea. Someone with cancer may use meditation or guided imagery to deal with the toxicities of chemotherapy or radiation. These situations illustrate instances where alternative treatments can be used to complement Western medicine.

If you are basically healthy, you may choose to see an alternative healer for advice on vitamins, herbs, nutrition, and exercise or for treatment of minor symptoms. But an alternative healer will not be able to immunize you against hepatitis or influenza or set your broken arm or fix your ruptured appendix. So even if you are healthy and are more comfortable with an alternative medicine, it's still wise to also have a relationship with a physician practicing Western medicine.

Some of my patients, in addition to seeing me, visit a variety of alternative practitioners who provide valuable services to them. For example, a number of my patients have found that acupuncture relieves various symptoms such as pain or nausea. Hypnotherapy has helped many of my patients stop smoking. Naturopathic physicians advise some of my patients regarding nutrition, either as a way to achieve weight loss or gain or to identify and control food allergies or to choose a reasonable program of vitamin and mineral supplementation. Some of my patients see Chinese herbalists for remedies for various maladies.

There are also situations where Western medicine has little to offer, and alternative therapy has more benefit. I have seen patients with arthritis pain, headaches, or fatigue that could not be alleviated by any treatment known to mainstream medicine. Yet in some cases these symptoms were helped by acupuncture, herbal therapy, or Reiki, for example. Ideally, Western and complementary traditional healers should be able to work together to help a patient get well.

A Warning About Miracle Cures

If you have a serious illness, be wary of alternative healers who make exaggerated claims, such as having a potion or a technique that will cure a fatal illness or offering a treatment that is effective for multiple diseases (cancer and AIDS, for example). Such claims sound too good to be true, and they usually are. They are easy to find all over the Internet. Do a Web search using the term *DHEA,* and you'll see what I mean.

Before there were effective treatments for HIV, some of my patients would occasionally seek maverick healers who offered a cure. The healer would frequently claim that their cure was being suppressed by the AMA because it also cured cancer and heart disease and would put doctors out of business. Often testimonials of individuals were produced, claiming to have been "on my deathbed" until Dr. Jones's treatment "cured me, and now I am HIV-negative." Patients of mine flew to Mexico or Bermuda or Switzerland and paid large amounts of money for these treatments. It was sad, and it was not a surprise that they did not work.

If a claim seems miraculous, and especially if the proponent claims it has been "suppressed" by powerful organizations, then it is probably not true.

Preventive Care and Fitness

Live long and prosper! As a doctor, I'd much rather help my patients stay well than to see them get sick. Being sick is a drag, as everyone knows. Besides, treatment for an illness can be can be uncomfortable, inconvenient, and expensive. It makes so much more sense to prevent a medical problem, or at least detect it early, than to wait until it hits you in the face. Of course, some problems just can't be prevented.

My heart sinks when I see a man with a condition that could have easily been avoided by making some lifestyle changes. It makes me sad to see someone with an advanced problem that could have been dealt with more easily if caught earlier.

Healthy patients sometimes apologize to me for "wasting" my time working on preventive care with them when I could be seeing people who are really sick and "need a doctor more." But my attitude is that preventive care is just the opposite of a waste. It's an investment that pays off many times over.

Staying healthy takes some work, a little luck, and the right genes. When we are young, it's easy for us to take our health for granted. That's the best time to develop healthy habits, to get the proper vaccines, and to screen for potential future problems.

Early is best, but it's never too late for screening and prevention. I see 19-year-olds getting their first adult checkup, and I see 50-year-olds getting theirs. Proactive health care is important, whatever age you are.

Even though prevention takes some effort, it's still true that many health problems are much easier to prevent than to treat. Or if a problem can't be prevented, it often can be managed or cured more readily when still in the early stages.

Every man is ultimately responsible for his own health, but by working with his doctor, he can learn how to give himself a better chance of maintaining this priceless asset. And I do mean priceless. There is nothing more valuable than one's health. Ask anyone living with an incurable illness.

In the following sections we will describe what goes on during a screening, or preventive, visit with your health care provider. I will discuss the immunizations that all gay men should consider having. There is a section on how to stay healthy during travel, which can be a little trickier than when you're home. Finally, there are sections on general fitness, healthy eating, and exercise.

Health is sometimes defined as "the absence of disease," but really it is more than that. Just as the word *peace* connotes more than simply "the absence of war," the word *health* brings to mind a state of vigor, of feeling good in body and mind. Similarly, the word *fitness* describes an optimal state of physical health, a goal for most people of all ages. It is my hope that the information in the following sections will help you stay healthy and fit.

Getting a Checkup

The Periodic Health Exam

Preventive care should be a collaboration between you and your health care provider. There are many things that the two of you can do to give you the best chance of staying healthy. One of the most important is a regular visit to your doctor to go over your general health and lifestyle and to see what you can do to maintain and improve them. People refer to this as a "checkup" or an "annual physical." The current medical term is *periodic health exam*. Not everyone needs one annually.

Although part of this checkup involves the doctor examining your body, from head to toe, this is probably not the most useful component of a screening/preventive visit. Of more importance is the time you and your doctor spend discussing your health habits, and how you might change your lifestyle to make it healthier. Other preventive and screening activities include immunizations, as well as laboratory tests, such as blood analysis.

How often should you have a maintenance visit to your doctor? There is no set rule, and it should be decided on an individual basis, depending on various circumstances.

In general, if you are fortunate enough to have no ongoing medical problems, and don't need any regular screening tests, it's good to see your doctor every three to five years until the age of forty. After that, an annual checkup is recommended for anyone, mostly to screen for heart disease and certain cancers and to review health habits.

For a sexually active gay man of any age, unless he is truly in a mutually monogamous relationship, I recommend an annual visit. The goal here is to screen for sexually transmitted diseases, including HIV, and to discuss safer sex and STD prevention. If a man is concerned that he may be having risky sex, this screening should be done even more frequently. Every six months is a good interval.

What Is Involved?

A complete periodic health exam consists of several parts. First there is the discussion of your lifestyle, health habits, and medical history. Then there is a physical exam. Finally comes blood testing and sometimes other tests, such as an analysis of a urine sample or an electrocardiogram (heart rhythm tracing).

Let's pretend that you, like many adults, have never had a checkup. For the remainder of this section, I'll walk you through a make-believe periodic health exam, so that you'll know what to expect or ask for when you get one from your own health care provider.

As with all medical encounters, a checkup starts with some chat. In some offices you will be asked to fill out a questionnaire about your health and past and present medical problems. I prefer gathering this information directly, by an interview before the exam. It's easier and more appropriate to do this while your clothes are on. You probably wouldn't want to be sitting there naked while a doctor or nurse is asking you a bunch of questions. If someone tries to interview you with your clothes off, and it makes you uncomfortable, tell them.

After we introduce ourselves to each other, first I'll want to know if there are any particular problems bothering you right now, or if you have any particular questions about your health. If you have a list, that's great; otherwise, it's easy to forget specific things you want to discuss. We'll talk about whatever may be on your mind with regard to your health, and we'll set goals for the visit.

Next we'll spend some time discussing your health habits. A healthy lifestyle includes regular exercise, eating right, avoiding excesses with alcohol and drugs, not using tobacco, and always wearing seat belts in a car and a helmet when on a bicycle or motorcycle.

Everyone knows this, but we all need to be reminded at times. And studies show that a doctor's advice can have a big influence on a person changing their habits in the right direction. So I'll try not to nag, but at the same time I'll try to help you work on any less-healthy habits you may have and get you started with changing them in the right direction. This is all common sense stuff, and it's covered in detail in other sections of this book.

As a gay man, sexual safety is by far—by *far*—the most important health habit you can have. HIV infection is your very biggest health risk. Have you heard the 50-50 prediction? At current rates of HIV exposure in North America, the average a 20-year-old, sexually active gay man has a 50% chance of catching HIV by the time he turns 50.

Guys, this is just *not* acceptable! Once you are infected, there is no going back. Enjoy sex, have fun, but learn how to do it safely, and do it that way every time. It was one thing to get infected when we didn't know any better. Now we all should know better. So be careful.

To get an idea of what a discussion of safer sex might consist of, please refer to the section on that topic in this book. Notice I didn't say "safe" sex, I said "safer." Any sexual interaction with another person involves some degree of risk of infection. But by practicing careful sexual habits, you can greatly reduce your chances of catching HIV or any number of other nasties. So decide where your personal boundaries of safety are, and stick to them. Don't become part of that 50% statistic, and let's try to drop that number to 10% or 1% or even zero, OK?

During this introductory part of the visit, we'll also get a detailed personal health history, to find out what kinds of problems you may have had in the past. Any hospitalizations, operations, immunizations, allergies? If you have any chronic (ongoing) medical conditions or are on any type of medication, we will discuss that. We'll also go over any medical problems that might run in your family, so that we can pay special attention to screening and prevention of those.

We'll find out a little bit about your life. What do you do for work? For relaxation? Are you single, or do you have a partner? How is your relationship with your family? Are you out to them? How is your support system? Any major changes or stresses in your life lately? Who would you want to be there for you if you became ill? Do you have a satisfying home life? Social life? Sex life? Do you have any trouble sleeping? Are your moods OK?

Although these might not seem like medical topics, this line of questioning is getting at your psychological health, which is just as important as your physical health. The two can have a great impact on each other. And it's very helpful for your doctor to have psychosocial information about you in order to take care of you as a whole person with a full life and not just a body with medical concerns.

The Exam

After the health interview it's time for the physical exam. This is the part you need to get undressed for, and this can be embarrassing or anxiety-provoking for many people. If that happens to you, just try to detach yourself emotionally, and pretend it's like bringing your car to the mechanic for a tune-up.

The exam involves a careful scrutiny of your entire body, from head to toe. The doctor will look, listen, feel, poke, and prod at you. Don't take it personally. No judgment is being made.

Important parts of the exam include: your weight, blood pressure, and pulse ("vital signs"); a look over your skin for any suspicious moles; examination of the thyroid and lymph nodes; a check inside your mouth; a quick check of heart, lungs, and abdomen; genital exam, including a check for hernias and for testicular cancer; and the anal/rectal exam, externally to look for warts and other lesions and internally to check for warts, hemorrhoids, as well as cancer of the rectum or prostate.

During the exam, if you have any questions or concerns about various parts of your body, this is the time to point them out. For example, if there is a mole you've been wondering about, or if one of your testicles seems different from the other, point it out and ask about it.

Guys have a tendency to make jokes when I examine their genitals or rectum. I can almost predict what they'll say. It's usually something along the lines of, "Gee, usually I get taken out to dinner before this part." This reflects the sexual tension that is an inevitable part of the exam. It's natural. We're not used to anyone touching us "down there" except in a sexual situation. But a physical exam is not a sexual situation. So just close you eyes and think about something mundane like walking the dog or doing your laundry, and it'll be over in a minute.

It's certainly your right to decline to have any part of your body examined. Occasionally a patient will not permit me to examine his genitals or anal area, and I respect his wishes. Touching someone against his will is battery—even in a medical situation.

But it's important to realize that the below-the-belt part is one of the most important parts of the screening exam, for a gay man especially. Often a man is unaware that that groin lump is a hernia or that rough spot on his penis is really a wart that is contagious to others. And it's difficult to examine one's own anus, yet that is an area that frequently gives us problems that need treatment. Countless times I have found anal warts or hemorrhoids in a person who was completely unaware he had a problem back there.

Wrapping Up

After the exam has been completed, it's likely the doctor will want to take some blood. Various blood tests might be performed. If you haven't had your cholesterol tested recently, that can be done. If you've had sex with anyone over the past year, or if it's been more than a year since your last test, your blood should be tested for syphilis and for HIV.

Remember, though, that it is illegal for you to be tested for HIV without your permission. So you and your doctor should discuss this, and you should only be tested if you are prepared to hear the result, whatever it may turn out to be. If your doctor offers to do "routine blood work," that does not automatically include an HIV test unless you specifically request one. A much more detailed discussion of HIV testing can be found in the section on HIV in this book.

If you don't know whether you've even been exposed to hepatitis A and/or B, or if you have had a hepatitis vaccine and want to know if it took, those things can be determined from the same blood sample.

Other types of test—for prostate or colon cancer, or for diabetes, for example—may be performed, depending on your age and on other factors such as symptoms or family history.

Finally comes the fun part—the shots. I usually save the shots for the very end. There are several kinds of immunizations that might be offered. None of these, by the way, involve infecting you with live viruses or bacteria. Instead, they consist of killed germs or synthetic proteins developed to help you become immune to a particular kind of bug without giving you a full-blown case of that infection. We'll discuss whatever immunizations you might need, and give them to you. The next section describes these immunizations.

Once you've had any shots you may need, we're nearly done. We'll wrap up by summarizing what I have found during our encounter. We'll talk some more about your overall state of health and how to optimize it. If you have habits that are unhealthy, we can talk about how you might change them. We'll arrange to meet again or talk on the phone once the results of any tests we've taken are back. Otherwise, that's it until next time.

You should leave the doctor's office feeling a sense of accomplishment, with the knowledge that you have done yourself a favor by actively working on your health. You should promise yourself that you'll work harder at staying healthy in whatever ways that applies to you. It may be by quitting cigarettes, exercising more, losing weight, developing a plan for sexual safety, or any number of goals that you and your doctor have come up with for you to work on.

Whatever your health situation, do remember that preventive care doesn't end when you leave the doctor's office. On the contrary, your visit with the doctor is just where it begins. After that, staying healthy is up to you.

Immunizations for Gay Men

Vaccines are a great way to keep from getting sick. Lots of people don't particularly like needles, but it's so much more pleasant to get a shot than to get some nasty infection. There are a host of infections that are preventable by vaccines, and scientists are working on more.

If you were born and raised in the United States, you probably had some vaccines in infancy and childhood. Most children are now routinely immunized for diseases such as polio, measles, mumps, rubella, chicken pox, hemophilus, diphtheria, and tetanus. Hepatitis B was added to the list a few years ago.

As an adult, there are fewer vaccines you'll need, but they are very important. Some are more important for you as a gay man than for others.

Everybody should have a diphtheria-tetanus booster every ten years. This will protect you from tetanus (lockjaw), a life-threatening infection that causes paralysis and can occur when you get a dirty wound (the proverbial stepping on a rusty nail is an example). It will also prevent diphtheria, a now-rare throat infection that can be very severe and that, like tetanus, can cause paralysis.

You may want to get an annual flu vaccine. These are given annually from October through December. There are many strains of flu, and every year the powers that be decide on the three strains most likely to cause an epidemic 18 months hence (that's how long it takes to make up a batch of vaccine).

A flu vaccine is only good for a year, and sometimes it's no good at all because the strains that come around that year are not the ones in the shot. In any case, it does no harm to get a flu shot. If you are young and healthy, it is optional

If you are over 65 or have a chronic condition like HIV, asthma, or diabetes, flu shots are strongly recommended. If you are the care giver of someone with HIV, you might also want to get a shot. And if you work with the public—for example, as a teacher, flight attendant, waiter, nurse, hairdresser, or doctor—you too might want a flu shot.

There is a "pneumonia vaccine," that protects against many strains of a common bacterium, pneumococcus, which is a leading cause of pneumonia. Pneumococcus can infect anyone, but it hits hardest those who are over 65 or have lung problems or have HIV. If you are in one of these groups, you should have a pneumonia vaccine every five years or so.

Finally, there are the hepatitis vaccines. You'll find detailed discussions of hepatitis A and B in the section on hepatitis. The viruses that cause these illnesses are the only sexually transmitted agents for which we have vaccines. Gay men are at particular risk of hepatitis, so you owe it to yourself to take advantage of the opportunity to be protected. The only drawbacks are the cost and the inconvenience.

Each dose of hepatitis A or B vaccine costs $50 to $70. Hepatitis B immunization requires three shots over a six month period, while hepatitis A immunization requires two shots, six to twelve months apart.

Note that many gay men are already immune to one or both of these viruses, and most are unaware of that fact. If you might have already been exposed, this can be determined by a blood test. If you find that you are already immune to hepatitis A and/or B, you have saved yourself the cost and hassle of several shots.

My wish for the near future is that we'll be able to give you vaccines for herpes, syphilis, and of course HIV. Much research is being done to develop vaccines for these infections, but at this point they are only a dream. Alas.

Travel Health

We live in an incredibly mobile society. Modern transportation allows a person to travel almost anywhere in the world with relative ease, for business or pleasure. Medical complications can be a traveler's worst nightmare. When traveling you can be exposed to various exotic illnesses. If you have a chronic medical condition, such as HIV infection, or if your health is fragile in any way, then travel has even more risk and uncertainty. But anyone can develop a new health problem at any time, and traveling is a most inconvenient time.

So before taking a trip of any distance, it's a good idea to plan ahead. Depending on your destination and your current state of health, you may want to get some medical advice before you leave so that you can ensure that health problems do not interfere with your trip.

Your pre-travel medical visit should be at least a month before departure, to give time for any immunizations to take effect. Some factors to consider are the following: Do you have any chronic medical problems? Do you take any medications regularly? Do you have any allergies or sensitivities? Are your routine immunizations up to date? Where are you going and for how long? Will you be staying in an urban or rural area?

The Traveler's Kit

Whatever your state of health, it always makes sense to pack a small first-aid kit. This should include a few adhesive bandages, some acetaminophen or aspirin for pain or fever, a good sunscreen, antibacterial ointment, hydrocortisone cream for rashes or stings, some loperamide (Imodium) for diarrhea, and perhaps some Dramamine if you are susceptible to motion sickness.

If you tend to suffer from jet lag, it can help to bring along some over-the-counter or prescription sleeping pills for the trip. Diphenhydramine (Benadryl) or melatonin (low dose: 1 milligram or so) are available without a prescription for this purpose. Triazolam (Halcion) is an excellent fast-acting sleeping pill available by prescription.

Bowel irregularity, either diarrhea or constipation, can be a problem for travelers. For many it helps to take a daily dose of fiber supplement (e.g., psyllium, or Metamucil) during a trip. Severe diarrhea while traveling is often a sign of a bacterial infection, especially if the diarrhea is watery or accompanied by cramps, blood, and/or fever. It is a good idea to bring a bottle of antibiotic pills (ciprofloxacin is standard), to be started in case of infectious diarrhea. In such cases, an antidiarrheal (such as loperamide) can help reduce the volume of stool, and it is also important to drink plenty of fluids to avoid becoming dehydrated. The antibiotics may also be used if another type of infection, such as bronchitis or a sore throat, occurs during travel.

Contents of the Basic First-aid Kit for Travelers

- ☐ Adhesive bandages
- ☐ Aspirin, acetaminophen, or ibuprofen
- ☐ Antinausea medication: Dramamine or Bonine
- ☐ Hydrocortisone cream 1% (for rashes or stings)
- ☐ Antibacterial ointment for wounds (e.g., Polysporin)
- ☐ Sleeping medication: diphenhydramine, melatonin, triazolam* (Halcion)
- ☐ Fiber supplement: psyllium (e.g., Metamucil)

- ☐ Antidiarrheal: loperamide (Imodium)
- ☐ Antibiotic for diarrhea or other infections: ciprofloxacin*
- ☐ Decongestant: pseudoephedrine (Sudafed) tablets, oxymetazoline (Afrin) nasal spray
- ☐ Epi–Pen* (if history of severe allergic reactions)
- ☐ Sunscreen with SPF 15 or greater

*Doctor's prescription required

If you are prone to upper respiratory tract problems, some decongestant pills, such as pseudoephedrine (Sudafed) and/or oxymetazoline nasal spray (Afrin) can help keep your ears from getting blocked during plane flights. People with a history of severe allergic reactions, either to insect stings or certain foods, should bring an emergency injector of epinephrine (Epi-Pen) to be used in case of a problem. Everyone's travel bag should include some good sunscreen (SPF 15 or greater), especially for those who are visiting tropical latitudes and/or anticipating much sun exposure. Some medications, such as the sulfa drugs used commonly by people with HIV to prevent pneumonia, can make a person more sun-sensitive, so if you are on any ongoing medications, ask your doctor if you need to avoid sun exposure.

Some Special Considerations

If you are dealing with an ongoing health problem or problems, travel requires additional preparation. I frequently encounter that situation with HIV-positive folks. There is no reason why a person with HIV/AIDS should not be able to travel with the proper advance preparation and a bit of luck.

A few narrow-minded countries (Russia, China, Egypt, Saudi Arabia, and the United States, for example) officially restrict entry of HIV-positive persons. Some require proof of a recent negative HIV test; others just do spot checks. If your agenda includes one of these countries and you are HIV-positive, you are at risk of being turned away at the border and sent home. However, you can sometimes take your chances and get in, especially if you do not appear ill. To be safe, contact your destination country's local consulate to find out if there are any restrictions on HIV-infected people entering the country. But don't raise a flag by giving your name.

Two patients told me the following stories within the past year. I have changed the details, but not the country, which we usually think of as not particularly AIDS-phobic:

Dino: *I have AIDS, and I planned a vacation in Australia. I know that they don't restrict people with AIDS from visiting, but just to be safe I checked with the local Australian consulate. I told them about my situation and asked them if I needed to do anything special in order to get a visa. Even though it was just going to be a two-week trip, they made me fill out pages of forms about my health status and my destinations. I had to provide blood work, a chest X ray, and a full medical report.*

My trip was postponed twice while the Australian authorities decided whether I could go. Finally, they decided not to give me the visa. They said it was not specifically because of I have AIDS, but because I might get sick while in Australia and put a strain on their health care system.

Rick: *I have AIDS, and my company sent me to Australia for a business trip. I figured my health status was none of their business, and I didn't mention it. No one asked. The trip went fine.*

So it seems the rule here is "don't ask, don't tell." If you are HIV-positive and plan a trip abroad, try to find out discreetly about the policies of the country your are visiting. If it looks like things will be OK, then don't rock the boat.

Bringing Your Medications

Many people take daily prescription medication for a chronic medical condition, whether it be HIV, high blood pressure, diabetes, or something else. Missing just one dose of medication can be dangerous or even life-threatening. When you travel, make sure you have enough for your entire trip, plus a few days' worth in case you get stranded. Likewise, if you wear glasses, it's a good idea to bring an extra pair and a copy of the prescription.

It is very important to carry your medication(s) on your person. Do not—I repeat—*do not* put them in checked baggage. Checked baggage can disappear, and Murphy's Law ("if something can go wrong, it will") says that if your meds are in a checked suitcase, the suitcase will not be there when you reach your destination. Just ask my patient who paid hundreds of dollars to have replacement doses of his experimental HIV medications airlifted to him in Mexico!

Also, keep your pills in their original bottles, which have the prescription label stating your name, your doctor's name, and the name of the medication. Customs officials tend to be suspicious of unlabeled pills and are likely to confiscate them. If you depend on the medications for your health, the rest of your trip could be in jeopardy.

In case something happens and your pills are lost, some people recommend you obtain fresh written prescriptions for all of your medications and keep them in your wallet while traveling. This makes sense as an extra security blanket, but no patient of mine has ever needed it. In addition, the names of medications may be different in a foreign country, and a local physician or pharmacist may not understand the prescription.

On occasion I have written a letter on behalf of a patient who is on daily maintenance medication. The letter is to be carried by the patient to ensure that his meds are not confiscated at a border. Usually the letter will identify the person as my patient and will state that he is bringing these medications with him and that they are essential for his health. I do not identify the health condition involved. Even with the letter it is still important to leave the pills in their original containers when traveling, as proof of their identity. And do not offer to show your pills or letter to the immigration officials unless they ask. Why invite trouble?

If you lose your medication or have a new health problem while you are abroad, consider contacting your doctor back home. Remember that worldwide communication is easy these days. In the past year I have received E-mail from a patient in Croatia, faxes from Costa Rica and Thailand, and a phone call from Australia. These modes of communication are inexpensive and efficient ways to communicate with your doctor back home.

Health Risks While Traveling

Even if your health is perfect, while you are traveling you may be exposed to various new health risks, and precautions are important.

Surprisingly, the most common cause of serious health problems in travelers is road accidents. Be particularly careful when driving outside the United States. Remember that traffic laws and customs are different in every country, and you are at increased risk of an accident when you drive in a foreign country. Of course, wherever you are you should not drink and drive.

Second to accidents, infections are the most common health hazard for travelers. These come most frequently from drinking impure water or from having sex.

Many parts of the world have bacteria, parasites, or viruses in their drinking water. Unless you are in a "Westernized" locale (North America, Western Europe, Japan, or Oceania), you should not drink the water. Instead use bottled water, boiled water, or canned carbonated beverages. Nor should you consume salads or raw fruit or vegetables or have a drink containing ice cubes. If you do, you are putting yourself at risk of bacterial diarrhea and possibly other infections, such as giardia or hepatitis A. Fruit that you peel yourself should be safe. Remember this slogan about fresh produce: Peel it, cook it, boil it, or forget it!

Regarding sex, the safest policy is to bring your sex with you in the form of a traveling companion or your trusty right hand. If you anticipate having sex with a new partner, make sure you have condoms. Remember that sex as a tourist, especially in certain parts of the world, is a bit riskier than sexual activity at home. Other countries have different customs and laws with regard to gay sex, so be careful. You may run the risk of getting assaulted, robbed, imprisoned, or all of the above. Even if you are confident that you will not get into trouble, be careful not to give or get any nasty germs. Use those rubbers.

Make sure your routine immunizations (diphtheria, tetanus, hepatitis B) are up to date. Now that a vaccine for hepatitis A is available, most travelers get their first shot before embarking. A second shot six to 12 months later will provide lifetime protection. More information on hepatitis prevention can be found in "The ABCs of Hepatitis" section of this book. For many parts of the world a booster of the inactivated (Salk) polio vaccine is also recommended.

> **Vaccines to Receive (or Update) Prior to Travel**
>
> ☐ Hepatitis A
> ☐ Hepatitis B
> ☐ Diphtheria-Tetanus
> ☐ Polio (Salk)
> ☐ Flu (if in season)
> ☐ Others (typhoid, meningococcus, etc., depending on destination)

Some places have problems with exotic infectious diseases such as malaria, cholera, or yellow fever. These can be prevented with proper precautions, which include preventive antibiotics or vaccines, use of insect repellents, and avoidance of swampy areas where such diseases are spread. If you may be traveling to an area where malaria occurs, your doctor can give you pills to take while away that should prevent you from catching the disease.

To get advice on the particular risks of your destination, ask your doctor, or call the local Health Department or public Travel Clinic. The U.S. Public Health Service has information bureaus in several major cities (see Appendix). Incidentally, all preventive antibiotics and vaccines used for travelers are safe for HIV-positive as well as HIV-negative individuals.

If you do have a medical problem while traveling, where should you seek care? If it's just a question, remember that you can first try contacting your primary care doctor back home. If it's more than just a simple question, keep in mind that North America and Western Europe have similar medical systems, and if you are traveling within that part of the globe, my advice is to go to a local doctor.

If you are visiting a more remote part of the world, I suggest you contact the local U.S. Embassy for advice. Often they will have a medical practitioner on staff who can help you, or they can direct you to a local Western-type doctor. If the problem can wait until you return home, be sure to tell your doctor where you have been, to help the doctor consider what you might have been exposed to.

Cruises

John: I just got back from a one-week cruise, and I've been sicker than a dog. My emphysema has been under control pretty well, but after a couple days on the ship I started having these violent coughing spasms, then fevers and shaking chills. I couldn't eat anything and could barely keep water down. There was a nurse on the ship, and he told me I probably had bronchitis, but there were no antibiotics on the ship. I just stayed in bed the whole time.

John immediately came to see me after returning from his cruise. A chest X ray revealed he had a serious case of pneumonia. If he had been able to start on antibiotics sooner, his pneumonia would not have been nearly as bad. As it was, it took him two weeks to recover.

Cruises can present some unique challenges if health problems occur. Gay cruises are becoming more and more popular. Be careful, though, if you have a chronic medical condition like AIDS, emphysema, or diabetes. Cruise ships may or may not have a doctor on board, and the medical facilities may be very limited or nonexistent. In fact, no U.S. or international law requires that cruise ships have any type of medical facilities. Every year, dozens of cruise ship passengers die at sea, and many hundreds are airlifted off the ship for medical reasons—a very expensive undertaking that is not covered by insurance.

Before deciding on a cruise ship vacation, check out what medical facilities will be available. Will there be a doctor on board? What is that doctor's background? What kind of emergency medical equipment is available? If you become ill while the boat is at sea, you may have a rough time until the boat reaches port or you are airlifted off. If your health is delicate, another type of vacation might be less risky.

I hope that this section has been helpful in planning your trip. The bottom line is, you should be able to travel just about anywhere and enjoy yourself safely—with a bit of foresight and planning. Bon voyage!

General Comments on Fitness

mericans are obsessed with fitness and nutrition, and yet our overall fitness is abysmal. According to the Centers for Disease Control, 33% of American men are overweight. The National Center for Health Statistics puts the figure much higher: 59%.

Over half of us are sedentary, which means we do not even participate in some moderate physical activity each day. We are constantly dieting and planning to exercise, yet as a population, our overall level of fitness is declining, not improving.

The energy we take in in the form of food must equal the energy we burn in our daily activities. Otherwise we gain weight. It's a simple law of physics.

There is a fairly broad range of what is considered healthy when it comes to body weight, though. Many people are not harmed by carrying a few extra pounds. Sure, a sensible diet is important for everyone. But if you are ten pounds overweight and don't exercise regularly, your priority should be to add some exercise to your daily routine rather than going on a restrictive, short-term diet.

A Weighty Problem

On average, Americans gain a pound a year throughout their adult lives. Some of this is because of what we eat. Our average diet is too high in fats and animal proteins and too low in carbohydrates and fresh fruits and vegetables.

Some of our weight gain is because of sedentary habits. People who are overweight tend to move more slowly and use energy more efficiently. They burn fewer calories during their daily activities. As a result, they tend to continue gaining. It's a vicious cycle. On the other hand, those who are not overweight tend to be more active, burn more calories, and not gain weight. Seems a little unfair, but that's the way it is.

Most out-of-shape men understand that by consuming fewer calories and by exercising more they can lose weight and become more trim. Knowledge is not as much of a problem as motivation. My goal in these sections is to describe the basics of a healthy diet and exercise program and to help motivate you to incorporate these into your life on a permanent basis.

Motivation to Get and Stay Fit

Attractiveness is one big motivator to get in shape and stay in shape, especially for some gay men. This has become a political issue in the gay community. Our magazines are filled with images of unrealistically muscular, trim, young bodies. Many critics, gay or not, say that our community is too obsessed with looks and with conformity to an unrealistic body type. They say that we have a tendency to be ageist and "looksist."

There is nothing wrong with wanting to look attractive. Anything that motivates a person to take better care of himself is a good thing on some level. But a person should not feel unattractive just because he doesn't look like the guys in the magazines. Attractiveness should not be the only reason for wanting to get into shape and stay in shape.

So I have mixed emotions when I hear a story like the following:

Jim: *I gained 40 pounds in my last relationship, and I really let myself go to pot. Now that we've split up, I've gone back to the gym, and I'm tanning, and I'm on a strict diet. Gotta be buffed for the beach this summer! Besides, I'm back on the market, and who is going to be interested in a fat, pasty guy?*

I guess Jim's recent lover was not interested in a fat, pasty guy. What does it say about Jim's respect for himself and for his lover that he let himself go to pot when he was in the relationship? I guess I'm glad Jim is now trying to take care of himself, though I may not agree with the details of his approach. And I wonder how long he'll stay in shape once he finds another boyfriend.

Healthy Reasons to Get and Stay Fit

Let's look at the medical reasons to get in shape and stay in shape. Men who are significantly overweight have a shorter life span. They have an increased risk of developing diabetes, high blood pressure, high cholesterol, heart attacks, arthritis, and even colon cancer.

Men who are not overweight and who exercise have a lower risk of all of the above problems. In addition, men who are in shape have more energy and endurance, sleep better, and age more slowly. Guys who are fit may be attractive because of their physical appearance, but more importantly, they are healthier, feel better physically, and have better self-esteem. And those attributes are very attractive.

Good health habits—a sensible diet and regular exercise—should not be viewed as special efforts. Jim is a terrible role model. Fitness is not a temporary condition. It is not a means to achieve a short-term goal, like looking good at the beach or disco in order to attract a boyfriend.

No one should feel like he is depriving himself by dieting or flogging himself by exercising. Such a person is eventually doomed to failure in his efforts because short-term deprivation does not lead to a lifetime of healthy habits. People who binge on fitness tend to bounce back to unhealthy habits as soon as the pressure is off.

Instead, every man should incorporate some sensible, healthy habits into his routine of life. These habits include 20 to 30 minutes of relatively vigorous exercise daily. They should include a sensible pattern of eating, which reduces the risk of heart disease, high blood pressure, and obesity. Healthy habits tend to increase a person's physical and emotional well-being. In the following sections we'll discuss diet first and then exercise. Both are important.

Healthy Eating

The majority of Americans weigh more than we would like. We are influenced by fashion, ads, and the media, where slenderness is synonymous with attractiveness. At any given time millions of Americans are "on a diet." This means they are restricting the type and/or quantity of food they eat, sometimes in a bizarre way, on the advice of a magazine article or book, in hopes of rapidly losing pounds that may have taken years to accumulate. They weigh themselves compulsively, and they are crushed if they don't lose those "excess pounds."

People who are dieting constantly tend to feel deprived. Even if they do lose weight, the chances are overwhelmingly high that it will not stay off. Within a year or two at most, they are exceedingly likely to be at or above their prediet weight.

Most fad diets do not lead to a lifelong pattern of healthy eating. The main benefit of fad diets is to make millions of dollars for the author of the latest diet book or the producer of the latest weight-loss supplement. At the same time, the dieter feels like a failure and a fatty. Eating sensibly should not be a fad. It should be an ingrained habit for everyone.

Healthy Eating Habits

This section contains information on eating sensibly to maintain a healthy weight. Healthy eating habits should help an overweight person normalize their weight. Even for those of us who do not have a weight problem, healthy eating can reduce our risk of developing various medical problems.

However, if you are ill and are losing weight because of your illness, ignore the dietary advice given here. You should consult your health care provider and/or a dietitian to discuss ways to gain weight. If you are trying to gain weight for health reasons, you should do it by using high-calorie "real" foods rather than synthetic or packaged dietary supplements if at all possible.

Eating sensibly means eating a variety of foods, and avoiding high-fat foods and concentrated sweets. The U.S. Department of Agriculture has an educational tool called the Food Guide Pyramid. This describes the proportions of various foods in their idea of an ideal diet.

At the base of the pyramid are starches—grains, bread, pasta, potatoes—which are recommended to make up the majority of calories taken each day. Just above the starches are fruits and vegetables. It is recommended that we each consume at least five servings of these daily. High-fat foods, such as meats and cheeses, are near the top of the pyramid, which means they should not be consumed in high quantity. Pure fats and oils, such as butter, should be used very sparingly if at all. They add only calories. The small amount of fats our bodies need we get as part of other foods.

I see things even more simply. I tell people that starches, fresh fruits, vegetables, and juices should make up most of what a person eats. High-protein foods, such as fish, chicken, or tofu, should be consumed in modest quantities and in forms that do not add a lot of extra fat.

A type of diet approach called The Zone has been popular lately, and some of my patients have been doing well with it. This type of diet recommends more protein and fat and less carbohydrate than the current USDA recommendations. Unrefined carbohydrates, which retain the fiber of the original whole grains, are favored. It takes some studying and some effort to follow this diet, but it can work well for those who put in the energy.

What about Supplements?

With a prudent diet including a variety of starches, fruits, and vegetables, nutritional supplements should not be necessary. Most men can get everything they need from this diet.

If you want to be sure, it is fine to take a daily multiple vitamin and mineral supplement, but no one has proven that this is necessary for a healthy person. The mineral supplement should include zinc, which men sometimes need. It should not include iron. Healthy men do not need iron supplementation, and too much iron may lead to heart disease. Vitamins C and

E and selenium, which are antioxidants, may be helpful in preventing heart disease and certain cancers. Good studies have shown that beta-carotene, another antioxidant, is not helpful and may be harmful, so I advise against taking it.

Juice bars are popular in the trendy (gay) sections of some cities. It feels magical to be able to drink juice freshly squeezed from fruits, vegetables, and wheat grass. Nutritionally, it is the about the same as eating fresh fruits, vegetables, and sprouts. It's good food because it's low in fat and not dense with calories or protein. But fresh juice has less fiber than the original fruits and vegetables it's made from—and there is nothing truly magical about it.

Avoiding Unhealthy Eating

Our typical American diet provides us with a ridiculous amount of fat and plenty of protein. High fat foods—such as cheeses, red meat, butter, and oils—should be consumed only as a small part of a meal. Otherwise we tend to take in far more fat than we need.

Some people pretend that snacks and desserts do not count toward their daily calorie quota. Of course these items—including potato chips and other fried snacks, doughnuts, ice cream, cake, and pie—are very high in fat and calories. They should not be part of a person's regular diet. If you are a sucker for ice cream, chocolate chip cookies, or corn chips, then don't buy them because if you do, you'll eat them! Think of it not as "dieting" but as making a permanent change in your shopping habits.

Restaurant meals are another reason we have trouble controlling our calorie intake. If you prepare your food yourself, you can choose the ingredients and be sure that there is not too much fat in what you eat. But nowadays we all tend to be too busy. It is much easier to stop by the fast-food restaurant on the way home.

A typical cheeseburger, fries, and milk shake from a fast-food establishment has more than your daily allotment of fat in it—just in that one meal. Other restaurants tend not to be much better. It is very hard to eat sensibly if one eats out. A few places are beginning to offer more sensible menu items, but they are the exception.

Portion size is also important. It is easy to gain weight—even on a low fat diet—if one eats too much. Restaurant portions tend to be too large. This is hard for those of us whose mothers taught us to always clean our plates. Ask for a "doggy bag" and take home leftovers to make into another meal. At home, use a moderate-sized plate, and dole yourself out sensible portions. Eat slowly, and you'll have a chance to feel full before you run and get a second helping.

Alcohol provides empty calories. If your weight is currently stable, adding one glass of wine to your daily calorie intake will give you enough calories to gain a pound a month; in ten years you'll have gained 120 pounds! It is acceptable to consume small amounts of alcohol regularly, but remember, moderation is the key.

Diet Pills

Dennis: *I just can't control what I eat, and I know I have to lose weight. Can't you just prescribe me some diet pills? Why are you doctors so stingy with those pills? I know they work.*

Actually, there is probably no safe, effective weight-loss remedy currently available by prescription. Besides, a pill is no substitute for healthy habits.

A combination of pills, fenfluramine and phentermine—nicknamed "fen-phen"—was recently popular and did help people lose weight temporarily. However, a significant number of those people developed heart valve abnormalities, some of which were fatal. For this reason fenfluramine and a related drug, dexfenfluramine, were taken off the market in mid-1997. Phentermine is still available.

A related drug, Meridia (sibutramine), has recently been released. There is not yet enough experience with this medication for me to judge its safety or effectiveness, although it appears safe from the studies that were done prior to Food and Drug Administration approval. I wouldn't get my hopes up, though. Remember that fenfluramine and dexfenfluramine, which work in a similar way, were found to be dangerous not long after they were approved and released.

A newer type of diet pill prevents the body from breaking down and absorbing the fat that a person eats. This drug, called Xenical (orlistat), is awaiting FDA approval. Xenical blocks an enzyme, lipase, in the small intestine, which normally aids in the digestion of fat. As a result, much of the fat is not absorbed, and the person does not gain the calories from it. Instead, the fat passes harmlessly through the digestive tract.

Well, not so harmlessly. A high fat content in the stool can cause diarrhea, stool leakage, and excessive flatulence (farting). For this reason, people who take Xenical are "punished" if they eat too much fat, and they learn how to eat a low fat diet so that they can avoid social embarrassment. Xenical may be a safer drug for weight loss, and it may help people learn to eat a more healthy diet, though how well it works for long-term weight loss is not yet clear. FDA approval has been delayed because of a possible increase in cancer risk with this drug.

Much research is currently going into what makes people gain weight. Several genes and hormones have been discovered that influence body weight in laboratory animals and humans. These may lead to better medications for control of appetite and weight gain. Until then, we are left with the simple advice: Eat sensibly, and exercise regularly.

When Eating Becomes a Medical Problem

Some gay men have eating disorders, meaning that they have a pathological relationship to food and are unable to control what they eat. They may starve themselves or eat too much, then induce vomiting or abuse laxatives. The typical individual with an eating disorder tends to be a young woman, but among men with eating disorders, a large proportion are gay. A person with an eating disorder may be of average weight, underweight, or overweight.

Anorexia nervosa is the term for the condition affecting those who starve themselves, and the word *bulimia* has been used for those who binge and purge. In reality, the two disorders overlap. The more general term *eating disorder* is the best way to describe the problem.

I have seen several men with eating disorders in my practice. Their condition is serious though treatable. Various techniques may work, depending on the symptoms and the individual patient. These include individual psychotherapy, group therapy, enrollment in an eating-disorders program (a self-help group called Overeaters Anonymous) and a type of antidepressant medication such as the drug Prozac (fluoxetine). Usually a combination of treatments is necessary.

Being extremely overweight, termed *morbid obesity,* can severely jeopardize a person's health. If someone is extremely obese and all efforts at weight loss have failed, then there are surgical procedures that can help.

Surgery for obesity entails shortening the digestive tract in order to reduce the absorption of calories or reducing the capacity of the stomach to permit the consumption of only small amounts of food at a time. (Liposuction is not a treatment for obesity; it is a way to remove an unwanted deposit of fat from one particular part of the body.)

Obesity surgery has short- and long-term risks and is only performed on people whose obesity is a serious medical problem and who have no alternative. If this applies to you, I recommend a careful discussion with your doctor about the surgical options.

Exercise

Many gay men were traumatized during childhood by competitive sports. We may have hated physical education classes, and maybe we were the last to be picked when the class was divided into teams for softball or soccer. And now that we've grown up, why should we choose to exercise when we don't have to?

Well, we should choose to exercise because it's good for us in a lot of ways. Regular exercise is very important for health. Only a minority of Americans get enough exercise. As a doctor, I talk about exercise every day to my patients, but I find it's as hard to get a couch potato to consider exercise as it is to get a nicotine addict to stop smoking. Or even harder.

Morey: *Exercise? Just the thought makes me want to go take a nap!*

Morey, believe it or not, exercise is good for you, and people who exercise tend to feel better, healthier. It may seem like a paradox, but vigorous exercise actually makes a person have more energy, not less. People who exercise tend to sleep better at night. People who are fit are better in bed. Exercise is an excellent stress reducer. And it helps a man feel better about his body. It's much easier to maintain a stable weight if you exercise regularly or to lose weight if you are overweight. Exercise lowers the chances of heart attacks and diseases such as diabetes.

Make Exercise Part of Your Daily Routine

Dwight: *When I was a teenager I hated phys ed class. I knew I was a sissy, and I accepted that, and I didn't like sports. I did whatever I could to get out of PE. The other guys teased me—*

"You throw like a girl!" I was very self-conscious. After high school I told myself no one could ever make me exercise again.

But then in my 20s, when I started dating, I realized that my posture was bad and that I had a doughy body and was getting paunchy. In my 20s! I really enjoyed feeling the hard bodies and washboard stomachs of some of the guys I went to bed with, and I wanted my body to be like that.

So I joined the Y and took a weight training class and then aerobics and then swimming. I was pretty lame when I started out, but no one teased me or made fun of me. I got hooked. Now, even though I have a demanding job, I still exercise every morning before work. Swimming is my favorite, and I've joined a gay swim club.

Exercise is like an addiction, but it's a good one. Now that I'm pushing 50, I feel much younger than lots of other men my age, and I'm sure it's because of my exercise habits. Some guys that are younger than me look old and tired. I don't.

Dwight is a lucky man. He got into the habit at a young age, and he has kept it up. More commonly I talk to men who keep meaning to get started but just never seem to get around to it. How many guys have a fancy exercise machine they bought so they could look just like the hunk who demonstrated it on TV, and now it's a $1,000-dollar clothes rack sitting in their bedroom? Or what about all those expensive gym memberships going unused?

Everybody is too busy. We work long days, we have a grueling commute home, then we collapse in front of the TV. Over and over people tell me, "My life is too busy. I just don't have the time to exercise."

Well then, make the time. Saying "I just don't have the time" really means "Exercise is not as important to me as these other activities in my life." But that's giving exercise a lower priority than it deserves. Exercise is one of the most important parts of a healthy life. And it shouldn't take that much time out of a busy schedule. The specific recommendations seem to change from year to year. A current standard is 30 minutes of moderate exercise daily, and that can be broken up into smaller blocks. Moderate exercise means brisk walking or the equivalent.

You would be amused at the excuses I hear from people about why they don't exercise. Sometimes they're even funnier than the "my dog ate my homework" stories we used to tell our teachers when we were kids. "I like to walk, but right now it's too cold/hot/rainy/snowy." "Why should I walk to work? My job has free parking." "Swimming would be fine, but I don't have a bathing suit that fits." "I bought a gym membership, but I'm waiting for things to quiet down at work." "I can't afford to join a gym." "I bought an exercise machine from one of those TV infomercials, but I haven't had the time to assemble it." "I don't have the energy to exercise." "I don't need to 'exercise'—I'm up and down from my desk to the copy machine at work all day." And on and on.

The point is that exercise should be a priority, and everybody can make time in his schedule if he wants—before work, during lunch hour, after work, or even during the work day. Exercise need not cost anything; in fact it can save you money.

Suggestions for Getting Started

Walk or bicycle to work. Use the stairs at work, rather than the elevator. Go to the gym over lunch, for a swim or for an aerobics class. (Just sitting in the sauna and checking out the other guys doesn't count!) If you like to walk and the weather's bad, go to a mall. Many malls open an hour early for "mall walkers," and it's free. Whatever you do, integrate exercise into your daily schedule. Don't make it a special event that you have to add to an already busy day, or it'll never happen.

There are two main categories of exercise. Aerobic exercises involve brisk movement so that you build up a sweat and your heart beats faster. Resistance exercise involves lifting weight in order to strengthen muscles. Both are important. After age 50, resistance exercise is more important because it helps to preserve the strength and agility that otherwise tend to decline with age, and it helps keep bones strong and prevent fractures.

> ### Exercise Tips
>
> ☐ Find an activity or activities that you enjoy.
> ☐ Set aside regular time in your daily schedule, or integrate the exercise into your routine of life.
> ☐ Consult your doctor prior to starting an exercise program if you are older than 40 or have a medical problem or a family history of cardiovascular disease.
> ☐ Start slow; don't overdo it.
> ☐ Remember that you are never too old to start

With any type of exercise a brief period of warm-up and stretching is a good idea before each session to prevent pulling a muscle. If you do pull a muscle or strain a joint, stop what you're doing, and apply ice to the area. If possible, wrap it with an Ace bandage, and elevate it to keep the swelling down. The word to remember for first aid is *RICE:* rest, ice, compression, and elevation. If you have an injury that produces severe pain, swelling, or bruising, you should see your physician.

Unless you're planning something simple like walking or cycling, you should consider taking an exercise class. The instructor will teach you how to perform the activity correctly with maximum benefit to you and minimum risk of injury. A class is a good way to see whether a given type of exercise appeals to you. If you are over 40, it is a good idea to consult your physician before embarking on a new exercise program.

Choosing a Type of Exercise

What type of exercise is best for you? Whatever type you can do most regularly. If you enjoy a solitary activity, consider swimming, running, walking, tai chi, yoga, weight lifting, or using a treadmill, stair climber, rowing machine, or stationary bicycle. If you like your exercise to be more social or competitive, join a group or league. There are hundreds to choose from.

Many larger cities have networks of gay sports leagues and clubs, ranging from bowling to swimming, softball, or hiking. (Some of them have great names. My favorite is Seattle's gay scuba club, called the Bottom Dwellers.) Of course, you always have a choice between a gay-oriented exercise environment, which has its social advantages, or a mixed one.

Dancing (folk, ballroom, western, square—even disco) is excellent exercise that can be so much fun that it's almost effortless, though very few people go out dancing every day. If you dance a few times a week and walk 30 minutes a day the rest of the time, there you are. Again, whatever program of exercise you choose, try to incorporate it into your life schedule so that it is a part of your daily routine.

For people who are ill or frail, exercise is still very important. The exercise need not be rigorous. Yoga, tai chi, light weight lifting, swimming, or walking are good choices. People with chronic fatigue syndrome often have more energy if they can be persuaded to participate in some sort of regular exercise program. Folks who have had heart attacks can attend special cardiac-rehab exercise classes. People with AIDS-related weight loss may preserve or even gain muscle mass with resistance exercising.

As we age, our exercise needs change. People over 50 should try to avoid high-impact exercise, such as running, which is hard on the hip, knee, and ankle joints. Instead they should concentrate on lower-impact activities. In addition, resistance (weight) training becomes more important as a person ages to counteract the natural loss of muscle bulk that accompanies growing older.

A few words to the gay bodybuilders or potential ones. Remember the Charles Atlas ads in the comic books? This muscular hunk telling the story of how he was a 90-pound weakling, and when the bully kicked sand in his face, he decided to become a bodybuilder and show him? That story means a lot to some gay men who grew up being nerdy sissies and as adults realize that they can become muscular hunks if they want to. Bodybuilding, via weight lifting, is a popular activity for some gay men. There is nothing inherently unhealthy about bodybuilding, and the exercise, if done right, can be a good combination of resistance and aerobic training. It certainly gets a guy into good shape.

If you plan to take up bodybuilding,or currently enjoy it, keep in mind a few things:

First, do it right. Take a class or engage the services of a personal trainer to guide you on technique and help you with your progress. It is easy to injure yourself by throwing weights around improperly.

Second, be careful with your diet. Some bodybuilding lore promotes exotic diet supplements, which may be very expensive. Real food is fine. You may need extra protein to help build muscle, but avoid taking in extra fat. Some of those muscular bodies have arteries that are pretty clogged with cholesterol. A muscular body isn't much good if you die of a heart attack at age 40. Supplements like creatine may or may not have value. There is no proof either way. If you take them and they seem to help, fine.

Third, consider carefully before taking anabolic steroids. They are readily available in the bodybuilding underground, and lots of bodybuilders use them. Personal trainers often offer them to my patients. Anabolic steroids do help a man put on muscle, but they have several downsides. They are illegal. You can get an infection, especially if you share needles used for injecting them. They can cause liver problems. They can cause personality changes. And they tend to make your testicles shrink and your breasts grow. Think about it.

Grooming

If you're looking here for beauty secrets for gay men, you've got the wrong book. There are aspects of grooming, though, that have medical implications. Grooming involves taking care of the surface of your body, your skin and hair. Healthy skin not only feels good, but it also makes a good first impression. Read the sections on grooming and on self-diagnosis and treatment of common skin problems to help you keep your skin in good shape.

Most men shave daily without giving it much thought. Then when they have a problem related to shaving, they don't know what to do about it. A section on healthy shaving is therefore included here.

Baldness is usually not a medical problem. It is a natural phenomenon. Society creates a problem by making baldness seem undesirable. Nonetheless, baldness has been medicalized, and there are medical treatments for it. Many gay men go to great lengths to deal with their hair loss. Prevention and treatment of baldness are covered in the final section of this section.

Take Care of Your Skin

hat is the biggest organ in your body? No, no, very funny. Don't you wish. Actually, in terms of surface area, it is the skin. Skin problems can be annoying, painful, itchy, unsightly, and sometimes deadly. Even if you take good care of your skin, problems can occur.

Healthy skin is attractive. It makes a person look robust, vigorous, and youthful. Be good to your skin. Once it's damaged, it's hard to repair. You can keep your skin healthy by avoiding too much sun, not smoking, and staying away from harsh soaps and cosmetics.

Protect Your Skin from the Sun

Our society seems to value a tanned look among light-skinned people. Models in men's fashion magazines tend to have a deep tan. Pale skin is seen as sickly-looking. But actually, the opposite is true. Tanning is bad for you. The same ultraviolet rays from the sun that make your skin tan also damage the elastic fibers in the skin, causing wrinkles. Sunlight can also damage the skin cells and lead to freckling, age spots, and skin cancer. My recommendation is to avoid sunbathing, or tanning, altogether. If you must do it, then do it in moderation.

If you are going to be out in the sun for very long, use a sunscreen. Sunscreens are creams that contain chemicals that absorb harmful ultraviolet rays before they damage the skin. Every sunscreen product is labeled with a sun protection factor number, or SPF. The higher the number, the better protected your skin will be. It used to be that the most potent sunscreens were SPF 15. Now there are much stronger ones available, and I recommend that you use a sunscreen rated at a minimum SPF of 15. They go up to 45 or higher. Don't sunbathe, but use a sunscreen when sun exposure is unavoidable.

I remember realizing for the first time that I was bald when I sunburned the top of my head marching in a gay-pride parade. I never knew it was possible to sunburn the top of your head, but I guess it makes sense when there's no hair there. The next year I wore a hat, but I also wore shorts, and the backs of my calves got sunburned. So the following year I used sunscreen on any exposed skin and wore a hat, and I managed to get through Pride Day without getting burned.

Ditch Those Cigarettes

Another way to be good to your skin is not to smoke. Smoking, like ultraviolet rays, damages the elastic fibers in your skin, making it lax and wrinkly. Smokers wrinkle earlier, and more heavily than nonsmokers. Studies have shown that smokers are perceived as five to ten years older than nonsmokers of the same age. If you smoke, maybe the threat of lung cancer or a heart attack hasn't been enough to scare you into quitting. I hope that the threat of premature wrinkling and unattractiveness will be better motivation to quit.

Treating Wrinkles

If you have wrinkles that you're unhappy with, there are various cosmetic products that can plump up the skin and fill the wrinkles out, but they only work temporarily. Nothing short of surgery can eliminate wrinkles, such as crow's feet or "laugh lines" around the mouth. However, a prescription drug called tretinoin (sold as Retin-A, or Renova), has been shown to smooth out crow's feet–type wrinkles when applied daily. It is not known how long this effect lasts or if it is lost when the treatment is stopped.

The best and healthiest way to deal with wrinkles is to avoid tanning and avoid smoking cigarettes. Not only will you have fewer wrinkles than the guy who tans and smokes, but you'll be less likely to get skin or lung cancer.

Be Gentle to Your Skin

The cosmetics industry would like us to be buying all kinds of expensive soaps, shampoos, moisturizers, and scents. Most people do not need these. Simple, inexpensive bath soap and shampoos are fine. Scents are not a medical issue, but it is my bias that a clean person should not smell of anything, and when a man hasn't bathed in a while, a healthy male odor is expected.

If your skin is sensitive, that is, if you develop rashes or skin irritation easily, avoid harsh soaps and cosmetics. For bathing, use a pure, hypoallergenic soap such as unscented Dove. Many people think Ivory is mild, but in fact it is quite harsh, as are most deodorant or antibacterial soaps.

After bathing, pat yourself dry, and leave your skin be. Most people's skin does a fine job of taking care of itself without the routine addition of powders, creams, or oils. Our skin has glands that moisturize and lubricate it naturally. Cosmetics, if anything, interfere with that process. If your skin is particularly dry, a mild, unscented moisturizer such as Eucerin may be helpful.

Some men's feet or groin tend to get too damp and sweaty and hence are susceptible to fungal infections (athlete's foot, jock itch). These infections are not transmitted from one person to another or from locker-room surfaces to a person. Instead, the spores that cause them are in the air and on our skin all the time. They grow where they find moist, warm skin. They can be prevented by using powders such as cornstarch or antifungal powders (Tinactin, Cruex) after bathing. They can be treated with antifungal creams, such as clotrimazole (Lotrimin) or prescription products. More detail can be found in the next section.

A Few Words About Deodorants

The one cosmetic product used by nearly all men is underarm deodorant. It is an expectation in our society that we not smell sweaty, although this is not a health issue per se. Deodorant products inhibit the growth of bacteria in the armpits and hence prevent the body odor that these bacteria produce. They usually also contain some kind of scent, which is not necessary but helps cover any odor that may occur.

Frequently I see men with rashes caused by harsh deodorants. If a rash occurs, stop the use of all deodorant for several days. One percent hydrocortisone cream applied lightly twice a day may help the rash clear up sooner. Try a different deodorant product once the rash is gone. An unscented antiperspirant will do fine and is less likely to be irritating to the skin. The "crystal" antiperspirants, which look like a big piece of quartz, are not hypoallergenic. On the contrary, they are the culprit for many cases of underarm rash I have seen lately.

Deodorant tastes awful. If you are showering in preparation for a date or for sex, it's a nice gesture to avoid putting on underarm deodorant after the shower, just in case your date or boyfriend wants to lick those armpits. Besides, the deodorant may cover up the pheromones that help turn him on.

Rashes, Lumps, and Bumps

I n this section I will discuss the most common skin problems that I see in my practice. Some of these you can diagnose and treat yourself without seeing a doctor, while others require professional medical evaluation and/or a doctor's treatment. If you have a skin problem that you don't know what to do with, the first provider you should consult is your primary care physician. Don't spend money on a dermatologist unless your primary physician feels you should see one.

Dandruff and Seborrhea

Dandruff is a flaky, sometimes itchy condition of the scalp. Besides being annoying, it is unsightly, especially if you wear dark shirts or suits.

Madison Avenue makes sure we are aware of what dandruff is because treatments for it are a big business. Several different types of medicated shampoo are effective for dandruff. Examples include zinc pyrithione (Head and Shoulders), selenium sulfide (Selsun), coal tar (Denorex), and ketoconazole (Nizoral; prescription only in the United States). These work by killing yeast that live in the skin of the scalp and/or by helping remove the flaky, dead layer of skin.

In choosing a dandruff shampoo, just take into account the cost (Head and Shoulders least, Nizoral most) and how caustic the product is (Denorex most caustic, Nizoral least). And see what works for you. If you are subject to dandruff, once you get it controlled with a few daily shampoos with your product of choice, it should only be necessary to repeat the treatment twice a week or so.

Seborrhea is a condition causing flakiness, redness, and sometimes itching on various parts of the face, most commonly in the eyebrows and over the bridge of the nose, sometimes in the mustache, beard, or elsewhere. It is probably the same basic condition as dandruff only not on the scalp. It is best treated either by washing the affected area with Nizoral shampoo or by applying one or both of the following creams twice a day: 1% hydrocortisone (no prescription required) and 2% ketoconazole (prescription required).

Both seborrhea and dandruff tend to be chronic. That is, they can be controlled, but not cured, so they recur when treatment is stopped. They are common in anyone but particularly common in HIV-positive individuals. They are not hard to treat. Most people find them unappealing and are happy to be rid of them.

Yeast Infections

Jock itch (tinea cruris) is a red, itchy rash found most often in the crease between the upper thighs and groin. It usually consists of a generally red area extending out onto the thigh, with a sharp margin, and sometimes with a few scattered red spots outside the margin. It may occur in the crack between the buttocks as well.

Athlete's foot (tinea pedis) is a similar rash to jock itch. It is red and itchy and is most frequently found between the toes but can affect any part of one or both feet.

Contrary to popular belief, one does not "catch" jock itch nor athlete's foot from another person or from the floor of the locker-room shower. Spores of the fungi responsible are around everywhere. They take hold where the skin is particularly inviting to them, and that usually means skin that stays moist.

That's why these problems are more common in summer, and they are more common in men whose footwear or underwear does not allow the skin beneath it to breathe or dry out. I see plenty of guys who go barefoot in the showers of the gym and never get athletes foot and others who have never set foot in a public shower yet have a rip-roaring case. It does seem that these types of infection are somewhat more common and pesky in HIV-infected people.

Both jock itch and athlete's foot are easily treated by any number of over-the-counter antifungal creams. Clotrimazole (Lotrimin) comes to mind, but there are others. Antifungals are also available as a spray or powder, but I have found the creams to be more effective. There are stronger, prescription-only creams that can be used if the nonprescription ones fail.

Once the symptoms are gone, the best way to prevent recurrence is to keep the area dry. Wear loose-fitting underwear, and make sure your shoes and socks can breathe. Cornstarch powder or talcum powder can also help keep the vulnerable skin dry.

Tinea Versicolor

Zachary: *I was so glad it was finally summer so I could go to the beach, but I was lying there the other day, and this friend came by and accused me of having leprosy! I know he was joking, but he pointed out these big white splotches on my chest and back and shoulders that I had never noticed before. It looks like I have some awful disease! I didn't notice it I guess because it doesn't itch or anything. What is it and how can I get rid of it?*

Zachary has a very common problem called tinea versicolor. For such a common problem, it's odd that it doesn't have a common name, but so be it. Tinea versicolor is caused by a fungus growing in the top (dead) layers of skin. The fungus is harmless and usually causes no symptoms. But it acts as a sunscreen, preventing the skin below from tanning. So when a man with tinea versicolor tans, he ends up with paler splotches wherever the fungus is growing.

Fortunately, tinea versicolor is easy to treat. Selsun Blue shampoo, sold as a dandruff treatment, will kill the fungus. What I recommend is to rub some Selsun Blue into all the pale spots one evening, then shower it off the following morning. That's all there is to it. The fungus is now dead (and the spots may turn red for a few days in response), though the spots will take weeks or months to become the same color as the surrounding skin. If Selsun Blue does not work for you, then ketoconazole (Nizoral, available by prescription), either in cream or pill form, should do the job.

Acne

Most of us have been through acne. It comes in various forms, but it usually consists of red bumps or whiteheads on the face, upper chest, or upper back. It is the typical adolescent skin problem, but it can occur at any age. Contrary to myth, chocolate and greasy foods do not bring on acne. Often there is no specific cause. Male hormone surges, as happen at adolescence or with the use of anabolic steroids, can cause acne to blossom.

Acne can be treated topically, with lotions or creams, or systemically, with various pills. Over-the-counter acne creams generally have benzoyl peroxide as the active ingredient. Prescription creams contain antibiotics such as clindamycin (Cleocin-T) and metronidazole (Metro-Gel) or the vitamin A analog tretinoin (Retin-A).

More severe cases of acne may respond to a daily dose of an oral antibiotic such as a tetracycline or erythromycin. Cystic acne, the kind that makes pits and scars, can be treated with Accutane (tretinoin). This is a potent oral medication that can have significant side-effects and toxicities. However, it is generally safe when the treatment is monitored carefully by a physician and it is taken for a limited period of time, generally 90 to 120 days. If your acne is bad enough, Accutane can be a godsend. When it works, it prevents some pretty nasty scarring.

Contact Dermatitis

An itchy red rash in only one, well-defined area is often a contact dermatitis, or an allergic reaction to something the skin is in contact with. Some common examples are: a rash under the watchband, caused by a reaction to the leather of the band; a rash under the watch face, caused by a reaction to the metal in the watch; a rash around the waist, corresponding to the elastic band in the underwear and representing an allergy to the elastic; and an armpit rash in response to deodorant. The rash of poison ivy is also a type of contact dermatitis.

If you think you have contact dermatitis, try eliminating the offending exposure, and treat the area with some 1% hydrocortisone cream twice a day. See your doctor if the rash fails to respond in a few days.

Various cosmetics can cause contact dermatitis. For example, I didn't recognize my patient Harold when he walked into my office recently. Although only 30 years old, Harold had had steel-grey hair for as long as I had known him. But the man walking into my office had shoe-polish black hair and around the edge of his hairline the skin was red and flaky.

Harold: *I got laid off from my old job, and when I started looking for a new one, the employment counselor told me that my grey hair made me look too old. She suggested I dye my hair. So I went to the drug store and got a bottle of hair dye, which I used the other night. I know it looks silly, and I'll let it grow out once I get a job again. But in the meantime, is there anything I can do about this rash?*

Obviously Harold was having a reaction to the hair dye. I gave him some hydrocortisone-containing lotion to sooth the irritation of his scalp caused by the dye. I told him I hoped he found a new job soon so that he could stop dying his hair. I suggested that if he had to give himself a touch-up, he should look for another brand of dye or go to a professional who might be able to use a less irritating product.

Miscellaneous Rashes

Various rashes may take a doctor to diagnose, but you can begin to try to figure them out yourself:

If a rash is very itchy and it gives you tiny bumps that you scratch open, most commonly on the backs of the hands, the arms, and around the belt line, then it's probably scabies, which has its own separate section under "Sexually Transmitted Diseases." You'll need to see your doctor for treatment.

If you suddenly get large itchy welts over a large area or all over your body, that's probably hives. This is an allergic reaction to something, often a food or a soap or laundry detergent. Think back, and try to remember if you've been exposed to anything new lately in those departments. Often the cause is never found. Over-the-counter antihistamines, such as Benadryl or Chlor-Trimeton, can be used to treat hives. If the hives persist, see your doctor.

Moles

Moles are a common cause of worry. Sometimes they bother a person because they are unsightly. Other times the person is worried that he may have skin cancer. A detailed discussion of the types of skin cancer is beyond the scope of this book. But here are some clues that may make you want to show a mole to your doctor. A mole is worrisome if it:

- has an open part that won't heal
- is black or very dark
- is growing or changing
- has multiple colors in it
- has an indistinct border around it

If in doubt, show it to your doctor. Melanoma, the worst kind of skin cancer, can be deadly but is often curable if caught early enough. If you have a large number of dark moles and especially if you have a family history of melanoma, you will probably need periodic visits to a dermatologist. There you will have your moles checked, possibly photographed, and removed and/or biopsied if need be.

Warts

Common warts are hard, calloused bumps on the hands or fingers. They can be distinguished from calluses because they do not occur in areas of pressure and they are round in shape. They are caused by a virus and can spread within one person or from one person to another. The same warts, when found on the feet or toes, are called plantar warts. There they can cause pain due to the pressure of being walked on.

Common warts and plantar warts are found more frequently and tend to be more severe in people with HIV infection. These warts are distinguished from venereal warts, which are softer and frillier, and which are mostly found on the genitals, anus, face, and mouth. These latter warts are described in the section on sexually transmitted diseases.

Common, or plantar, warts can be treated with over-the counter caustic preparations containing salicylic acid. This substance is either sold in a liquid form that is painted on or as impregnated plasters that are applied to the area. In either case, the medication is left on overnight, and then in the morning the area is scrubbed to remove the medication and the dead skin that has dissolved. The process is repeated until the wart is gone.

Often this is not enough to totally get rid of the wart. In that case, a doctor can often finish it off by freezing it with liquid nitrogen. More extreme measures—such as cutting the warts out, vaporizing them with a laser, or injecting them with little bits of chemotherapy drugs to kill them—are performed by specialists such as dermatologists or podiatrists.

Shaving

Shaving is an ancient custom, practiced daily by many men worldwide. It consists of scraping the hair off the face (or other body part) with a sharp tool or razor to produce a smooth, hairless appearance to the skin. There is nothing new about the habit—it was practiced by ancient Greeks, Babylonians, and Egyptians. Today, the majority of men in Western cultures shave daily.

Facial hair can dramatically change the way a man looks. Usually, a man with facial hair is seen as rougher, older, or (some would say) more masculine. The amount and length of facial hair growth also changes the texture of a man's face. A clean-shaven face can feel as delicate and smooth as a baby's bottom; a day or two of beard growth and it's more like sandpaper; a full growth of hair and it feels soft and furry.

Shaving is an engineering challenge that we tend to take for granted. You may be surprised to learn that dry hair is as hard as aluminum, while the skin underneath is as soft and fragile as, well, a baby's bottom. A razor must slice through the hairs while leaving intact the delicate skin below. To complicate matters further, facial skin has normal folds and creases that can get in the way of the razor.

How to Shave

Who taught you how to shave? Your father? A high school buddy? Remember the first time you shaved? Are you sure you learned to doing it right? Do you cut yourself frequently? Does your skin burn afterwards? Do you get bumps and rashes where you shave?

Here are some tips to make your shaving experience as satisfactory as possible:

■ Start by washing the area thoroughly with soap and water, to remove dirt and oil from the skin and hair shafts.

■ Then rinse with warm water for one to two minutes. This allows the hairs to absorb water and soften, so that they are no longer as hard as aluminum, but as soft as, well, wet hair.

■ Rub shaving cream into the area for a few more minutes, to further soften the hair and smooth the path of the razor.

■ Wet the razor blade with warm water, to lubricate it. Keep the blade wet during the shaving process.

■ Begin by shaving the more easy-to-shave areas, leaving the tougher areas for last, so that the hair there will be at its softest.

■ If you strive for too close a shave, you can irritate your skin or cause other problems, so don't be overzealous.

■ Once you are done, rinse thoroughly. Pat your skin dry.

Medical Complications of Shaving

Several problems can arise from shaving:

Razor burn: If you pull the skin too tight when shaving, the skin at the base of each hair shaft will pop up, and it will be nicked by the passing razor (ouch!).

Solution: don't pull the skin so tight.

Razor bump: In men with very curly hair, particularly African-Americans, closely shaved hairs curve back and grow into the skin, irritating the skin and causing painful bumps, which may or may not become infected.

A similar problem can occur in any man who shaves too close. If the newly shaven hair retracts below the skin surface, it can grow out through unbroken skin rather than through the natural opening at the base of the hair shaft.

A good solution to this problem is to not shave at all, since the irritation is caused by newly shaven hairs growing through the skin. However, this is not practical for many men whose jobs require that they be clean-shaven.

The next best solution is to avoid too-close shaves, by using an electric razor, for example. Antibiotic lotions or pills may also help if infection is part of the problem. They will kill the bacteria that cause whiteheads, but the problem will recur as long as hairs are cut so that they grow through skin and irritate it.

Skin infections: Some people get whiteheads where they shave, even if they do not shave too close. This occurs if they have a bacterium called staphylococcus living on their skin, which many of us carry, usually without being aware of it. Staph can infect the skin if it is traumatized, making little pustules. A similar bacterium, streptococcus, can cause a more crusty type of skin infection (impetigo).

Both staph and strep can be spread by shaving. The razor sweeps the bacteria across the skin surface and deposits them in micronicks, where they begin to grow and cause infection.

Warts are a viral infection that, like staph and strep, are spread by shaving.

Solutions: Avoid shaving, if possible, until any skin infection is cleared up. Staph and strep can be treated with oral antibiotics or with antibiotics applied to the skin or both. In addition, antibacterial soaps (Dial or Lever 2000) can help inhibit the growth of these bacteria on your skin.

Have your doctor freeze or burn warts off your face. Try to avoid shaving areas where there are warts, to prevent spreading the virus to other parts of your face.

Never share a razor. Consider it an intimate, personal item like your toothbrush. Other nasty bugs—such as the viruses that cause hepatitis B, HIV, and warts—are carried by razors.

Finally, if shaving bothers you or gives you skin problems, then consider giving up the practice. Many men seem never to have considered this option, but speaking as a man who has worn a beard for years, I don't miss shaving one bit. Besides, the preppy look is out, the bear look is in—and think of the money you'll save on razors and shaving cream!

Some Notes on Shaving Other Body Parts

Shaving your scalp or your body is not that different from shaving your face. Men shave their bodies for various reasons—for sports such as swimming or cycling, to show off their muscle definition, for simple vanity, and for various sexual reasons.

If you shave part of your body, you might try "dry shaving"—using a sharp razor on clean, dry skin. You won't get as close a shave, but you might avoid some of the problems described above with facial shaving, and it will itch less growing back. For example, this works well when shaving the genitals, where the skin is especially sensitive.

Waxing is also used to remove hair from body parts. This involves applying melted wax to the skin, then peeling it off and taking the hair with it. It sounds painful, but people who wax regularly say that it gets easier and easier and the hair gets softer and softer each time they do it.

Skin infections after shaving seem to be more common on shaved body parts other than the face. For example:

Wayne: *What is this terrible rash on my thighs? I shaved my legs for a bicycle race, and it's always itchy as hell after I do that, but I never got zits all over my thighs before.*

I obtained some of the material from one of the white pustules on Wayne's thigh, and sent it to the lab for culture. It turned out to have staph bacteria in it. The "rash" was actually a skin infection called folliculitis, or infection in the hair follicles. It cleared up with a short course of oral antibiotic capsules (cephalexin, to be specific).

Folliculitis is not a rare sight on a cyclist's or swimmer's shaved legs. It doesn't look or feel great there—or on a bodybuilder's shaved chest or on the sides of the scalp of a guy with a Mohawk, either. Over the years, I've seen all of the above.

If you get whiteheads in an area you have shaved, they should probably be treated with an antibiotic that you can get with a doctor's prescription. I generally prescribe cephalexin, but any number of different antibiotics will do. A prescription antibiotic cream, Bactroban (mupirocin), also works well. Washing with antibacterial soaps, such as Dial or Lever 2000, and not shaving too close can help keep the infection from recurring.

Hair Loss

I first realized I was going bald when I sunburned my scalp marching in a gay pride parade. Now I wear a hat, and I have a T-shirt that says I DON'T HAVE A BALD SPOT. IT'S A SOLAR PANEL FOR A SEX MACHINE. Every hair on your body grows in cycles. An individual hair grows for several months, then that hair is shed, and that follicle rests for a while. We are all losing hair constantly, but new hair grows to replace the lost hair. That is, except for on the tops of our heads. There, for many men, the hair is gradually lost for good as the years go by, and we become [*shudder*] bald.

Losing the hair on top of the head is a normal process for men. Most men, though not all, experience this phenomenon as they get older. That's why it's called *male pattern baldness,* or *androgenetic alopecia,* to use a fancy medical term.

Other forms of hair loss, either patchy or total loss of hair, are not due to male hormones. They can be caused by medication (such as chemotherapy for cancer) or by illness (such as thyroid disorders) or autoimmune illnesses going by the name *alopecia areata.* If you are having hair loss in an unusual pattern, you should see your doctor to determine whether this might be due to a medical problem.

What's Wrong With Being Bald?

Going bald on top is not a medical problem. It just means that you are a man with lots of male hormones, which are the trigger for male hair loss. So why isn't it OK to go bald?

Well, some men would say it is OK and even attractive. Just look at a recent photo of Sean Connery or of Patrick Stewart if you want to see a sexy-looking bald man. But usually our society, and especially our gay men's culture, puts a higher value on youthfulness. And baldness just doesn't say "young." It says "mature."

If your image of yourself is a young stud or a preppy collegiate type, then you might be unhappy losing your hair and looking like a daddy. Unless, perhaps, you look like Sean Connery.

In addition, there is lots of money to be made in treating baldness. Hair replacement for men is a huge industry, and the pharmaceutical companies are pouring millions of dollars into researching treatments for hair loss. So these folks have a big stake in making sure that men continue to be unhappy with losing their hair, and their advertising campaigns tell us just how much happier, wealthier, more attractive, and more sexually successful we men can be with a full head of hair.

Dealing With Baldness

You can do various things to prevent, or reverse, baldness. Castration is the most effective option. No more male hormones, no more male pattern baldness. For obvious reasons, most men are not interested in being gelded in order to keep their hair.

Medical Treatment of Hair Loss

Another way to prevent or reverse balding is to apply a topical medication to the scalp. Only one, minoxidil, sold over the counter as Rogaine and other various generic versions, has been proven to alter the natural progression of male hair loss.

Minoxidil works for some people, to some degree. In a minority of cases, men experience some hair regrowth, and in more cases the balding process will slow down or stabilize. But the medication needs to be applied to the scalp twice a day, every day, and if you stop, all the hair that has been gained will fall right out.

Minoxidil does not work on the front of the scalp, only on the back part of the top of the head, the vertex. A new, stronger concentration of minoxidil works a little better than the original strength, but still it's no miracle cure for baldness.

Other topical medications are currently in various stages of testing. Some of these may prove to work better to regrow hair, either used alone or in various combinations. For example, tretinoin (Retin-A or Renova), which is used to treat acne and wrinkles, may help when mixed with minoxidil.

We now have a systemic medication, a pill that is taken once a day by mouth, to treat male pattern baldness. The drug finasteride has been sold for several years, under the name of Proscar, as a treatment for enlarged prostate symptoms. It works by preventing testosterone from being converted to dihydroxytestosterone, or DHT, which is the hormone that actively stimulates hair loss in the scalp.

Some men taking Proscar for prostate problems noticed that they had less of a problem with pattern baldness. Now the manufacturer has received approval to market smaller doses of finasteride as a treatment for male pattern baldness, under the name of Propecia. The major side effect—reportedly occurring in just a few percent of users—is a diminished sexual ability. In addition, the drug interferes with the ability to test the blood for prostate cancer. But why worry about these things if you can have a full head of hair?

Surgical Approaches to Hair Loss

Hair transplants are an effective way to have some hair growing in the bald part of your head. A surgeon removes some skin, complete with hair follicles, from elsewhere (usually the back of the head, just above the nape of the neck, where baldness seldom reaches). The skin is divided into little "plugs" that are planted in the bald part of the scalp.

A bad hair transplant is not particularly attractive or convincing. The little plugs are obvious: they look like the tufts of bristles on a toothbrush. More sophisticated techniques use "microplugs" of hair follicles, which do not show as much. The advantage of a hair transplant is that the result is usually permanent, and it is a perfect match for the other hair on one's head.

Hair transplants are not cheap. The cost runs in the several thousand dollar range. If you consider this option, you would be advised to shop around. In addition, you should meet with people who have had the procedure done by the doctor you are considering, to get an idea of what the result will look like.

Scalp reduction surgery can shrink your bald spot. Crudely put, this procedure involves removing some or all of the skin over your bald spot and then stretching the hairy part of your scalp to cover it up. If it's good enough for Michael Jackson (who had it done after burning his scalp while filming a Pepsi commercial), well, maybe it's good enough for you.

Scalp reduction has the advantage of a more natural distribution to the hair follicles, as compared to a hair transplant. If you have a large bald area, it is not feasible for scalp reduction to completely cover it over, but in such cases the surgery may be used in conjunction with hair transplantation.

Cosmetic Approaches to Hair Loss

If you don't want medication or surgery for baldness, you can always get a toupee. The technology of wig making is improving constantly, and even I have been fooled, but you'll have to spend a lot of money on a toupee good enough to fool your doctor.

Good wigs cost a lot of money and require more upkeep than your own hair. They may be glued or anchored onto your scalp or your remaining hair so that you can swim or shower with them. In my opinion, if you get a toupee, it's not worth getting anything but a very believable one. What is the point of pretending you have a full head of hair when everyone can tell you're pretending? To me that would be far more embarrassing than being bald.

There is also the "comb over," in which a long fringe of hair from one side of the head is combed over the top of the head. In Japan, the term for a man who does this is "Uncle Bar Code." Usually a comb-over does not disguise baldness, but rather it draws attention to it. It is not clear to me why someone would want to do that.

Hair transplants, salves for a bald scalp, hormone-blocking pills, wigs—some men sure make a large effort, and spend a lot of money, to hide their normal male baldness. The easiest way to deal with baldness is to accept it and be proud that you are a normal healthy male with lots of male hormones. You'll be just as popular and a lot less poor. If you want, you can buy one of those "solar panel for a sex machine" T-shirts. Or wear a hat. I hear hats are coming back into fashion lately. Besides, unlike Rogaine, a hat will keep your scalp from getting sunburned when you march in the parade.

Body Modification

Each of us inhabits a physical body, the shell that holds our spirit, and we bring it with us everywhere we go. We adorn and groom ourselves in ways that are pleasing to ourselves and to others. We exercise and diet, to change our shape. And sometimes we want to customize our body by altering it in a more permanent way, for instance with a tattoo, a piercing, or cosmetic surgery.

People seem to have an innate desire for body art. It is practiced in all human cultures. People modify their bodies for many reasons. They may like the appearance. They may want to become more attractive to other people, or they may want to shock them. Peer pressure has a role in some people's choices. Some decide to modify their body to conform to a certain societal ideal of beauty.

Body modification may not seem like a medical issue, except perhaps in the case of cosmetic surgery. But it actually is a frequent topic of consultation between doctor and patient. For example, a man may consult his physician for advice on the risks in getting a tattoo, for treatment for an infected piercing, or for a referral for liposuction or a chin lift.

Body modification is the ultimate statement of one's ownership of his body. As gay men, we already behave sexually with our bodies in a way that makes us outlaws in the eyes of some people, religions, and jurisdictions. The practices of tattooing, body piercing, scarification, and branding are not usually illegal, but they definitely have an "outlaw" flavor to them. These ways of customizing one's body are not particular to gay men, but they are becoming more and more popular in certain segments of our community.

Plastic surgery, as performed by a doctor, is just another kind of body modification. What is the philosophical difference between a gay man getting his nipple pierced and a woman getting breast implants? In both cases, the body is being modified from its original state purely for the preference of the person involved and for no medical or therapeutic purpose.

There is nothing inherently wrong with any form of body modification that can be done safely, provided that it is done after careful consideration. A given act of body modification, whether it is a hair transplant, liposuction, a tattoo, a penis piercing, or a facelift, can be a wonderful gift you give to yourself. It can also be a mistake that you will regret for the rest of your life. None of these procedures can easily be undone. They should be considered permanent. So before you go under the knife or needle, ask yourself these questions:

■ Am I really sure this is what I want?
■ Am I doing this for myself, or for my partner or friends?
■ How will I feel if people react negatively?
■ Will I be happy with this decision five, ten, or 20 years from now?

If after careful consideration you decide that this is something you really want, then go for it, and enjoy the results. If you are not sure, then postpone the decision and think about it some more.

In the following sections, we will discuss various types of permanent body modification: cosmetic surgery, permanent hair removal, piercing, tattooing, branding, and scarification. Some of these procedures are performed by medical doctors, while others are performed by other trained professionals—or sometimes by amateurs. My goal is to provide you with enough information to help you weigh the pros and cons of any of these procedures.

Cosmetic Surgery

osmetic surgery is body modification that is done by a doctor. Sometimes it is done to correct a birth defect, remove or modify a scar, or correct a deformity resulting from an accident or injury. Other types of cosmetic surgery are more elective, such as when a person wants to change the natural appearance or shape of his body. This may involve removal and tightening of tissue (e.g., eye-lift, face-lift, chin-lift, tummy tuck). Or it may entail the implantation of foreign material into the body (e.g., cheek implants, pectoral implants, calf implants, collagen injections into the lips).

The term *liposuction,* like the term *implant,* refers to a technique, not a particular operation. Liposuction is often done in conjunction with other surgery to tighten the skin in the area involved. Contrary to what some would like to believe, it is not a treatment for obesity.

Liposuction is used by cosmetic surgeons to remove excess fat from places where it is causing unsightly bulging. A suction device is inserted through a small incision, and fatty tissue is sucked out. Many lay people think this is a simple procedure, like vacuuming dust out of a corner. Actually, liposuction is serious surgery and can have serious complications, including bleeding, infection, and occasionally death.

Raoul's Story—A Tummy-Tuck

Raoul came to me for a complete exam, as a new patient. As I examined his abdomen, I noticed that there was something unusual about his navel. It was smooth and shaped more like a little slit than a normal navel. I must have stared at it because he started to talk about it.

Raoul: *Actually, that's not my navel. It's a fake. A few years ago, when I turned 60, I decid-*

ed I was tired of my love handles. I had them removed by liposuction. But then I had all this loose skin around my waist, which was just as bad. So I had a tummy tuck. The plastic surgeon made an incision across my groin, from one side to the other. He pulled all the loose skin from my belly down into my groin, cut off the excess, and sewed it back together, below my bikini line. The skin he removed included my belly button, so he made me a new one. I'm very happy with my flat tummy, and people don't seem to notice that my belly button is a little unusual.

Planning Cosmetic Surgery

A person seeking cosmetic surgery is usually motivated by the desire to look younger, more attractive, or both. Sometimes the result is neither. The best one can say is that the person looks "different" after the surgery.

Before you consider cosmetic surgery, do some soul-searching. Ask yourself what is really motivating you to seek this surgery. Is it to help you get a boyfriend or to pretend that you are younger than you are? Consider whether it is possible for you to become comfortable with your body in its current state or if there are other ways to improve your appearance, self-image, and dating success. Ways that don't involve surgery.

Al: *I always hated my big, hooked, Slavic nose. The only reason I never got a nose job was because I never had the money. But right now I'm having a real intense affair with this man, and he really blew me away the other day. We were in the shower, and he started staring at my face, and he said, "You know, you have the greatest nose!" I couldn't believe it. I still think my nose is ugly, but if he likes it, I'll keep it.*

Remember also that cosmetic surgery is not without risk. It may sound funny, but it's really tragic to hear that a drug lord or some celebrity's spouse or a gay personal fitness trainer has died after extensive liposuction and/or facial plastic surgery. Fatalities are the exception, of course, but worldwide there are a number of deaths annually from cosmetic surgery. In addition, cosmetic surgery is painful, and it can be complicated by unwanted scarring or infection. If a general anesthetic is used, there is additional risk. Ask yourself if these risks are worth the result you desire.

I have certainly seen some excellent cosmetic surgery. And there are cases where it really helps a person's body image. For example, some men have relatively large, loose breasts. A good plastic surgeon can shrink these and tighten them up. There are many other examples where a person is unhappy about a particular aspect of his appearance, and a little cosmetic surgery can do a lot.

But I have also seen face-lifts that give a person little, flat eyes and a tight, expressionless mouth. And why anyone would want collagen injections in their lips is beyond me. But to each his own, and if your dream is to have big fat lips, and you have the cash, then the technology is there to make your dream come true. After all, you only live once.

Be sure to shop around before hiring someone to operate on you. Many cosmetic surgeons advertise, but never choose one just on the basis of an ad. A better way to find one is to ask friends who have had cosmetic surgery about their experiences. You can also ask your primary care doctor to give you some names.

Meet with your prospective cosmetic surgeon and find out all you can about the procedure. How long does the surgery take? What risks are involved? Will general anesthesia be required, or can it be done under a local? How painful is it afterwards? How much aftercare is required, and how long does it take to heal? What will you look like during the healing process? Will you have to wear a paper bag over your head?

Usually the doctor will be able to give you some written material and provide you with some before-and-after photographs of some of his patients. Ask for the names of patients who have had the procedure done by the same doctor. Contact them, and see if they are happy with their results.

Many people are very pleased with the outcome of their cosmetic surgery. It can be a great gift to give yourself if it's something you really want. Just don't rush into it. Do some research in advance. Make sure you are doing it for the right reasons. After all, it's your body.

Genital Enhancement

Penis Lengthening

S urgery to enlarge the penis is a special type of cosmetic surgery that has recently been developed. We all know that penis size is the measure of a man, right? No, seriously, many guys are hung up (no pun intended) about the size of their member. They want it to be larger and will go to great lengths (no pun intended) to do so.

Vacuum pump devices are advertised in gay men's magazines as a way to increase penis size. These machines certainly can help pump a reluctant cock into an erect state, as discussed in the "Sexual Dysfunction and Its Treatment" section of this book. A Plexiglas cylinder is placed over the penis and connected to a pump. The air is pumped out of the cylinder, and the resulting vacuum sucks blood into the penis, engorging it. To maintain the engorged state, an elastic band is rolled onto the base of the penis. The resulting "artificial" erection can be used quite satisfactorily for sex.

The ads for these devices claim that regular pumping can permanently increase the size of your penis, and they sometimes quote testimonials to that effect. I know of no proof that that is true. I guess that repeated pumping can stretch the penile tissue so that it is longer when flaccid, sort of like a rubber band that has been stretched beyond its point of elasticity. Anyway, pumps are not a medically accepted way to increase penis size. But they are perfectly safe to play with if used as directed.

Surgery is the only medically accepted method to enlarge your penis. Two techniques are used: one to lengthen the organ and one to make it fatter.

The penis-lengthening procedure takes advantage of the fact that the base of your penis is buried, or anchored, inside your body. Where the penis meets the groin, it takes a 90-degree turn downward, below the scrotum. Next time you have an erection, feel the area below the scrotum. You will notice that it is hard, just like your penis. That is because the base of your penis, complete with erectile tissue, is there under the surface. This anchor helps your erect penis stick out at an angle to your body.

The internal part of the penis is held in place by bands of fibrous tissue called the suspensory ligaments. If these ligaments are cut by a surgeon, the base of the penis is freed up and more of the penis hangs out of the body. The gain in length is usually an inch or so.

But there is a trade-off. A penis with its suspensory ligaments cut is no longer anchored. When erect, while just as hard as it ever was, it will flop around at the base rather than sticking out at an angle. If you want to screw someone, you will probably need to hold the base of your erect penis with your hand to stabilize it. Just like the guy with the gigantic penis in the porno movies. (No, I don't know if he has had this surgery.)

Honestly, penis-lengthening surgery is really useful only for those rare men who have an abnormally small penis, one that is otherwise too small for sexual penetration. For such men, surgery can help produce a much more satisfying sex life. For the vast majority of men, though, a longer penis will not lead to greater sexual pleasure for them or their partners. Those who undergo the surgery for that reason are bound to be disappointed.

The main beneficial effect, if any, is on the man's self-image. And perhaps that is better addressed with a little psychotherapy than with an expensive, potentially damaging operation.

Penile Fat Injections

Doctors have also devised a way to make a penis fatter, although I have seldom heard a man complain that his penis or his partner's was too "skinny." This penis-fattening procedure involves using liposuction to remove fat from elsewhere in the body, usually the lower belly. This fat is then injected under the skin of the penis, which normally does not have a significant amount of fat. Now the penis has a layer of fat, so it is wider.

However, the injected fat is unstable. It can coalesce into lumps or accumulate at the base of the penis, and it often is reabsorbed over time. I do not recommend this procedure.

Many men who have had their penises fattened are unhappy with the resulting lumpy penis, generating a number of lawsuits. In fact, my malpractice insurance company recently informed me by registered mail that they were adding a rider to all of their policies, stating that they would not cover claims resulting from injecting fat into the penis. As if I were planning to add this to my professional repertoire. Anyway, my advice on penile fat injections is: Avoid them.

Foreskin Restoration

Another type of penis modification is foreskin restoration. Some circumcised men feel cheated that their foreskin was cut off before they were old enough to decide for themselves. They want their foreskin back.

To restore the foreskin, the skin of the penis is first stretched over the head. Medical tape is used to keep the skin stretched. Under constant tension, the skin grows, becoming more and more redundant until it covers the head of the penis, the way a natural foreskin would. This can be done gradually, on one's own, over a period of months to years. Various devices are available to facilitate this. It is completely safe but takes a great deal of patience and self-discipline.

My description makes foreskin restoration seem much easier and simpler than it really is. It is a challenge, but for those who have done it, it is worth the effort. There are good books, Web sites, and Internet discussion groups with loads of information on this subject. The "before" and "after" photos can be quite impressive. If you are interested, I recommend you explore this area. Do not try foreskin restoration on your own without first consulting some of these sources, which can be found in the appendix to this book.

Foreskins can also be restored surgically. This usually involves a graft of skin from elsewhere in the body. The advantage is that it does not take the months or years of nonsurgical restoration. There are several disadvantages. It is expensive, painful, and somewhat risky. Not everyone who undergoes surgical foreskin restoration is happy with the result. It is very important to find a surgeon who has done a number of such surgeries and who can put you in contact with men who have had the procedure. Be careful. This is a situation where money may not be a substitute for the patience and effort needed for a nonsurgical approach.

Permanent Hair Removal

Electrolysis

The time-tested way to remove hair permanently is with electrolysis. In this procedure, an electrologist uses a tweezer to grab the base of a hair shaft, then sticks a tiny needle into the pit that the hair grows out of. An electric current is briefly passed through the needle, permanently killing the root of the hair. It tends to hurt. A lot.

Why would anyone want to do this?

It's actually quite popular. Some men have very hairy bodies, which bothers them. The hair can be thinned or removed from any body part. Thick beard growth can be thinned, or straggling hairs around the edges of the beard can be removed. Electrolysis is also an important part of male-to-female sex reassignment, where extensive work is done to remove or reduce facial and body hair.

Jean-Michel: *I naturally have a pretty smooth, hairless body, and I am happy with that. Except for my upper back, which is positively furry! For my birthday my lover bought me a year's worth of electrolysis sessions. I go every Tuesday after work. The electrologist says my back sure won't be hairless after a year, but it'll be a lot less furry than it is now.*

Electrolysis is a very painstaking, time-consuming procedure. Every hair root must be zapped individually, and there may be upwards of 600 hairs per square inch in some areas. Only a small area of skin can be done at one time because of the pain and the time involved. People who undergo the procedure usually have no more than one to three hours of electrolysis per week, for reasons of tolerability and cost.

Usually the same patch of skin must be redone a second or third time—or more—as hairs that were dormant earlier begin to grow out.

Electrolysis is painful. Some people can endure it without outside help, but many tolerate it better with some sort of painkiller. Nonprescription medications—aspirin or Tylenol, for example—often aren't strong enough. For my patients getting extensive electrolysis, I prescribe narcotic pain relievers—such as Vicodin (hydrocodone) or Darvocet (propoxyphene)—with instructions to take one pill before each session. Another helpful prescription medication is a cream called EMLA, which contains a mixture of local anesthetics. It is applied to the skin in the area to be treated, 30 to 60 minutes before the session, and does a good job of numbing it for a few hours.

Electrolysis is permanent. Once the hair follicles are destroyed, there is nothing—I repeat, *nothing*—that will bring them back. Consider yourself warned. If your current lover prefers the smooth, hairless look, your next one may favor a hairy, bearish appearance, so beware. If you get electrolysis, do it because you want it, not to please someone else.

Some people develop scars or pits from electrolysis. Some electrologists are more "gentle" and leave fewer scars, but their work may be less "clean," with more hair regrowth. Again, it helps to talk to satisfied (and less-than-satisfied) clients of a prospective electrologist, before you take the plunge.

Electrologists are trained, certified, and licensed. Don't go to one who isn't. If you care enough about your appearance to get electrolysis, you won't want a practitioner who leaves your skin pitted, scarred, or just as hairy as before. My favorite electrologist is the character played by Carroll Baker in the movie *Andy Warhol's Bad*. Great movie. If you've never seen it, you must rent it and watch it. But don't worry. Unlike the Carroll Baker character, most electrologists do not run all-female murder squads on the side.

An Alternative Method of Permanent Hair Removal

Some cosmetic dermatologists have recently begun using lasers to remove unwanted hair. A light-absorbing cream is applied to the hair-bearing area, and a laser is swept over the site. This procedure potentially has an advantage over electrolysis in that each hair does not need to be zapped individually. A given session takes much less time than a typical session of electrolysis.

The laser procedure kills a proportion of the hair follicles, but no one knows yet how complete or permanent the effect is. It will likely need to be repeated several times, at intervals, in order to get rid of all unwanted hair growth in a given site. Right now it is quite expensive, but then again so is electrolysis. The costs of each procedure are probably comparable for what you get.

Body Piercing

I f you are considering a body piercing, you should start by talking to someone who has had that kind of piercing for a while. Ask him what it was like to get the piercing and what it feels like now. For many people, a piercing will increase the sensitivity and erogenous potential of a body part; but occasionally, a piercing will actually reduce the sensitivity. Most people are very happy with their body piercings, but a few people regret getting them. So give it much careful consideration before you take the plunge. People have different experiences with body piercings, as the following stories illustrate:

Dyer: *It took me a long time to get up the courage to get my nipples pierced. I brought my boyfriend along. It hurt like hell but just for a second. I screamed and squeezed my boyfriend's hand real hard when the needle went through, and then it was over. The pain of the healing process wasn't too bad, though I was pretty stingy with hugs for a few weeks. I took very good care of my piercings, and after six months they seem to be completely healed. I'm very proud of my pierced nipples. They have grown a lot since being pierced, and they are much more sensitive and fun to play with. I just went back and got my tongue done. Wanna see?*

Washington: *I didn't have much trouble getting my tit piercings to heal. I thought it would be great to have my tits pierced because they have always been one of my favorite erogenous zones. But the rings seem to be a turn-off to some of the guys I've slept with. In fact, they tend to avoid playing with my tits. They seem to be afraid of the rings, even though I tell them they can play hard with them. I may just take the rings out.*

What is Body Piercing?

Piercing involves using a sharp needle to poke through the flesh and implant a piece of jewelry. The jewelry is left in the fresh wound, which heals around it, forming a permanent hole in the flesh in which various pieces of jewelry can be worn. Placement of jewelry in the body in this fashion is an ancient art, practiced in many cultures.

Pierced earlobes have been accepted in our society for many years, but for a long time only women (and pirates) had their ears pierced. Gay men led the way for men to pierce their ears, and now men of all sexual persuasions have pierced ears.

More recently it became popular for gay men to get their nipples pierced. Although many other people have had this done, it has the reputation of being a "gay thing." What would TV news coverage of gay-pride parades be without the obligatory shots of men bearing their chests with their pierced nipples right after the shots of the Dykes on Bikes and the drag queens? There may be just as many women and straight men with pierced nipples, but if there are, they're keeping their shirts on, and we're not.

The term *body piercing* tends to refer to to any piercing other than the earlobe. In addition to the nipples, many other body parts can be pierced. As one piercer has overstated it, "If it sticks out, it can be pierced." Popular areas, in addition to the nipples, include: the top part of the ear, the eyebrow, the nostril, the nasal septum, the tongue, the lip, the navel, the penis (various ways), and the perineum (the place between the base of the scrotum and the anus). Some of these piercings are purely aesthetic, but many types of piercing have a role in enhancing sexual attractiveness, sensation, and enjoyment.

Some people, especially those of African heritage, tend to form keloids, or large lumpy scars that develop at sites of injury. If you are a keloid former, you might not want to get any type of piercing because the result might be quite unsightly. But a skilled piercer may be able to reduce your chances of getting a keloid. For example, an experienced piercer tells me that a keloid is less likely to form if a larger gauge of needle is used.

Reasons for Getting a Piercing

Why would anyone want to get a part of their body pierced? To some people, piercing seems like mutilation. Fine, that means it's not for them. For other people, it is very appealing. As noted above, some people get pierced for the look of it or for erotic purposes. One man, when asked how he possibly could have gotten his penis pierced, replied "I like Junior, so I gave him a ring."

For some men body piercings are a way to customize their bodies, asserting their uniqueness. For others a body piercing may symbolize their devotion to their partner or commemoration of an event or a person.

Bert: In honor of our fifth anniversary and our commitment to each other, my husband and I went out and got our nipples pierced. Now when I look down at those rings hanging there, I think of my man and my bond with him.

J.B.: I only get a piercing on Solstice. That is when the energy is right to put a new piece of jewelry in my body. Next Solstice, I plan to get my septum pierced.

Zack: When a dear friend of mine was ill and knew he was dying, he took all of his body jewelry out and gave it away. He gave me the Prince Albert ring that had dangled from the end of his penis for years. I had it sterilized, and then I installed it in my own Prince Albert piercing. It means a lot to me to have that ring in my body, the ring that was a part of my friend's body for such a long time. He is gone now, but that ring keeps his spirit living in my dick.

Piercings and Healing Times

Earlobe		6 to 8 weeks
Ear cartilage		3 to 12 months
Eyebrow		6 to 8 weeks
Lip		6 to 8 weeks
Tongue		4 to 6 weeks
Nipples		3 months to 2 years
Navel		3 months to 2 years
Penis:	Foreskin	6 to 12 weeks
	Urethra (Prince Albert)	6 to 8 weeks
	Frenum	3 to 12 months
	Head of penis	6 to 12 months
Perineum (Guiche)		3 to 12 months

Choosing a Piercer

Body piercing is very safe when performed by an experienced and skilled practitioner, who will know just where and how to pierce you safely. That part is key. Find a well-trained, professional piercer. You wouldn't let a friend attempt to practice liposuction on you with his vacuum cleaner. So don't ever let a well-meaning friend stick a needle into you.

And please, don't let your hairdresser go near your nipple with an ear-piercing gun because it won't work. Anyone who tries that doesn't know what they're doing, and they'll just make a bloody mess.

Finally, don't even consider asking your doctor to perform a piercing on you. Medical schools just do not teach body-piercing techniques. Believe me. I went to medical school, and I would have remembered that class!

How do you find a good piercer? Look for a professional, and be careful. It takes special expertise to properly pierce a body part. Fortunately, reputable body-piercing salons are opening up in major cities everywhere, with piercers who have undergone extensive training before setting up shop. Inspect the piercing salon, and ask about the piercer's training, experience, and other qualifications, before submitting to the needle. There's no rush. Be selective. It is not uncommon for a person to travel to another city to be pierced by the professional of their choice for the job.

Ask to see photos of the piercer's work if available. Ask if the piercer has any references, any clients who would be willing to talk to you about their satisfaction with their piercings.

A good piercer will always use sterile needles and jewelry and wear rubber gloves to prevent infection. If you see evidence to the contrary in a piercing salon, run, do not walk, out the door. If a needle were reused or nonsterile jewelry used, transmission of blood-borne diseases such as hepatitis B or C or HIV could occur.

Most jurisdictions do not regulate or license body piercers yet, so as a consumer, it is up to you to protect yourself. There is a movement afoot to have piercers licensed by the states. A license would at least ensure that minimal sanitation efforts are being made. The Association of Professional Pierces is active in ensuring that piercing is done safely and skillfully. Membership in this association is evidence that your piercer cares about these issues.

Choice of Jewelry

Piercing needles and jewelry are usually made of surgical stainless steel, which is hypoallergenic. Do not consider cheaper metals, which may contain nickel , to which many people react badly. However, some people cannot even tolerate surgical steel. Gold is even more inert than surgical steel, though more expensive, and it is less likely to cause a reaction.

The jewelry for most body piercings is of a thicker gauge than earlobe jewelry. Too-thin jewelry will cut through a piercing. Ever seen anyone with slits in their earlobes where the piercings used to be? Then you know what I mean. Think of a wire cheese cutter—it slices right through a hard piece of cheese, but a chopstick on its side would never be able to slice cheese. Similarly, a thicker-gauge ring can't slice through your flesh the way a thin-gauge ring would. So don't be tempted to ask for a thin-gauge piece of jewelry in a body piercing. It won't hurt any less going in, and it may slice through the piercing, and a good piercer would probably refuse to do it.

Jewelry comes in various shapes, usually variations on two themes: rings or studs. Some piercings heal more easily with a ring, others with a stud in place. Your piercer will tell you which shape is most appropriate for your new piercing. After the piercing has healed, you may wear a variety of types of jewelry in it.

Aftercare

Once a piercing has been done, the original jewelry must be left in the piercing for a period of time—weeks to months—in order for the piercing to heal. If the jewelry is removed too soon, the hole will heal shut and the piercing will be lost. A fresh piercing can be cleaned with an antiseptic solution, and the jewelry should be turned in the piercing to get rid of any crusted material that accumulates.

If excessive discharge is present at the site of a piercing, it may be infected. A triple antibiotic ointment, such as Neosporin, applied two or three times a day and worked into the piercing, should take care of this. If swelling and pain occur, it may be a sign of a more deep-seated infection, and oral antibiotics may be in order; see your doctor. Remember that most doctors are not knowledgeable about body piercings, so expect a reaction of surprise.

The doctor may first suggest that you remove the jewelry. Actually, that is the last thing you want to do. The jewelry helps keep the piercing open and allows infected pus to drain out. Removing the jewelry may cause the piercing to seal shut, trapping the pus inside and prolonging the course of infection.

Incidentally, don't be too bothered if your doctor seems judgmental about body piercings. Remember that it's your body, and it's your right to adorn it as you like. As body piercings become more popular, I see my medical colleagues becoming more relaxed and less freaked out when they see a patient with them. The sight of nipple-ring shadows on a chest x-ray used to be trigger giggles in the radiology department, but now they practically go unnoticed, at least in the hospital where I practice.

Your piercer should be able to advise you on details of aftercare and help with any questions you have. I suggest you ask your piercer rather than your doctor, again because the doctor may just not be very knowledgeable about piercing and may react judgmentally and just tell you not to do it.

Frequently Asked Questions About Piercings

Will my boyfriend freak out?

Why don't you ask him? If you have a boyfriend, part of the deal is that he gets to play with your body. So if you are going to get yourself pierced, you should make sure he's comfortable playing with a body that has jewelry in it. If body jewelry is a big turn-off to him, you might think twice. Besides, he should be available to hold your hand when the needle goes in. If he is unsupportive of your getting pierced, you might keep the issue open until he comes around.

Can I damage my body with a piercing?

Depends what you call "damage." You'll be making a new hole in your body, a hole that you weren't born with. If that bothers you, don't do it. Otherwise, a reputable piercer will not intentionally do a piercing that will cause damage to you.

What about metal detectors at airports?

Usually they don't detect body piercings. The metal is not massive enough. In those rare cases when you might set off a metal detector, be frank. They'll run their little wands over you and that should satisfy them. Otherwise, offer to strip for them right there. They will tend not to take you up on this.

What about medical X rays or magnetic resonance scans?

Metal body jewelry shows up on X rays. No big deal. On the other hand, the powerful magnet used in an MRI scanner could theoretically rip the jewelry out of your body. Before an MRI scan the technician will usually ask if you have any metal in your body. You will be asked to take the jewelry out before you are scanned.

I am a model-actor. What about me?

Avoid body piercing unless you plan to never take your clothes off professionally or unless you are planning to do only pornography, in which case body jewelry might—I repeat, *might*—be OK.

Will it hurt?

Well, yes, sure, but just for a few seconds while the needle is going in. An experienced piercer can whip that needle and piece of jewelry into you before you know it. Afterwards it may smart a bit, but it shouldn't be too bad. Local anesthetic should never be necessary for a piercing. Besides, injection of a local anesthetic distorts the tissue, preventing the piercing from going in straight. During the healing process, the pain should not be bad enough to require medication other than perhaps Tylenol. If a new piercing starts to hurt more, that may mean it is infected.

How long does it take to heal?

Body piercings can take anywhere from a month to over a year to heal, depending on the person and on the site pierced. They require special care during the healing process; the piercer should provide aftercare instructions. A table of common piercings and healing times is included.

There is crusting at the edges of my piercing. Does that mean it is infected?

Not necessarily. Signs of infection include redness, swelling, increasing pain in the days after a piercing, and a profuse, green-colored, and/or foul-smelling discharge. If you think you have an infected piercing, see you health care provider, or ask your piercer if you're not sure.

Tattooing, Scarification, and Branding

Tattooing

Tattooing is an ancient art. Many cultures have long traditions of tattooing. It has always enjoyed some degree of popularity, but lately tattooing seems to be having a renaissance. The process of tattooing involves using a needle to deposit a tiny bit of colored pigment under the skin. The pigment makes a permanent mark. A tattoo artist uses this technique to draw a design on the skin. Many colors are available, though some pigments have a tendency to fade or blur more than others.

If you are considering a tattoo, spend some time thinking about what design you want and where. To help with your decision you can buy temporary tattoos to test-drive your new adornment, or you can draw on yourself with marking pens. You can also talk to friends who have tattoos.

Never get tattooed when you are drunk or stoned. A reputable tattooist will refuse to go near you in this state. An impulsive tattoo serves mostly as a reminder of a crazy day you'd rather forget. Why carry that around for the rest of your life?

As with piercing, tattooing can spread infection if nonsterile needles are used. For that reason—and because tattooing is permanent—it is important to seek an experienced and skilled tattoo artist. Some locales license and regulate tattooists to ensure safety. Others simply make tattooing illegal, which does not make it safer but drives it underground, making it less safe.

You should ask to see photographs of the tattoo artist's work and ask for references from satisfied customers. Membership in the Alliance of Professional Tattooists, which works to ensure that tattooing is carried out safely and ethically, is a good clue that your tattoo artist cares about their craft.

Tattoos have few complications. Of course, sterile needles must be used to prevent transmission of diseases such as HIV, hepatitis B, or hepatitis C. For this reason it is imperative to have your tattoo done by a reputable tattoo artist. Bacterial infection of the tattooed skin is a very rare complication. I have never seen it happen, though it is theoretically possible. Antibacterial ointment, and possibly an oral antibiotic, should take care of the problem if necessary.

Getting a tattoo can be somewhat painful, but people who have been tattooed usually tell me that the pain is easily tolerable, and pain medication is not necessary. Some parts of the body are more sensitive than others. Your tattoo artist can give you an idea of whether the site you have chosen is particularly tender.

Some people have an allergic reaction to certain pigments, causing itching and/or swelling at the tattoo site. Hydrocortisone cream, available without a prescription, can take care of this. Sometimes stronger, prescription-strength creams are necessary. A skin moisturizer can be helpful during the healing process. Tattoos, like some other kinds of art, tend to fade in the sun, so avoid strong sunlight on your new adornment.

If you are tired of that tattoo you got on an impulse or if it contains the name of an old boyfriend that you'd rather forget, you might want to get it removed or altered. A tattoo artist can often cover over or remodel a tattoo you want changed.

A tattoo can often be faded or "removed" by a dermatologist, using a laser. But the process is time-consuming and expensive and is not covered by insurance. A series of low-dose treatments are usually necessary to avoid burning the skin with too intense treatment all at once. Removing a tattoo takes longer than getting one. Also, removal is seldom complete, depending on what pigments were used in the tattoo. A better choice is not to get the tattoo in the first place, unless you are quite sure you want it there for the rest of your life.

Scarification

Scarification is another ancient art that is still traditionally practiced in some tribal societies. This involves making cuts in the skin and then rubbing an irritating material, such as ashes, into the cuts. The resulting wounds heal as lines in the skin that are pigmented, raised, or both. Healing time is usually one to two months.

Some urban tribal people—particularly gay folk and particularly in the leather community—are experimenting with scarification. I have had some patients visit me to show me their scarifications, usually on their upper back. It certainly gives a very "tribal" look. Like other forms of body modification, it should be considered permanent, so think carefully before you go for it. The only way I can imagine "undoing" a scarification would be to have plastic surgery.

Branding

A local body piercer informs me that branding is becoming more popular lately. A design is fashioned in surgical steel, which is then heated and applied to the skin to make a scar. It does sound painful, but there should be little danger to it, so if it is something you really want, go for it. You'll probably be the only branded man on your block. Again, remember there is no easy way to undo a branding, so make certain it is what you want before taking the plunge.

Substance Use and Addiction

Even though the HIV/AIDS epidemic may be the biggest health threat the gay community has ever faced, the disease of substance use and addiction was here first. It will be haunting many of us long after the cure for HIV is found. Right now our resources are directed to the battle against AIDS, but we must not let ourselves ignore other threats to the health of our community, such as drugs.

Are gay men more prone to addiction than other people? That depends on the drug, and the group of gay men studied. What is important is that for many gay men substance use is intertwined with their gay lives.

There are many reasons a gay man may use drugs. We belong to a stigmatized group, and we are under siege from such enemies as religious bigots, opportunistic politicians, gay bashers, and HIV. It is difficult to live with such pressures. Drugs can be an escape, a way for some of us to ease or numb the stresses in our lives.

In addition, drugs are an accepted part of many of our gay social institutions. Gay men frequently gather in settings where the use of alcohol, tobacco, or illicit drugs, such as crystal methamphetamine, are popular. Peer pressure, the need to belong or fit in, is a powerful influence.

Finally, for many men sex is connected with the use of certain drugs, such as cocaine, amphetamine, inhaled nitrates ("poppers"), alcohol, and tobacco. These substances are used to relax inhibitions, increase sex drive, enhance sexual pleasure, or simply add to the "atmosphere" of the sexual experience.

Defining Some Terms

What is addiction? Medically, an addiction is defined as a chronic, progressive disease, involving excessive and persistent use of psychoactive substances and leading to negative social, psychological, and/or medical consequences.

Abuse is more difficult to define, and it is more subjective. The line between *use* and *abuse* is fuzzy. What is simply use to one person may seem like abuse to another. One might say that drug abuse involves the use of a mind-altering substance for pleasure despite awareness of negative health effects. I tend to prefer the term *drug use* to *drug abuse* because the former is less judgmental.

The Process of Addiction

How does someone become addicted to a substance? Mood-altering drugs, whether legal (alcohol, nicotine) or illegal (marijuana, methamphetamine, heroin), generally give an immediate reward, a "high", when they are taken. Afterwards, the person remembers that pleasurable feeling and wants to have it again, so he takes another dose of the drug. Once this pattern has gone on for a while, it becomes a habit. The drug may also become associated with other activities, such as socializing or returning home from work or the end of dinner or sex. Each of these activities may remind the person it is time for another dose of the drug. That "habit connection" is the basis for psychological addiction.

In addition, many drugs have a definite withdrawal syndrome. This consists of various unpleasant physical or emotional sensations, such as nausea, abdominal pain, tremor, anxiety, fatigue, or fear, which occur after the person has been without the drug for a period of time. These feelings are accompanied by an intense craving for the drug, which the user knows will relieve the symptoms. The drug is taken and the symptoms go away. This cycle of use, abstinence, withdrawal, craving, and renewed use comprises the process of physical addiction. Most—though not all—drugs of abuse are both physically and psychologically addictive, at least to some degree.

Acknowledging the Problem

People who use drugs or are addicted are not evil or immoral or weak. They have a habit or illness that they have little control over but that is morally neutral. The problem for the addict is that the drug rules his life. When drug use becomes a problem, the addict generally needs some sort of outside help to get the drug out of his life or at least to regain enough control so that he can use it in moderation.

The man who habitually uses mind-altering substances is often ashamed and/or defensive about his habit. But it is very important to be able to speak frankly about substance use with a doctor because the subject is very relevant to one's health. Doctors really try to be helpful and nonjudgmental. The point is to help the drug user get better, not to punish or criticize him. Physicians do not report illicit drug use among their patients to law enforcement officials. If drug use is a problem for you or someone you love, you should be able to talk to your doctor in confidence, without fear of being judged or penalized.

We must acknowledge that substance use and addiction are definitely problems for many gay men. We need to swallow our gay pride and realize that we are just as susceptible to addiction as other people, if not more so. Some studies have found higher rates of alcoholism, nicotine addiction, and abuse of certain illicit drugs (crystal methamphetamine, for example) in some groups of gay men, in some parts of the United States. It is hard to know whether this is true of gay men in general or just a certain subculture of the gay male population. That is because often the study samples are gathered from settings such as bars, where substance use is encouraged.

Special Considerations for Gay Men

The gay male drug user has his own particular set of potential health problems and concerns. Many studies have shown a connection between the use of recreational substances and risk of exposure to HIV and other sexually transmitted diseases. Use of alcohol, poppers, cocaine, or methamphetamine by gay men during sex are all associated with an increased risk of developing HIV infection.

Often the substance use takes place in a bar or club, which may be the man's primary social outlet. Later, in recovering from addiction, the addicted man needs to develop new ways of socializing with other gay men.

For some men the stresses of being gay in an unsupportive society or the resulting self-esteem issues have helped pushed them into substance use. As part of the recovery process, individual or group psychotherapy may be called for to help such men develop pride in their gay identity and enable them to do without their chemical crutch. Obviously, for such men a gay-supportive recovery program is essential for success in developing and maintaining freedom from drug use. The program need not be specifically gay-oriented to be gay-supportive. But any attempt to help a gay male user get clean must honor and respect his gay identity, or the treatment is likely to fail.

David: *I remember the first time I went to an inpatient alcohol treatment center. My counselor there told me I should not mention my lover during group sessions because it would upset the other clients and interfere with their treatment. My lover could visit, but we could not show affection in front of the other clients. The homophobic atmosphere definitely interfered with my treatment. After I relapsed I made sure the next treatment facility would accept me for who I am as a gay man.*

It does not help that tobacco and alcohol companies are now targeting gay men specifically with their advertising, even though we may be flattered by their attention. It does help that there are many gay-run, or at least gay-supportive, substance abuse programs throughout the United States. In addition, many "mainstream" programs have realized that they cannot treat their gay clients with any less respect than their straight ones. So most gay men who want to give up an addiction can find the appropriate help. Of course, the first step is to acknowledge that there is a problem at all.

Hitting Bottom and Heading Back Up

By the time an addict is ready to seek help, he may have developed serious medical and/or emotional problems from the use of his drug. In some cases he may have lost his job, his friends, or even his home. Alcohol, tobacco, and illicit drugs can cause severe physical and/or psychological damage to those men who abuse them. This sort of individual tragedy, called "hitting bottom," often has a positive side in that it can lead to the person's acknowledging the problem, which is the first step on the road to recovery.

Once the problem is recognized, the next step is getting help. A doctor can provide advice on the negative consequences of a given drug and information on how to reduce or stop one's use. Usually, however, more than just the advice of one's health care provider is needed. This help may come in the form of peer support, such as Alcoholics Anonymous or Narcotics Anonymous. There are gay sections of such groups in many locales. For a few people, participation in such groups is all that's needed for recovery.

In most cases, however, recovery from a serious addiction requires the professional help found in a drug-treatment program. Treatment may occur either in a residential (inpatient) or day-treatment (outpatient) setting. It involves detoxification from the drug(s) of abuse, education on the addiction and recovery process, evaluation and treatment for any coexisting psychological and medical issues, and development of ongoing support systems to maintain the drug-free state after the initial phase of treatment is past. Frequently this means that the addict must find a whole new set of nonusing friends in order to maintain his sobriety.

Relapse is a common event for all recovering addicts. It must not be seen as a failure but rather as a natural, though unfortunate, part of a lifelong illness. If someone relapses, the proper response for him is to dust himself off, get clean and sober again with whatever help is necessary, learn from the experience, and move on without recrimination.

In addition, many drug users have a psychiatric disorder, such as depression or anxiety, which is often undiagnosed and may be masked by the drug(s) taken. These folks are said to have a "dual diagnosis," and recovery involves treatment of their substance abuse as well as their psychiatric disorder.

What's Next

In the following sections, I will address the important features of each major drug of abuse. The most common substance problems among gay men include alcoholism, tobacco use, and illicit drug use. Incidentally, although tobacco and alcohol are legal for consumption by adults, they cause more people more harm than any of the illegal drugs. If tobacco and alcohol are recognized as the addictive, harmful drugs that they are, then most users have a "polydrug" habit, meaning they use two or more drugs regularly.

In addition to discussing specific substances of abuse, I will devote some attention to the phenomenon of codependency. This is an essential part of the addiction process in many cases, and it needs to be addressed whenever addiction is addressed.

For each drug, I will describe its mind-altering effects, how (or whether) it causes addiction, the consequences of continued use, how to recognize that there is a problem, and how to try to conquer the habit. My hope is that the information will provide motivation for some readers or their loved ones to get help in overcoming their drug habit. Drugs take a huge toll on our community, and we must deal with this problem to maintain and improve our health, individually and collectively.

Alcohol and the Gay Community

O ver 15 million Americans abuse alcohol, though most do not realize or acknowledge it. Many of these alcoholics—perhaps a disproportionate number—are gay men. Since much gay socializing goes on in bars or lounges, where the point is to buy and consume alcohol, it makes sense that there may be more alcoholism among gay men. However, there are no good statistics on the actual number of gay male alcoholics. Suffice it to say that too many gay men have a problem with this drug.

There is little harm in consuming small amounts of alcohol. A habit of up to two drinks a day of wine, beer, or hard liquor is probably not a bad thing for most healthy men. A daily glass of red wine or perhaps other types of alcoholic beverage may even offer some protection against heart attack and stroke, perhaps by reducing the ability of the blood to clot. A drink or two at the end of the day helps many people relax and unwind. But if someone drinks more than that or repeatedly drinks to the point of drunkenness or gets in trouble because of his drinking, then it is a problem.

What is Alcoholism?

When does one cross the line between *social drinking* and *problem drinking*? The boundary is blurry. There is no agreed definition of alcoholism. Sometimes, as with an advanced alcoholic sleeping on the sidewalk, the diagnosis is obvious. But often, especially in its early stages, the disease of alcoholism goes unnoticed both by the person involved and his loved ones. One simple definition of an alcoholic is a person who continues to drink despite experiencing problems (whether social, psychological, or physical) caused by his drinking. This definition applies to many early-stage alcoholics who are in denial about their condition.

The following questions can help you determine whether you or someone you love may have a problem with alcohol:

- Have you ever felt you should cut down on your drinking?
- Have people annoyed you by criticizing your drinking?
- Have you felt guilty about your drinking?
- Have you had an eye-opener, a drink first thing in the morning to steady your nerves or get rid of a hangover?
- Are you drinking more than four drinks at a sitting—or 12 or more a week?

If the answer is yes to two or more of these questions, then drinking is probably a problem.

Murray: *Ever since my lover died, the lounge is my main social outlet. After work I usually stop there for a drink on my way home. Then I have dinner there, and usually I run into friends and hang out for the evening. I don't think I drink too much—maybe one or two drinks an hour. I know that adds up to seven or eight drinks by the time I leave, but I never feel drunk, and I have no trouble driving home.*

Is Murray an alcoholic? Almost certainly yes, though his life seems stable and he doesn't seem to be having any negative consequences from his drinking. Yet.

The Medical Effects of Alcohol

Alcohol is one of the most toxic substances that can legally be sold for human consumption in the United States. After ingestion, it is absorbed directly into the bloodstream through the stomach lining. It acts on the brain to produce a typical "buzz." In low doses, it can produce the desirable effects of calming anxiety and relaxing inhibitions. But in higher doses and/or with repeated consumption it causes a great deal of harm. Both naturally brewed alcohol, such as wine or beer, and distilled liquor, such as vodka or whiskey, are equally toxic; the only difference is in the amount of alcohol per serving. If a person only drinks beer or wine, he can still be just as much of an alcoholic as one who drinks vodka.

Acute alcohol intoxication, or drunkenness, causes severe impairment of perception and judgment. It is the leading cause of traffic fatalities in the United States. Alcohol itself is very toxic. Coma or even death can result when an inexperienced person rapidly consumes a large amount of alcohol, for example on a dare or as part of a fraternity initiation.

Another deadly consequence of alcohol use is HIV infection. Many gay men enjoy having some alcohol when they go out to the bars because it relaxes their inhibitions and allows them to meet other men more easily. The flip side of this is that it can relax their inhibitions so much that they become careless about sexual safety. I have met a number of HIV-infected men who were so drunk the night they got infected that they don't even remember the encounter. This phenomenon, where a person who has been drinking acts as if he is awake yet has no memory the next day of that period of time, is called an "alcoholic blackout." Anyone who drinks enough to suffer an alcoholic blackout is very likely to be an alcoholic.

Alcohol causes damage to many parts of the body. It is broken down by the liver, and it injures the liver cells as it passes through them. The liver is very good at regenerating itself, but over time or with heavy alcohol consumption, the harm is more than can be repaired. A scarring process, called cirrhosis, occurs. This ultimately leads to destruction of so much liver tissue that liver failure, and ultimately death, result.

The stomach lining can be damaged by alcohol. This can cause generalized inflammation (gastritis) or discrete gaps (ulcers) in the stomach lining. Alcohol can numb the pain of ulcers, so the alcoholic will sometimes have another drink to quell his stomach pain, which only makes the ulcer worse.

Long-term alcohol consumers have higher rates of cancer of the throat, esophagus, and liver than light drinkers or nondrinkers, the first two cancers being especially common in alcoholics who also smoke cigarettes.

Alcohol causes a disturbance of sleep. Even though the initial response to a drink or two is a sense of relaxation, the drug prevents a person from entering normal sleep phases. This tends to make the person want to have "just one more drink" to relax, which only makes the problem worse. Some alcoholics drink until they pass out each night, but they are not getting normal, restful sleep this way.

Finally, alcohol can cause irreversible damage to the brain and spinal cord. Over years of drinking, enough degeneration occurs in these areas that the alcoholic can develop a form of dementia similar to Alzheimer's disease. The short-term memory goes, and in addition, problems with balance and walking develop.

Social Consequences of Alcohol Use

Alcohol use can cause a person social problems. Despite his best efforts to deny or cover up the problem, an alcoholic may lose his job, his relationship, or his social standing due to the effects of his drinking. In a relationship, alcohol is a tough rival. Often the nonalcoholic partner recognizes the problem before the alcoholic himself can admit that anything is wrong. The following is a not uncommon story:

Mutt: *After 15 years, I have decided I am going to leave Jeff. I used to be able to talk to him, but lately he is already drunk when I get home from work, and he has been passing out during dinner. I can't remember when we last had sex. We have lost most of our friends. I'm tired of calling Jeff's boss in the morning with some excuse about why he can't come in to work, when really he is just too hung over to get out of bed. I've tried and tried to talk to him about all this, but he just tells me he's fine and to mind my own business. I can't compete with the bottle, and I need to have a life. The only way I can do it is to leave. Maybe some day he'll realize he has a problem and get some help.*

Self-preservation. That's one way to deal with a loved one who is an alcoholic. The partner of an alcoholic may also find some support from peers in a group called Al-Anon, which is like Alcoholics Anonymous but for the families and friends of alcoholics. There are gay and lesbian Al-Anon groups in many cities, and mainstream groups may be supportive of gay participants. Al-Anon is listed in the phone book.

Another way to deal with an alcoholic loved one is to perform what is called an "intervention." This involves bringing together several important people from the alcoholic's life—friends, family, coworkers—and confronting the alcoholic with his situation. The intervention should be planned and orchestrated by an experienced substance-abuse counselor. Sometimes if the alcoholic's problems are thrown in his face this way, he may be willing to get treatment for his addiction. Prior to the intervention, a bed at a treatment center should be reserved so that the alcoholic can go straight into treatment if he is willing.

Recovery From Alcoholism

Treatment for alcoholism is a long process. Many would say that recovery is lifelong. The process starts when the alcoholic at last acknowledges he has a problem. The next step is getting help getting sober. And finally there is maintenance of sobriety. A few recovering alcoholics can later return to drinking in a controlled fashion, but this is unusual, and it is risky to try.

Some problem drinkers are able to quit cold turkey, without help, and suffer no ill effects. More commonly, if someone is truly addicted to alcohol, he will require medical and psychosocial support during the short-term and long-term withdrawal process.

Detoxification from alcohol can be dangerous or even life-threatening to a heavy drinker and must be done under medical supervision. Often this is done most effectively as part of an overall treatment program that deals with all aspects of the addiction. A person undergoing alcohol withdrawal may develop vomiting, confusion, agitation, insomnia, and seizures. Medications such as diazepam (Valium) and its relatives can help control these problems. It is possible for most people to safely detoxify at home, but in severe cases hospitalization is required.

Alcohol treatment programs can be inpatient or outpatient. The trend—for economic reasons—is toward shorter and shorter inpatient stays. Treatment involves educating the alcoholic about the drug, the disease, and all of its medical, social, and psychological complications. Some treatment programs use other techniques, such as aversion therapy.

Usually a peer support group, such as Alcoholics Anonymous, is part of treatment. There are many gay AA groups in large and medium-sized U.S. cities. For a man who is used to socializing in bars, gay AA is an excellent way to socialize with other gay people in a sober setting and to find new, sober friends to replace those old drinking buddies.

Most treatment programs stress total abstinence from alcohol and other addictive or mind-altering substances. Some, however, subscribe to a "harm reduction" model that allows for a small, controlled amount of drinking, or occasional, nonaddictive use of other substances such as marijuana. Many treatment professionals, however, feel that this is risky and that it encourages a relapse back into active alcoholism.

A gay man will not do well in alcohol treatment unless the program acknowledges and respects his particular needs as a gay man. This does not necessarily require attending a gay-run treatment center, although those work very well. Many "mainstream" treatment programs are now very gay-supportive.

But choose carefully. I have seen situations, for example, where a gay man was not permitted to visit his partner in treatment. This is absolutely wrong because the support and understanding of an alcoholic's partner or spouse are an essential part of treatment. And I have had gay patients go through treatment and tell me they were advised not to come out to the other clients because it would upset them and deflect the focus away from alcohol issues. Such an attitude is very harmful and disrespectful to the gay client. It dooms his treatment to failure because he is unable to address the role that alcohol plays in his life as a gay man.

Staying Sober

Once an alcoholic is detoxified and out of the first stages of treatment, maintaining sobriety is the next challenge. Old patterns and habits, old ways of socializing, need to be changed to the extent that alcohol was a part of them. Some gay men need to make an entirely new circle of sober friends because all their old friends were alcoholics, and the bottle was all they had in common.

A newly sober alcoholic is emotionally frail and vulnerable. He often suffers from insomnia and depression. In a sense he is grieving the loss of his closest friend—alcohol. He may require some medical attention for these problems. Relapse is always a risk, and upwards of 50% of alcoholics relapse at some point after treatment. If relapse occurs, the best thing is to accept the relapse as part of the disease, move on, and get sober again.

Relapse can be avoided in several ways. The first is to make sure that the recovering alcoholic has adequate support from partner, friends, coworkers, and sober buddies. AA has what is called a "sponsor" program through which a long-term AA member acts as sort of a "big brother" to newer members.

Many gay men prefer a gay male sponsor. If you are a new AA member, be careful when choosing a sponsor. It is sad but true that some established gay male AA members are notorious for sponsoring and sexually preying on newly sober members. The AA term for this is the "13th step" (AA has 12 standard steps to recovery). Because of this—and to avoid any sexual tension—some gay men prefer a female or a straight male to be their first AA sponsor.

There are medical ways to help the alcoholic avoid relapse. An old drug, disulfiram (Antabuse), which must be taken every day, causes severe symptoms (headache, violent vomiting) if one drinks while on it, which is a strong incentive not to drink. However, Antabuse can be thwarted if the person skips a dose in order to drink the following evening. It works best as part of an overall treatment program in which the recovering alcoholic takes his daily dose of Antabuse under the observation of a pharmacist or counselor.

A newer drug, naltrexone (ReVia), helps reduce the cravings for alcohol in newly sober individuals. It is not a cure for alcoholism, however, and it is best used as part of an integrated program to treat all aspects of the disease. If you feel you have a problem with alcohol, don't just ask your doctor for a ReVia prescription. Get help from a reputable alcohol-recovery program.

Tobacco

C igarette smoking is the largest preventable cause of premature death in the United States. It is also the single largest cause of cancer, lung disease, and heart disease. Cigarettes are simply a very efficient way to rapidly deliver nicotine, an extremely addictive drug, into a person's system. The drug reaches the brain only seven seconds after cigarette smoke is inhaled. Nicotine addiction is the most common form of drug dependency in the United States. Nicotine is also a deadly drug. In pure form, it is used as an insecticide. The amount of nicotine in a pack of cigarettes—if eaten all at once—is enough to kill a person.

Some surveys indicate that gay men are much more likely than straight men to be cigarette smokers. For gay men, however, HIV and AIDS are the biggest enemies right now, and perhaps that gives some of us a "so what" attitude about the dangers of cigarettes. But it would be a tragic irony if many of the current generation of gay men escape HIV infection only to end up dying early from the effects of cigarette smoking.

Smoking has many serious, long-term health effects. It pains me when I see a gay man smoke. Every smoker eventually suffers the consequences of this addiction. It is interesting to note that there are very few smokers over the age of 70. Most smokers who reach that age have quit; others have died before getting that old. It has been said that cigarettes are the only consumer product that when used as intended predictably cause disease and death in the consumer. Is that perverse or what?

Why would anyone want to smoke? Not only does it cause serious health problems, it stains the teeth and fingers, makes the skin wrinkle, and gives a person bad breath. But many smokers genuinely enjoy the way that smoking makes them feel, and nicotine is one of the most highly addictive substances known.

Dan: *I never considered quitting smoking until I had my heart attack at age 55. While I was in the hospital, the doctor told me I had to quit or I would have another heart attack. I was too busy dealing with all the tests in the hospital to even think about withdrawal, and when I went home after a few days, I told myself I was a nonsmoker. Quitting was easy! But then I was sitting at home with nothing to do but rest and recover from the heart attack, and there were cigarettes on the nightstand, and it was too easy to pick them up. So I started again. I tell myself it's my only vice. I don't drink alcohol or have sex any more. But I know I have to quit. Some day. Maybe if I have another heart attack...*

Most smokers become addicted by the time they reach their early 20s. If a person has not started smoking by then, he is very unlikely to ever become a smoker. The first time a person smokes it may make him ill. He may have uncontrollable coughing or even vomit. But if the peer pressure is strong enough, he will try again and soon will get over these initial negative effects. Thereafter, smoking may give him pleasurable sensations, such as a sense of relaxation and well-being, improved mood, and an increased alertness and attention span—mostly due to the effects of the drug nicotine.

Soon after a person takes up smoking, the cycle of psychological and physical addiction sets in. The smoker is reminded to "light up" many times during the day, such as when he gets out of bed, when he gets into his car, after a meal, and of course after sex. If he attempts to stop smoking, all these cues will nag at him to light up again. In addition, the symptoms of physical withdrawal from nicotine, such as anxiety, irritability, increase in appetite, and cravings for a cigarette, will occur. In other words, he is hooked. Ninety percent of people who smoke are physically addicted to nicotine.

The Adverse Effects Of Cigarette Smoking

Smoking has a huge number of negative health effects. It has immediate effects, including raising the blood pressure and increasing the level of carbon monoxide in the blood while reducing the level of oxygen in the blood.

Many of the health consequences of smoking occur only after years of the habit. Most people know that long-term smoking can lead to lung cancer. Smokers are also at risk of other types of cancer involving the mouth, throat, esophagus, stomach, pancreas, bladder, and kidneys. Smoking damages and weakens lung tissue over the years, eventually causing emphysema, a condition in which the lungs lose their natural elasticity. It also damages the blood vessels, leading to heart attacks, strokes, and loss of circulation in the feet or hands, sometimes resulting in amputation. And smokers with HIV have been shown to get sicker sooner than nonsmokers with HIV.

Preparing to Quit Cigarettes

So we all know how harmful smoking is and how addictive nicotine is. If you are a smoker, the question is, how and when are you going to quit? This question is very important, if not for yourself, then for the people who love you and care about you .

The first step toward quitting is recognizing that you are addicted and that you want to stop smoking. It may seem that most smokers should already be at that point, but it's surprising how many say "I could stop any time I want to. I just don't want to." Those are the words of an addict.

Roger: *I want to quit smoking, but I know I'll gain weight, and right now it's more important for me to stay thin.*

There's that addict talking again. Sure it's true that smokers gain an average of five to ten pounds when they quit. However, if the quitter exercises regularly, the weight gain can be reduced or eliminated. Besides, the health risks of continued smoking are much worse than the health risk of gaining that small amount of weight.

Once you decide you want to quit, you need to convince yourself that it is possible. You must know some ex-smokers. There are as many ex-smokers as there are current smokers in the United States, and 2 to 3% of all smokers quit each year, many without any outside help. So quitting is certainly possible. If they can do it, then so can you. If you have never tried to quit before, you should know that most smokers try several times before quitting for good. But maybe you'll be the lucky one who succeeds on the first try. If you have tried before, then maybe this will be the time that you quit for good.

Now you are determined to quit, so set a quit date. This should be at least a month in advance to give yourself time to prepare. Tell your friends about your plans so that they can encourage you. You may want to attend a smoking cessation program in preparation for quitting. There are many to choose from. The Lung Association offers frequent programs as do many community hospitals. There are also commercial programs, such as Smokenders. If you prefer, gay and lesbian addiction-recovery agencies and community centers in many communities offer smoking cessation classes. And if you are HIV-positive, some AIDS service organizations now have programs specifically targeted to HIV-positive smokers.

Bill: *My partner and I are both heavy smokers, and he has no interest in quitting. But when my mother developed emphysema, I decided I had to quit. I tried to convince Alex to go to a smoking cessation program with me, but he just would not. I told him it would be very hard for me to quit with him still smoking around me and that his secondhand smoke would be almost as bad for me as if I myself were smoking. So he has agreed to stop smoking inside the house or in the car, and now I have enrolled in a smoking cessation class and have set a quit date. And maybe if I do quit, he will eventually quit as well.*

In preparation for your quit date, start to cut down. There are two ways to do this. Some people switch to brands with successively less nicotine while smoking the same number of cigarettes per day. Others gradually cut down on the number of cigarettes per day.

The first strategy gets at the physical addiction, while the second addresses the psychological aspects more. I recommend the latter. If certain activities, such as driving to work or having sex, are an immediate trigger for you to light up, you need to break that connection. Every several days pick one situation during the day when you usually have a cigarette, and cut that one out for good. By the time your quit date has arrived, you will have eliminated many of the cues that remind you it's time to light up.

Social pressures are also helping people cut out cigarettes at certain times and in certain places. More and more, smoking is forbidden in various workplaces and other public places, such as restaurants and airplanes. Soon smoking will even be forbidden in bars, which have been the last public venue to permit smoking. This narrows the options for smokers to smoke and may make it easier to quit.

Social pressures within the gay community can also be an incentive to quit. Now that it is acceptable and admirable to be a nonsmoker, being a smoker can limit a man's social options.

Timothy: *I smoked for over 20 years. I tried to quit many times. Every day, to be exact. But I never was serious about it until last year when I finally quit for good. Why then? For one thing, I realized that none of my friends smoked anymore, so when I was with them I had to excuse myself to have a cigarette. And my workplace became smoke-free, so it was much more inconvenient for me to smoke during the day.*

But most importantly, I had met a guy that I really liked, and he was a nonsmoker, and I didn't want him to know that I smoked. So every time we got together, first I would shower, put on fresh clothes, brush my teeth furiously, and pop a mint into my mouth to get rid of the smell. I never let him come back to my smelly apartment—we always had to go to his.

Finally, when we started getting serious, I decided I had to quit. I fessed up to my boyfriend, and he was completely supportive. I ended up using nicotine patches for almost six months, but now I know I'll never go back to smoking. Those ads that make it look like a man is sexier and more popular have it all wrong. It's the other way around. Incidentally, I gave up my smelly, smoky apartment. My boyfriend's was big enough for the two of us.

Smoking Cessation Aids

In advance of your quit date, you should investigate some nicotine replacement therapy to help you through withdrawal. Right now nicotine is available as a gum or a skin patch over the counter and as a nasal spray by prescription. The idea is to give your body some of the nicotine it is missing so that you can get through the withdrawal period in one piece, without losing your sanity, and without losing all of your friends in the process.

Remember, nicotine replacement does not make you want to quit. It simply helps with the withdrawal symptoms after you do quit. So don't start on patches, for example, until your quit date, and don't rely on them to provide the motivation for you to remain a nonsmoker. That needs to come from elsewhere. Also, never smoke when you are also using the nicotine gum or patches. You could make yourself sick from a nicotine overdose. And besides, once you light up one cigarette after your quit date, you have relapsed, and your chance of remaining a nonsmoker in the near future are basically nil. You will need to start the quitting process all over again.

Nicotine patches are popular and have the advantage that they deliver nicotine into the bloodstream at a constant rate throughout the day. They come in various strengths to correspond with how heavy a smoker you were and can be tapered downward until you no longer need them. They do nothing for the habit part of cigarette addiction, however. You have to work on that part yourself.

Nicotine gum releases the drug into the mouth, where it is absorbed directly into the bloodstream. The idea is to chew a piece until the peppery, tingly nicotine is released, then to park the gum between the teeth and cheek for a while, then chew some more. It is like a plastic version of chewing tobacco. A person chews a piece every few hours, as a substitute for smoking, during the withdrawal period. This intermittent use may help with the habitual aspect of cigarette smoking.

Speaking of chewing tobacco, it is not a healthy substitute for cigarette smoking. It has nearly as many harmful health effects, it is just as addictive, and it is just as disgusting—or more so—to nonusers. So don't start it in an attempt to get off cigarettes. Many people have tried this, and they end up addicted to the chewing tobacco, no better off than when they they were smoking.

Nicotine nasal spray is currently available only by prescription. It comes as a bottle of liquid that is squirted into the nose at intervals. The nicotine is instantly absorbed and rapidly reaches the brain, so the effect is similar to smoking a cigarette but without the smoke. This nicotine delivery system may be helpful for some people as an aid to quitting cigarettes, but it appears to be rather addictive itself, and so if you start it, you may have some trouble getting off it. Still, it's less harmful to your health than smoking.

There are some nonnicotine drugs that your doctor may be able to help you with to ease the symptoms of withdrawal. Three different prescription drugs can sometimes be helpful. One is clonidine (Catapres), a drug intended to help lower blood pressure. It is available as a pill, to be taken a few times a day, or a skin patch, which is changed weekly. For some people it has a mild sedative effect and is helpful with the agitation that accompanies withdrawal. Another medication is buspirone (BuSpar), which is approved for the treatment of anxiety. This is a pill that is taken two or three times a day.

Perhaps the most promising nonnicotine smoking-cessation drug is Zyban (bupropion). This medication was originally approved (under the name Wellbutrin) for treatment of depression. Later it was found to have value as an aid to smoking cessation, and the FDA has approved its use for this purpose. Zyban is taken twice a day, starting at least a week before one's "quit date" for smoking. People who quit smoking with the assistance of this medication seem to have double the success rate of those who do not. Zyban should be continued for at least two months in order to reduce the risk of relapse to smoking.

The Process of Quitting

So let's say you've decided to quit, and now it's finally the evening before the big day. You really want it to work. Have your last cigarette. Invite a buddy over to share the ceremony.

Clean out all the ashtrays and get rid of them. Your friend can take them and dispose of them. Destroy your leftover cigarettes: shred them and put them in the trash. Set out your nicotine patch—or gum or spray—where you can get to it first thing in the morning. Then go to bed knowing that when you wake up you will be a nonsmoker.

The next day begins the really hard part: nicotine withdrawal. The first few days are the toughest. Irritability, insomnia, anxiety, increases in appetite, and cravings for cigarettes may make your life miserable. Do be prepared to gain some weight. The average person gains five to ten pounds after quitting smoking. The health consequences of this weight gain are trivial compared to the benefits of being a nonsmoker.

Help yourself get through these first few days by taking extra-good care of yourself. Get some exercise. It relieves stress, and it helps prevent weight gain. Drink lots of water to wash all the poisons out of your system. Make a commitment to staying smoke-free. Have your drapes cleaned. Wash out your car ashtray and stuff tissues in it. Reward yourself with a nonfattening gift, like a massage. Tell your coworkers and friends so that they can give you hugs of encouragement and support. It still won't be easy.

Once you get past the first few weeks of being a nonsmoker, the chances are smaller and smaller that you will ever resume. Many nonsmokers grow to hate the smell of cigarette smoke, and many are actually quite allergic or intolerant to it. No one is quite as militant about the evils of smoking as a reformed smoker, and why not?

But many other smokers remain susceptible to temptation, and relapse can occur even after being smoke-free for years. Heartbreaking but true. It sure is sad to see a 50-year-old man fall back into smoking after ten years of being a nonsmoker. So if you quit, don't be tempted to smoke that one cigarette someone offers you at the bar. It could start the process of addiction all over again.

The Health Benefits of Quitting

The benefits of being a nonsmoker begin to accrue as soon as you quit. Your risk of heart attack and stroke begin to go down within 24 hours after you stop smoking because the carbon monoxide level in the blood declines and the oxygen level increases.

Over the next few weeks the cilia, tiny hairs in the bronchial passages, begin to grow back. (Smoking kills the cilia, so smokers have a harder time clearing mucus out of their lungs.)

As the cilia recover they begin to sweep dirty mucus out of the bronchial passages and into the upper airway. Initially this may lead to an increase in cough, with lots of dark sputum as the clean-out process begins. After a few weeks the cough will decrease, and eventually the familiar morning "smoker's cough" will diminish or disappear entirely.

After several years the risk of heart attack will approach that of a nonsmoker, and after ten to 15 years so will the cancer risk. If the lungs have been damaged, they will never be as strong as those of a nonsmoker the same age, but they will always be in better shape than they would have been if you had continued to smoke.

Finally, if you put your mind to it, you can quit with no help at all. In fact, this is how the majority of people quit smoking. For example:

Marvin: *I never questioned why I smoked. I came out in my early 20s by going to the bars, and I started smoking because it was just something to do with my hands. Soon I was smoking when I wasn't in the bars too. When my 30th birthday was approaching, I decided to start taking better care of myself. I joined the Y, where I swim three days a week, and started walking to work instead of taking the bus.*

One day on the way to work I asked myself what I was doing with that cigarette in my hand when I was trying to get healthier. I decided that that would be my last cigarette, and it was. Now that I'm almost 40, I am so grateful to myself for quitting ten years ago. I feel good about my health. I see people my age who are still smoking, and they look old and tired.

Illicit Drugs

Numerous mind-altering substances can be obtained illicitly. These different drugs vary greatly in their potential for harm, addiction, or abuse. Some are quite popular among certain groups of gay men, and they are often used in sexual situations, either for relaxation of inhibitions or for their libido-enhancing properties. Often, use of these drugs is associated with a greatly increased risk of contracting HIV infection and/or other sexually transmitted diseases.

Many men have tried and enjoyed one or several of these drugs once or a few times, without having any significant adverse consequences from the experience. Some continue to occasionally partake of a drug without ill effect. The danger comes with frequent, repeated use, and/or use to the point of loss of judgment or control and/or administration by routes—intravenous or intranasal, for example—that can cause other health problems. In these cases, the user is likely to develop medical, psychological, social, and/or legal problems relating to his drug use.

Because most of these drugs are illegal, there is a chance of getting in trouble even with one episode of use. If the authorities are involved, it is more frequently the seller than the user of an illegal drug who gets arrested. But many employers now perform drug testing on their employees' urine, so the one puff of a joint you had last weekend could cost you your job. If you dabble, be careful.

Cocaine

Cocaine is the granddaddy of stimulant drugs. It is extracted from the leaf of the coca plant, which grows in South America. There the natives have traditionally chewed coca leaves in order to increase their energy. In this crude form, the drug does not seem to be par-ticularly addictive or harmful.

Purified cocaine, however, is another story. This is a highly addictive drug and a powerful stimulant. Cocaine hydrochloride, the traditional form of the drug, is sniffed or injected intra-venously. Crack cocaine, which is smoked, has lately become the more popular form because of its lower price, rapid action, and ease of administration.

Cocaine produces a euphoric feeling, or "high," with increased energy and libido. This effect peaks ten to 20 minutes after snorting cocaine and five to ten minutes after injecting or snorting it. It lasts for an additional hour or so. Injection or smoking cocaine produces a more intense high than snorting. Use of cocaine during sex is popular among some gay men.

Once the high wears off, the user may feel an unpleasant letdown feeling, or crash. This feeling makes the user want to repeat the high. The result can be a binge of continuous cocaine use, during which the user may not eat or sleep for days and may have intense libido, resulting in indiscriminate and often unsafe sex. For example, this man came in for an HIV test after being treated for cocaine addiction:

Geoff: *Normally I'm completely straight, but when I'm using cocaine I'm bi. In other words, I'll screw anything that moves. And when I'm in that state, forget about condoms. Now that I've been clean and sober for a month, I want to start having sex with my wife again, but we both agree that I should have a blood test first.*

Cocaine addiction has many serious health consequences in addition to the risk of sexu-ally transmitted disease. Snorted cocaine can eat a hole through the nasal septum, the wall between the two sides of the nose. If the user is injecting the drug, there is risk of infection, especially if he is sharing needles. Heavy users may lose tremendous amounts of weight and suffer from malnutrition. Sleep deprivation, coupled with the effects of the drug, can lead to irritability, violence, hallucinations, and paranoia. Some people suffer heart attacks or strokes while using cocaine because the drug can cause a rapid increase in blood pressure. The complications of acute cocaine intoxication sometimes constitute a medical emergency and frequently require hospital treatment.

Withdrawal from cocaine can produce lethargy, depression, and intense craving for the drug. There is no medication that will counteract these feelings, but they naturally diminish in time. People who are attempting to kick a cocaine habit can benefit from a substance-abuse treatment program. Recovery from cocaine also may involve group support through Cocaine Anonymous or Narcotics Anonymous. The ex-cocaine user must surround himself with supportive, clean and sober friends and eliminate the friends that provide him with his drug or encourage him to use, or he is at very high risk of relapse.

Other Stimulants: Amphetamines

Amphetamines are synthetic stimulants whose effects are similar to those of cocaine but last much longer. Drugs in this class include methamphetamine (Methedrine; crystal, ice, crank, or speed), MDMA (XTC, ecstasy), and methylphenidate (Ritalin). Depending on the form of the drug, it may be smoked, injected, snorted, swallowed, or inserted into the rectum. The effects of a single dose may last up to a day or more. Some drugs of this type are legally prescribed for the treatment of narcolepsy or attention deficit disorder.

"Crystal" methamphetamine is the most popular stimulant used by gay men. It is easily and inexpensively synthesized from legally available chemicals and is often made in impromptu labs set up in motel rooms. It is cheaper than cocaine, and the effect lasts longer. Use of this drug is increasing rapidly, especially in the western United States. It is most commonly injected and snorted. Crystal is more popular among West Coast gay men than those in the eastern part of the country.

Many gay men associate crystal with sex, and a drug binge is frequently accompanied by a binge of uninhibited sexual behavior. Gay men in Seattle or San Francisco who use methamphetamine have been shown to be many times more likely than nonusers to be HIV-positive.

In taking methamphetamine, the user is seeking a state of euphoria, stimulation, connectedness, and increased libido, which may last up to 15 hours or more. But often, in addition, he experiences restlessness, anxiety, headache, rapid heart beat, loss of appetite, and insomnia. With excessive or repeated use, paranoia, hallucinations, and violent outbursts can occur. The drug may have severe toxic effects, including seizures, stroke, heart attack, or sudden death. When usage stops, the person often suffers a "crash," characterized by extreme depression and lack of energy, leading to a craving for another dose of the drug.

Medical treatment may be required for acute methamphetamine toxicity. Tranquilizing drugs such as diazepam (Valium) are helpful in reducing the agitation and anxiety. They are sometimes obtained illicitly by speed users for this purpose.

Like cocaine, crystal meth can dominate and destroy a person's life. The addict may devote all of his time and energy to the drug. Other activities, such as eating, relationships, and self-care, are set aside. Taking medications for other health problems, such as HIV infection, becomes a low priority. In Seattle, where crystal meth is very popular, I have seen many gay men die from its direct or indirect effects.

Because of the rapidly growing popularity of methamphetamine, treatment programs designed specifically for crystal users have been set up in many cities. Often these programs target gay men as clients, and they are particularly sensitive to the needs of this population in dealing with this drug.

MDMA is another popular illicit stimulant though not nearly as popular among gay men as methamphetamine. It is taken orally. The effects of the drug may vary from batch to batch because it is often impure, but in general they are similar to the effects of methamphetamine. This drug is often used to enhance sex.

Methylphenidate, or Ritalin, is sold by prescription for various purposes but usually for treatment of narcolepsy or attention deficit disorder. The drug is diverted and sold to a small but dedicated group of users, who enjoy its stimulant-euphoriant effect. Ritalin users may take the drug orally or crush and dissolve the pills for injection. The side effects are similar to those of the other stimulants. In addition, people who inject Ritalin tend to develop severe lung disease, which is ultimately fatal.

Some drugs that are sold over the counter as decongestants or appetite suppressants are chemically related to amphetamines and have a similar but much weaker effect. These include ephedrine (sometimes sold as Herbal Ecstasy) and phenylpropanolamine. Occasionally a person will develop a habit of taking very large quantities of these drugs—hundreds of pills a day—for the stimulant effect. Deaths have occurred among heavy users of these drugs. Ephedrine is currently being more tightly regulated, and may be taken off the market.

Opiates

Heroin, a purified derivative from the seed pod of the opium poppy (Papaver somniferum), has been around for many years but has seen a resurgence in popularity during the 1990s. The price has dropped, the purity is higher, and the availability is greater. Although traditionally given by injection, it is becoming much more common for people to snort or smoke the drug, allowing some to become addicted who would otherwise shy away from needles. It is quite popular among certain circles of gay men, perhaps more commonly in the eastern United States than in the West.

Heroin is classified as a depressant, which means it makes a person drowsy, but it also produces a feeling of well-being, warmth, and relaxation. It works by mimicking the body's natural painkillers, endorphins, which are normally released at times of stress or traumatic injury. Heroin is highly addictive after only two or three uses.

After long-term heroin use, the high cannot be obtained any longer. However, after going without the drug for only eight hours or so, the heroin addict develops a very uncomfortable withdrawal syndrome, consisting of body aches, abdominal pain, insomnia, irritability, and intense craving. The addict must therefore "use" several times a day in order to be able to function, and the motivation for use is to prevent withdrawal rather than to get high.

It is not uncommon for a heroin addict to die of an inadvertent overdose. This is because the purity of street lots of heroin varies greatly from batch to batch. If the user injects his usual dose from a batch that is unexpectedly potent, the overdose can suppress his breathing and kill him. Other hazards of heroin use include infection from dirty needles, as well as the impact of having one's life ruled by a drug. Many heroin addicts' lives revolve around finding the next fix.

Treatment of heroin use first involves getting off the drug. The withdrawal syndrome is unpleasant but not dangerous or life-threatening, though few people are willing to go through it without help. In a jail where I once worked, heroin addicts were allowed to go through withdrawal untreated. This is called "cold turkey" because of the gooseflesh that is part of the withdrawal syndrome. They were miserable for a week or two, but then they were fine, and usually—to my surprise—they did not seem angry afterwards.

A prescription medication, clonidine (Catapres), sold for treatment of high blood pressure and available as a pill or a skin patch, can reduce the symptoms of heroin withdrawal and eases the way for some people. Recently some private clinics have been withdrawing people rapidly under general anesthesia, using a drug (naltrexone) that immediately blocks the effects of the heroin. The person awakens from the anesthetic with the withdrawal process well underway. The naltrexone in his system blocks the effects of any heroin he may try to take. This process is expensive, and its safety and long-term efficacy are uncertain.

Alternatively, a heroin addict may seek help by enrolling in a methadone program. Methadone is a synthetic relative of heroin that blocks the withdrawal syndrome without causing much of a high if any. It is given by mouth once a day, in place of heroin. Later, the methadone may be tapered off or the person may be maintained indefinitely on methadone. Although they remain addicted to methadone, some people on methadone maintenance do not have most of the usual negative health and social consequences of drug addiction, and they may lead active and productive lives. Methadone programs also provide ongoing drug counseling for their clients.

Although any doctor in the United States may legally prescribe methadone, it is only permitted for the purpose of controlling pain. The use of methadone to treat heroin addiction is restricted to licensed methadone clinics as part of an overall addiction recovery program. If you use heroin and are interested in methadone, your health care provider cannot prescribe it for you but can refer you to a methadone clinic.

Prescription painkillers—such as morphine, meperidine (Demerol), hydromorphone (Dilaudid), and oxycodone (Percodan)—are in the same family as heroin and have similar potential for addiction. It is very rare for a person to become addicted when these drugs are prescribed short-term for pain. However, they are sometimes diverted for street use to be sold to addicts. For some people, they are a "drug of choice" for abuse. They may be taken orally or by injection. The withdrawal symptoms are the same as those for heroin, and the treatment is the same.

Cannabis (Marijuana)

Marijuana, or pot, consists of the leaves and flower buds of certain strains of the hemp plant, *Cannabis sativa*. The plant material is dried and then either smoked or ingested. People have used marijuana since ancient times, for medicinal purposes, spiritual reasons, or just relaxation. The active ingredients of marijuana, which include tetrahydrocannabinol, or THC, and related compounds, produce a sense of relaxation in low doses; euphoria, comfort, and food cravings in moderate doses; and hallucinations and disorientation in high doses. Marijuana use is quite popular in the United States, with about ten million Americans smoking it once a month or more. There is no evidence that gay men are particularly higher consumers of this drug than anyone else.

Although classed as a narcotic with no therapeutic purpose and highly illegal, marijuana does not appear to be a particularly harmful drug. Many people appear able to use it infrequently, in small amounts, without becoming addicted or suffering health consequences.

Modern strains of cannabis are so potent that just a few puffs of a marijuana cigarette are enough to produce the desired effect of well-being and relaxation.

However, for about 10% of users, marijuana is definitely a drug of abuse, consumed daily and in large quantity. Such people appear to be truly addicted, in that they are unable to control or stop their use. (It is interesting to compare that statistic with tobacco, with 80 to 90% of cigarette smokers addicted.) Marijuana is also often part of the "menu" of a person who abuses multiple illicit drugs.

The long-term effects of daily marijuana consumption have not been defined. For example, we do not know if it causes lung disease after years of use, although it makes sense that it would. Neither has the withdrawal syndrome been well-described, though heavy users have reported to me that they develop anxiety and insomnia when they try to quit.

Since many people appear to use marijuana occasionally and without a negative impact on their lives, it may be hard to know when one crosses the line and the drug becomes a problem. I see marijuana addiction as similar to alcoholism, as one end of a continuum of use. There are many parallels between marijuana and alcohol use, and many physicians believe that the latter drug is far more toxic. Marijuana is a problem when the drug is ruling the person's life, that is, when the person persists in its use despite negative legal, social, economic, or health consequences.

Marijuana addiction is best treated by abstinence and group support along the lines of alcoholism treatment. Often people who have had a problem with alcohol find they are using marijuana in a similar way. Alcoholics Anonymous groups and alcohol treatment centers tend to be sympathetic to the analogy and deal with marijuana use almost as if it is a form of alcohol use. Treatment programs specifically targeted to marijuana addicts are being set up.

Marijuana may have legitimate medical uses. It appears able to alleviate nausea, pain, and anxiety in individuals with certain chronic illnesses, such as cancer or AIDS, although good, controlled studies have not been performed.

A synthetic version of THC, sold as Marinol and taken as an oral capsule, is available by prescription for treatment of nausea or loss of appetite associated with cancer chemotherapy or AIDS. Marinol is effective, but people who take it tend to report that it is different from smoking marijuana—that it does not work as well, that it takes longer to take effect, and that the dose is harder to control. Studies comparing the effectiveness of Marinol with that of smoked marijuana leaf have not been performed.

Various U.S. states have relaxed their laws penalizing the use of marijuana, especially with regard to its use by chronically ill people for symptom control ("medical marijuana"). However, the federal government is opposed to such efforts and is attempting to penalize doctors who recommend their patients use marijuana. This conflict may finally lead to some studies of the actual benefit versus risk of marijuana use.

Poppers (Amyl and Other Volatile Nitrates)

Amyl nitrate is a prescription drug that has been used for many years for treatment of angina, or chest pain, in people with heart disease. The prescription form of the drug comes as a liquid sealed in a little cloth-covered glass ampoule, which is broken (hence the term *poppers*) and then sniffed. The amyl nitrate is absorbed almost immediately from the lungs into the bloodstream, where it dilates blood vessels. By increasing blood flow to the heart, it relieves chest pain caused by lack of blood flow.

In the 1970s, gay men discovered poppers. Someone found that this drug could enhance sexual desire and promote more intense orgasms. The effect of one hit lasts only a few minutes because the drug is rapidly cleared from the system. Dizziness, palpitations, and headache are common side effects.

Private companies began manufacturing and bottling amyl nitrate for recreational use, under such names as "Locker Room" and "Rush," sold supposedly as "room odorizer." It became a common sight to see men sniffing out of these little brown bottles, on dance floors and at sex clubs.

Then in the early 1980s, AIDS hit. At first no one knew what was making gay men get sick all of a sudden. Researchers examined the lifestyles of sexually active gay men to see what they might be doing that might harm their immune systems. Poppers were immediately suspected as a cause of AIDS because they were used almost exclusively by gay men. Ultimately, their sale was banned by the government.

Although HIV has long since been accepted as the cause of AIDS, the stigma of poppers lives on. However, they have never been proven to be the cause of any medical problem, other than the occasional chemical burn caused by spillage onto the skin. Variants of amyl nitrate are available semi-illicitly in the United States (with labels such as "video head cleaner" or "carburetor cleaner"), and the original drug remains available without a prescription in many countries, for example Great Britain.

Amyl nitrate is not addictive, and it is not clear whether it causes harm with occasional use. It certainly is not the cause of AIDS, though its use may contribute to HIV transmission. However, amyl nitrate can cause dangerously low blood pressure—and possibly death—in a man who is taking Viagra to improve his erections. Do not use amyl if you have taken Viagra within the past 24 hours.

Dissociative and Hallucinogenic Drugs

Ketamine: Circuit parties, all-night dance parties held for gay men in various cities across the country, are a popular setting for the use of many drugs. One particularly strange one is ketamine, popularly known as "K" or "Special K." This drug is used by prescription as an anesthetic for people and animals. Commercial supplies are diverted for recreational use. It can be snorted, smoked, eaten, or injected.

Ketamine produces hallucinations and a dissociated state. In this condition, the user has little or no concern for his surroundings or his personal safety, and his sense of his body is altered. The man who is moving more and more slowly on the dance floor and ends up slumping to the floor while everyone else is dancing around him may have taken Special K. He may become completely unresponsive, a state referred to as a "K-hole."

Reactions to ketamine have led to some dramatic scenes at circuit parties when fallen party goers are taken away in ambulances. Coma and death can result from the use of this drug. I am curious as to why it appeals to people.

Little research attention has been paid to the issue of the use of ketamine by gay men. However, as its use increases I anticipate the appearance programs and campaigns addressing ketamine use.

LSD: An extremely potent drug, meaning that a very tiny amount has a powerful effect. It is both a stimulant, and a hallucinogen, producing sensations of altered reality, as well as frank hallucinations, in very low doses. LSD is taken orally. It has been illegal in the United States for many years.

LSD does not appear to be addictive, and there is no known withdrawal syndrome after prolonged use. An occasional individual will use LSD regularly for a period of time, but most will use it only very rarely, sometimes while dabbling with various other mind-altering drugs. LSD occasionally produces paranoia and/or violence. It has never been a very popular drug, either among gay men or in the larger population.

There are many other less common "street drugs" out there. I have attempted to describe the ones most commonly used by gay men. If you are curious about a drug that is not listed, let me know, and I will try to include it in the next edition of this book.

Codependency

rank: *Joe's OK, but in the last year he's discovered cocaine, and I'm beginning to worry about him. At first he just used it occasionally, and it seemed to give him more energy, and he really became an animal in bed. He got me to try it, but I didn't like the way it made me feel.*

Anyway, the past few months he's been using too much. Sometimes he's up all night and misses work the next day. Lately that's been happening once a week, or more. His boss is an old buddy of mine, so I've been able to persuade him not to fire Joe.

He doesn't eat right when he uses, and it's beginning to show. I've been cooking some of his favorite dishes, to try to help him put some flesh back on his bones. I know he's spending lots of money on coke because our checking account keeps getting overdrawn. Our salaries used to be enough to meet our expenses, but now I've had to transfer money from savings to keep the checking account in the black.

I'm afraid to confront Joe about this problem because he's been so cranky lately, and I love him, and I don't want to make him feel worse than he already does. I just don't know what to do. My last lover was an alcoholic. How do I end up with these winners?

A Codependent Relationship

Frank is a classic codependent, or enabler. As Joe's drug habit has progressed, Frank has done his best to protect him from its consequences. He's kept Joe from losing his job. He has tried to help him counteract the weight loss resulting from his coke use. He is even supporting Joe's drug habit financially by funneling money from savings into the account that Joe has been draining to buy cocaine. And he is afraid to talk to Joe about the situation.

Why is Frank doing this? Ostensibly because he loves Joe. Every little act is designed to protect or cushion Joe's life from the negative effects of his drug habit. Frank feels rewarded by taking care of Joe in this way.

But in the long run, Frank's behavior is very harmful to Joe's well being. By protecting Joe from the consequences of his coke use, he is preventing Joe from seeing how damaging his addiction has become to many aspects of his life. In doing so, Frank is facilitating Joe's drug habit. Which is just the opposite of what Joe needs.

What Joe really needs is to be hit in the face with the consequences of his cocaine addiction. He needs to take responsibility for missing work, even if that means he loses his job. He needs to see that the cocaine is damaging his health as he loses weight from not eating. And he needs Frank to stop paying for his drug and to start confronting him with what the drug is doing to his life and to their relationship.

This is very difficult. Codependency stems from the very human desire to be loved and needed. Frank gets off on taking care of Joe, on Joe needing him. But it is an unhealthy situation because it relies on Joe remaining ill with his drug habit, and it perpetuates and supports the habit.

A degree of mutual dependency is a part of all loving relationships. To depend on one's partner is not bad, per se. It's great when one member of a couple is supportive of the other and takes care of him in times of need.

The sickness we call codependency occurs when the relationship focuses on maintaining one member of the couple in an ill, dependent state. The caregiver appears to be supportive, but at the same time he is unconsciously working to perpetuate his partner's illness because he needs to be needed.

Many addicts, such as Joe, are very good at choosing partners who will support their habit or whom they can train to do so. They have a history of being with loving, codependent partners who help them remain addicts.

Likewise, many codependents end up with a string of drug-addicted partners. Usually the codependent man is a sweet, caring individual, and he can't understand why he ends up falling in love with (potential) addicts. The reason is that he needs to be in a helping role. Unconsciously he has chosen as a partner a man who will be dependent and needy. Or the addict has chosen him for the complimentary reason.

Codependency can involve any type of drug use. Although cocaine was the drug of choice in Frank and Joe's story, alcoholism is the classic scenario for codependency. Also, codependency need not be a one-way street. The two members of a couple may be mutually codependent, each supporting and perpetuating the illness of the other. It may also involve situations other than drug use, such as irresponsible sex, compulsive gambling, or even the medical illness of one partner.

For example, now that some people with AIDS are getting better with the help of new treatments, I am seeing some relationships end. In these cases, it seems that the whole relationship was based on the healthy partner taking care of the ill, needy partner. When the ill partner began to get better, the healthy partner lost interest and left because his need to be needed was no longer being met. Although it may not have been apparent, the relationship was a codependent one.

Getting Better

Let's get back to Frank and Joe. Both men need treatment. Joe needs treatment for his drug habit, Frank needs treatment for his codependency, and together they need to recognize that their relationship has begun to revolve around their mutual illness. A gay-supportive substance-abuse treatment program will recognize this. In such a program, both members of the couple will be treated. Otherwise the risk of relapse is very high.

If both Frank and Joe acknowledge their problems, and agree to face and deal with them, then the outlook is good, both for them as individuals and as a couple. After successfully completing treatment together, they can each begin to support the other in staying healthy rather than remaining sick.

Genitourinary Structure and Function

Our bodies are designed for multiple purposes. A man's urinary system and his genital system are intertwined, and they share some plumbing. The penis, obviously, is both the nozzle through which we pass urine and also an organ of sexual pleasure. So we refer to this part of our body as our genitourinary system.

It is impossible to discuss the sexual functions of the genitourinary system without considering the urinary function as well. This is a complex part of the body. It is richly endowed with blood vessels and nerve endings, and there is sophisticated plumbing built-in to control the flow of the various fluids that pass through it.

Many gay men also consider their anus and rectum to be an important sexual region. Like the penis, the anus has the dual functions of waste elimination and sexual pleasure. Also like the penis, the anus is richly endowed with blood vessels and nerve endings.

In addition to our male anatomy, various hormones flow through our bodies. They influence the structure and function of our sex organs and our brains, and they are an important part of our male physiology.

It's important for every gay man to be familiar with the way his male plumbing and wiring are designed, how they work, the ways in which things can go awry, and how to keep the system in good working order.

In the following sections we'll first discuss the variety of male hormones, both natural and synthetic. Next we'll explore the different parts of a gay male's sexual apparatus—the penis, the scrotum and its contents, the prostate, anus, and rectum—how they are constructed, and how they function. Sexually transmitted diseases often cause problems with the sex organs. These disorders have their own separate sections in the book.

Male Hormones

All human beings have sex hormones, which belong to a class of molecules called *steroid hormones.* Some sex hormones are more "male" (testosterone being the most important of these male hormones, or androgens). Some hormones are more "female" (estrogen is the classic female hormone). Everybody has both male and female hormones. Men have a lot more testosterone than estrogen, and for women it's the other way around.

Testosterone helps make our bodies male. An embryo starts out with the potential to develop either male or female sexual organs. In a boy embryo it is the testosterone that stimulates the development of the penis, testes, prostate, and the apparatus that connects them all together.

Later on, in puberty, rising testosterone levels promote the growth of facial and body hair, as well as the maturation of the sex organs. Throughout a man's life testosterone is necessary for the maintenance and function of these organs. There is no difference in testosterone levels between the average gay and straight man.

Testosterone is made primarily in the testes, from which it is released into the bloodstream to travel to the other parts of the body where it acts. Some testosterone is converted into dihydrotestosterone, or DHT, at the site of action. DHT is more potent but otherwise similar to testosterone itself. Castration (removal of the testes) eliminates testosterone and therefore prevents the effects of this hormone.

Androgens also do some things we would rather they not do. At puberty, rapid increases in levels of these hormones help trigger acne. Testosterone and DHT are responsible for promoting male pattern baldness, which affects most men over time. By continuing to stimulate prostate growth throughout life, these hormones are largely to blame for the symptoms of an enlarged prostate, which plague many older men.

Medications that block the conversion of testosterone to DHT have been developed in efforts to counteract these unwanted androgenic effects. Finasteride, or Proscar, is the first to be released. It is approved for treatment of the symptoms of an enlarged prostate and, in a weaker strength, as a therapy for male baldness (see also "Hair Loss").

Testosterone promotes muscle growth and a masculine body shape and fat distribution. This results in men's bodies having broader shoulders and narrower hips than women's. Testosterone tends to raise the cholesterol levels, including the LDL cholesterol, the type that is highly correlated with heart and blood-vessel disease. This is one reason why men have heart attacks earlier and more commonly than women.

Testosterone has effects on the psyche. If given to monkeys, testosterone produces aggressive behavior, so for a long time people have assumed it does the same thing for human males. However, recent studies in humans do not confirm that high testosterone levels cause aggressiveness or irritability.

It is unquestionably true, however, that testosterone stimulates the sex drive. A high testosterone level will make a man hornier, and if his testosterone drops too low, he'll lose all interest in sex, as well as any ability to function sexually. Incidentally, this seems to be true for women as well as men. Women seem to require some testosterone to have an adequate sex drive.

In the 1920s, when the sex hormones were discovered, a clever scientist wondered if maybe homosexual men were "that way" because they had too much estrogen and not enough testosterone. So he gave testosterone injections to a group of gay men in hopes of turning them straight. What he found instead was that all it did was make them hornier. They chased men that much more and continued to be uninterested in women. It's important to keep this in mind because it says that being gay has nothing to do with hormones. Hormones produce maleness, and they give us our libido but not our sexual orientation.

Androgen Deficiency and Replacement

Sometimes, for various reasons, some men stop making as much testosterone as they should. This happens most frequently in men with liver disease, alcoholism, or AIDS, but it can happen to a healthy man as well. The main symptoms of a testosterone deficiency are fatigue, loss of libido, and diminished erections. These can be corrected by testosterone replacement therapy.

Oral forms of testosterone are impractical as replacement therapy because the hormone passes through the liver after ingestion, and it is mostly destroyed before it reaches the bloodstream. So testosterone replacement therapy is best administered in such a way that it bypasses the digestive tract and liver.

The time-tested (and least expensive) method of testosterone replacement is to give it as an injection. The testosterone is bound to a fatty molecule and comes as an oily liquid in a base of cottonseed or sesame oil. Popular forms are testosterone cypionate and testosterone enanthate. A dose of one of these preparations is injected deep into the muscle of the hip or thigh every ten to 14 days. A man can be taught to give himself his own testosterone injections, or a friend or partner can do it, or he can get them at his doctor's office (which is more expensive and more of a hassle).

Recently two new delivery systems have been developed that administer testosterone directly through the skin. Both brands of testosterone patch are considerably more expensive than the shots.

The first testosterone patch to be released, Testoderm, is a soft, flexible square of cloth and plastic that is applied to the scrotum and changed every 24 hours. The scrotum must be kept shaved for proper contact, and the man may need to wear briefs to hold the patch on. The hormone is well absorbed through the scrotal skin, but many men find this device awkward and inconvenient.

Androderm is a testosterone skin patch that is applied to the trunk or a limb. The man wears one or two patches at a time and changes them every 24 hours. This device is less awkward than a scrotal patch, but the adhesive is very strong and frequently causes skin irritation.

Anabolic Steroids

Soon after all the various properties of testosterone were discovered, biochemists set out to create similar compounds that might have just some of these properties without the others. A series of drugs called *anabolic steroids* were designed to have only the muscle-building effects of testosterone without its other actions, such as stimulation of libido. Examples of anabolic steroids include nandrolone (Deca-Durabolin), given by injection, and stanozolol (Winstrol) and oxandrolone (Oxandrin), which are pills taken orally.

These drugs do seem to encourage growth of muscle bulk more than plain testosterone does, but they are not completely free of the other effects of testosterone. They have limited legitimate medical uses, mostly for people with muscle wasting due to chronic disease, such as AIDS.

Anabolic steroids are taken illicitly by many bodybuilders, weight lifters, and other athletes, as a way to promote more rapid and extreme growth of muscle mass in response to exercise. Generally these people use high doses of synthetic anabolic steroids as well as testosterone itself. The drugs are given in elaborate dosing schemes, called "stacking," to achieve the desired effect.

Note that anabolic steroids do not cause muscle growth all by themselves. Resistance training, i.e., weight lifting, is required. Weight lifters who have reached a plateau where they are unable to make further gains in mass often turn to anabolic steroids to give them a boost.

This use of anabolic steroids is illegal, and for this reason all anabolic steroids, as well as testosterone itself, have now been classified as "controlled substances" by the U.S. Food and Drug Administration. In addition, it is unethical to use these substances in preparation for athletic competition.

Anabolic steroids have several potential deleterious effects, many of which do not reverse when the drug is stopped. They may cause bloating, acne, and unwanted body-hair growth. They also may accelerate male pattern baldness. Notice the thinning hair on many competitive bodybuilders. Steroids also cause the testicles to shrink and the breasts to grow. They promote hardening of the arteries, which may lead to a heart attack at an early age. They can damage the liver or cause liver tumors, which may be fatal. They may effect the mood and/or libido. Anyone contemplating taking anabolic steroids should be aware of these effects.

DHEA

Dihydroepiandrosterone, or DHEA, is a naturally occurring androgenic (male-type) hormone that is made in the adrenal glands, near the kidneys, rather than in the testes, like testosterone.

All humans, both male and female, have DHEA, and the hormone is converted into both testosterone and estrogen in the body. Males have more DHEA than females, and levels of DHEA decline with age in both sexes.

Some people have postulated that low DHEA levels are the cause of many of the diseases of aging. DHEA has been called "the youth hormone." Several popular books have been written on the topic. Claims have been made that DHEA can increase energy, improve libido, build muscle, prevent various cancers, reverse heart disease, improve memory and mood, and extend life. None of these claims have been proven by rigorous studies.

It has become popular for people to self-prescribe and take DHEA. Because of a loophole in the law, DHEA may be purchased without a prescription as a "dietary supplement" in health food stores. Be aware that the purity of this product is not monitored by any outside agency and may vary from bottle to bottle.

Researchers actually don't know much about what DHEA really does. Few controlled studies have been performed in humans. Small doses, 25 to 50 milligrams daily, do appear to improve the sense of physical and psychological well being in some people over 40. It has not been shown that DHEA supplementation can slow the natural aging process, however, or reverse or prevent any disease. The long-term effects of taking DHEA are unknown. Some of my patients taking DHEA do not feel particularly better on it, but they continue because they feel it is good for them in some way.

Higher doses of DHEA may cause the same side effects as other male hormones: acne, shrinking of the testicles, coarsening of facial and body hair, acceleration of pattern baldness on the scalp. In addition, DHEA may stimulate the development or progression of prostate cancer.

It may be safe to try taking DHEA at up to 50 milligram daily, but if you do so, be careful, and let your doctor know you are doing it. If you truly feel better while on DHEA, you may choose to continue—with the awareness that there may be some unknown long-term consequences. If taking DHEA does not improve your energy, libido, or anything else, then I would suggest you stop taking it. Any man taking DHEA should make sure he is screened for prostate cancer annually.

The Genitourinary System

T he external genitalia of a man consist of the penis, the scrotum (ball sac), and the scrotal contents: the testicles, or balls, and the epididymis and vas deferens, which make up the tubing through which the sperm flow from the testicles up toward the prostate.

The internal genitalia include the prostate, an organ the size and shape of a chestnut. The prostate sits just inside the body at the base of the penis. As many gay men know, it can be felt by placing a finger inside of the rectum, and feeling the forward part of the rectal wall, toward the penis. Beside the prostate lie the seminal vesicles, elongated pouches in which are mixed the sperm (from the testicles) and seminal fluid (made in the prostate), which then sit there until they are expelled with the next ejaculation.

The urinary system is integrated into this system. Urine is made in the kidneys and flows into the bladder, where it is stored. It drains from the base of the bladder through a tube called the urethra, which passes through the core of the prostate, then through the penis and out.

When a man urinates, signals from the brain cause the bladder to squeeze, and the sphincter muscle at the bladder's base relaxes. Urine then flows through the urethra and out of the body. Urination is usually a voluntary act.

Ejaculation is a more complex and less voluntary process. The sperm, the little tadpole-shaped guys that swim around in the semen, are made in the testicles. The fluid that makes up most of the ejaculate is made inside your body, in the prostate. After a batch of sperm are made, they are transported through the epididymis and vas deferens, from the testicles, up into the body, where they are deposited in the seminal vesicles, one on each side of the prostate.

At the same time, the prostate is manufacturing a salty, sugary fluid that serves as a carrier and nutrient solution for the sperm. This seminal fluid is pumped into the seminal vesicles, where it is mixed with the sperm.

When orgasm occurs, a series of involuntary muscle contractions pump the seminal fluid–sperm mixture from the seminal vesicles, into the urethra, and out the end of the penis. A valve deep inside the urethra closes during orgasm to prevent the ejaculatory fluid from being pumped upwards into the bladder rather than out through the penis.

In the following sections we'll discuss separately the three main parts of the male genital system: the penis, the scrotum and its contents, and the prostate. Together they make an integrated system, but it is easier to understand their intricacies if each is discussed on its own.

The Penis

The penis (cock, dick, etc.) is an organ that has a dual purpose: to perform sexual functions and for urination. Most men consider their penis to be pretty important to them, and some men have been accused of thinking with their penis. In fact, the ancient Roman slang term for penis is the Latin word *mentula,* which means "little brain." Thinking with your penis can get you in trouble, so be careful. Use your brain for thinking and your penis for other things.

Every man knows what a penis is, unless he's from Mars, but let me describe it anyway. The penis is a fleshy appendage that hangs from the base of the groin. It is hollow because along its underside runs the tube called the urethra, through which urine and semen flow at the appropriate time for each. The urethra terminates at an opening, called the meatus, at the tip of the penis.

The penis is constructed of two main parts: the shaft, which gives the penis its length, and the head, whose purpose is most likely for sexual stimulation, since it is the most sensitive part of the organ and has no other apparent purpose. The bulk of the penile shaft consists of erectile tissue, which is spongy tissue that at times of sexual arousal fills with blood, causing expansion and hardening of the penis (an erection).

The Foreskin and Circumcision

In its unaltered and resting state, the skin of the penile shaft is loose and redundant. It extends over the penile head, forming the foreskin. In certain cultures, the foreskins of male children are routinely amputated. This process, called circumcision, originated as a religious and/or hygienic practice.

Circumcision has been adopted on a society-wide basis in some Westernized cultures, particularly in the United States, where the majority of male infants are circumcised by physicians, shortly after birth. The current medical justification for circumcision is that a circumcised ("cut") penis is easier to keep clean, is less susceptible to urinary tract infections during childhood, and is less susceptible to sexually transmitted diseases and cancer during adulthood.

Many physicians have begun to question the need for routine neonatal circumcision. It is not difficult to keep an uncircumcised penis clean, and with care, most sexually transmitted diseases can be prevented. Circumcision removes some of the most sensitive tissue of the penis, resulting—according to some—in a reduction in sexual pleasure. Some, myself included, feel it is unethical to permanently alter the body of a baby boy before he is old enough to consider the matter and make the decision for himself. Because of these considerations, routine neonatal circumcision is becoming less common than it used to be, though the majority of boys born in the United States continue to be circumcised.

Penis Size

Normal penises come in a range of sizes. Differences in the size of the flaccid penis tend to even out with erection. In other words, guys whose resting member is quite large often find that it does not get that much bigger when erect, while a penis that is fairly small in repose will enlarge relatively more with erection.

It is common for a man to worry that his penis is too small. Maybe this is because the penis tends to symbolize masculinity and power. Rich, powerful men tend to create immense penis-shaped objects, such as skyscrapers, monuments, and missiles, as if to say, "Look how big mine is!"

In reality, penis size is seldom a problem, except for those few penises that are unusually small or large. As a tool of sexual enjoyment, most any size of penis will do just fine, be it the man's own or a partner's.

Some friendly advice: Don't measure your penis. You'll probably be depressed if you do. The average size is smaller than you think. Disregard the claims of guys advertising in the personals. Any man who claims to have the proverbial 8-inch penis is either exaggerating, or a freak of nature. If yours feels good and does what it is supposed to do, it is the right size. For that reason, I feel it is inappropriate to give the dimensions of an average penis in this book. Sorry.

Very rarely a man will have an abnormally small penis ("micropenis") that interferes with sexual function. This situation can be improved with surgery (discussed in the section titled "Genital Enhancement"). Use of a vacuum pump (discussed in the section titled "Sexual Dysfunction and Its Treatment") is a good way to artificially produce an erection, and manufacturers claim that their pumps can permanently increase penis size, but as far as I know there is not good proof of this.

Erections

An erection is the result of a complex process resulting from sexual arousal, which comes from mental stimulation (the brain has been called a man's most important and largest sexual organ), physical stimulation, or both. Sexual arousal triggers signals to the nerves in the pelvis, which then direct an increase in the amount of blood flowing into the penis. When the rate of blood flowing into the penis exceeds the rate of blood flowing out, the penis fills with blood, expands, and becomes hard—in other words, an erection.

Some men enjoy wearing a type of device known as a "cock ring" during sex, to enhance or prolong their erection. This is a ring—made of metal, rubber, or leather—that fits around the base of the penis and scrotum or sometimes just around the base of the penis. By providing a little constriction in the area, a cock ring can still permit blood to flow into the penis through the arteries, which are fairly resilient. At the same time, the cock ring makes it more difficult for blood to leave the penis, through the veins, which are more easily compressed. Hence some men find a cock ring gives them a better erection. There is nothing harmful about using a cock ring if one uses it correctly.

Stan: *I had a new metal cock ring, and it was a little small, but I was doing a lot of crystal that night, and I didn't care—all I was thinking about was how horny I was. Afterwards, I just couldn't get the ring off. I tried and tried, and the more I tried, the deeper it cut into my skin. Finally, the next morning, I went to the emergency room, where they cut it off—the cock ring, not my cock! In the meantime, I found I was unable to pee because the pressure of the cock ring had damaged my urethra. I ended up having to have a catheter put up into my penis to drain my bladder for a week, until my urethra healed and I could pee on my own again.*

A cock ring must be the proper size. It won't work if it's too big in diameter. It should provide just enough constriction to do the job. If a cock ring is too tight, it can cut into the flesh or cause damage to the urinary tract. Stan's story really did happen, and he's not the only patient of mine who has had this kind of misadventure. Be careful of metal cock rings, which can be impossible to remove if they are too tight.

Sometimes a man just can't "get it up," or his erection doesn't get as hard as it needs to be in order to enter his partner's anus, or it doesn't last long enough or get hard enough to have satisfying sex. This problem is called *erectile dysfunction,* or *impotence.* The causes and treatments of erectile dysfunction are discussed in the section titled "Sexual Dysfunction and Its Treatment."

Bladder Problems

Men frequently develop problems involving their urination. Something is wrong if urination is painful, frequent, difficult, or some combination of these things. Some sexually transmitted diseases—for example, gonorrhea and chlamydia—can cause urinary symptomatology (discussed in the section titled "Bacterial STDs"). The term *urethritis* covers these infections. Here we will discuss urinary symptoms that are not caused by a sexually transmitted infection.

Mack: *Today when I got up to pee, it just burned like fire. I've urinated twice since then, and it still hurts, and it feels like I have to pee right after I'm done. Also, my urine is cloudy, and it smells terrible. And I've got a dull ache in my groin, which is worse when I try to pee.*

Mack has all of the symptoms of a bladder infection. These infections are not that common in men, but they do occur. Normally, urine is sterile and clean, and the downward flushing action of urination keeps it that way. A man's urethra is long enough that bacteria can seldom swim all the way up into it to infect the bladder.

A culture of Mack's urine confirmed that he did indeed have a bladder infection. He was better after a few days of taking antibiotics. But then he came back a month later, with all of the same symptoms.

Now, any man is entitled to have one bladder infection. But when he gets a second one, it's time to try to find out why. So Mack and I explored the possible reasons why he might be getting these infections.

Urinary Irritants

- Alcoholic beverages
- Chocolate
- Coffee (including decaf)
- Fresh fruit
- Fruit juice
- Spicy foods
- Tea
- Tomatoes
- Vitamin C

Mack told me he always drank plenty of water (good), and he was too young (30) to have any prostate problems, which can lead to urinary tract infections in older men; besides, he had no prostate symptoms, such as hesitant urination or a slow stream. But then he asked me if there could be any connection with the fact that both times he got a bladder infection he had been screwing his partner particularly vigorously the night before. Being in a long-term, monogamous relationship and both being HIV-negative, Mack and his partner were not in the habit of using condoms.

The answer, I told him, was yes, definitely. Prolonged intercourse can allow bacteria (and there are plenty inside a man's rectum) to swim into the urethra and up into the bladder, starting an infection. I suggested to Mack that he try to drink a lot of fluids before sex; that he use a condom for fucking, even despite what he told me about his relationship; and that he urinate immediately after sex. By following this advice, Mack has avoided further trouble with bladder infections. Incidentally, I have also seen men develop bladder infections after prolonged, heavy-duty sessions of oral sex, as well. Older men suffering from prostate enlargement may also develop bladder infections because they may have trouble emptying their bladder completely.

Frequent or painful urination can come from many other causes besides bladder infections, so it's good to see your doctor if you have these symptoms. For example, frequent urination can be the first sign of diabetes. A urinalysis will often reveal the cause of the problem. If you do have a bladder infection, you will receive an antibiotic prescription. If it's some other sort of problem, that will be treated as indicated.

Many times, it is a man's diet that is causing his urination to be frequent and/or uncomfortable. (See Sam's story in "Bacterial STDs") Acidic fruits, spicy foods, tea, and coffee are frequent culprits (see table). These, not coincidentally, are the same things that can cause anal itching or burning. Often, by just cutting down on intake of coffee and other acidic or spicy substances, and by drinking more plain water, a man can restore his urinary function to normal.

The Scrotum and Its Contents

hen I was in high school, a classmate used to use *scrotum* as an epithet. It was so bizarre it was funny. We use all kinds of sexual or excretory terms as epithets. I've been called an asshole, a dick head, a jerk-off—but a scrotum?

The scrotum may be funny-looking to some people, but it's a turn-on to some others, and it's a very important part of every man's sexual apparatus. It's the sac that holds your testicles—your balls—as well as other essential sexual parts.

The Testicles

The testes, or testicles, are the most obvious and familiar inhabitants of your scrotum. They make sperm, and they also make the male hormone, testosterone. It's hard to be a man if you don't have balls. In fact, *testicle* is Latin for "little witness" because your balls are evidence of your masculinity. They live in a sac that hangs outside your body because they need to have a cooler temperature than the rest of your body in order to properly produce sperm.

The wall of the scrotum contains an interesting layer of muscle, just under the skin, that contracts in the cold to bring your testicles up closer to the warmth of your body and relaxes in hot weather so that the testicles can hang lower and cool off a bit. Fear also makes the scrotum contract, to bring the little guys up closer to your body for protection. You know the feeling.

Other Scrotal Apparatus

Attached to the back of each testicle is a little rubbery structure called the epididymis, which stores the sperm that are made in that testicle. From the epididymis runs a tube, the vas deferens, which carries the sperm up into the body from the scrotum, to join with the seminal fluid from the prostate prior to ejaculation.

Accompanying the vas deferens are arteries and veins. In some men, the veins grow excessively, forming a varicocele, which feels like a bag of worms or spaghetti in the scrotum, usually above the testicle. There is nothing harmful about having a varicocele, but if it becomes too big or unsightly, it can be taken care of surgically.

In addition, the body makes some lubricating fluid for the inside of the scrotum so that the testicles can slide around easily in there. Occasionally the drainage mechanism for this fluid goes awry, and the scrotum enlarges slowly over time under the pressure of fluid being pumped in. This is called a hydrocele. It is not a dangerous problem, but it can be annoying unless, like some men, you enjoy having an extra-large scrotum. A hydrocele can be taken care of with a simple operation.

Pain in the Scrotum

Because our testicles are important, Father Nature wants them protected from injury. That's why he enables our scrotums to tighten up when danger is around. And to teach us to protect our balls, he has given them great capacity for pain when we are hit down there. You know what it feels like—I don't need to describe it to you—it's like, well, getting hit in the balls. Athletic supporters and protective cups were invented to protect us from this sort of problem during sports activities. Nevertheless, many guys enjoy having their balls played with during sex, gently or even roughly. Nothing wrong with that if that's what turns you on.

If your balls ache and/or swell and you have not been hit there, see your doctor as soon as possible. Chances are you have epididymitis, an infection of the epididymis and sometimes of the testicle itself. This causes terrible aching pain, as well as swelling and firmness of the epididymis, usually just on one side. You can examine yourself to check whether you might have epididymitis, although the doctor will probably insist in feeling down there too. Epididymitis is not uncommon and is easy to treat with a few weeks of antibiotics, though it takes longer for the swelling to totally go away, and the pain can linger for months.

A less common cause of pain and swelling of a man's testicle is called torsion, where the testicle twists inside the scrotal sack, pinching off its blood supply. This usually occurs in young boys, but it can occasionally occur in an adult. It must be dealt with rapidly or the testicle will become gangrenous from lack of blood flow, and it will need to be removed.

Cancer of the Testicle

Testicular cancer occurs mainly in men between the ages of 20 and 45, but it can occur at any age. Men who were born with an undescended testicle—that is, one that lives up inside the groin rather than down in the scrotum—have a much higher risk of cancer in that testicle, even if it was surgically brought down into the scrotum at some point.

Cancer of the testicle is nearly 100% curable if it is detected and treated promptly. Since the prime age range for testicular cancer is also the highest risk time for HIV, it is common for a man with HIV to develop testicular cancer. However, the two do not seem to be related; having HIV probably does not put a person at increased risk for testicular cancer. The cancer is no more serious in someone who is HIV-positive than it is in an HIV-negative man.

Testicular cancer shows up as a very hard lump, either attached to the testicle or within the contour of the testicle. Normally a testicle is rubbery, like an earlobe. Cancer is hard, like a peach pit. I see about three cases of testicular cancer a year, and what impresses me most is how very hard they feel. Incidentally, I am never the first to discover the lump on a routine exam. The patient or his partner always finds it first and comes in to have me check it out. Surprisingly, testicular cancer is usually not painful, though it can occasionally cause some discomfort.

All men should examine their balls regularly for signs of cancer. Familiarize yourself with the geography in your scrotum: On each side there is a testicle with its epididymis attached to the upper back surface and then a bunch of spaghetti-like tubing (the vas deferens, as well as veins and arteries) leading up from the testicle into the groin. A cancer would be part of the testicle, attached to it, and it would be hard like a stone rather than rubbery like everything else in there.

If you find something suspicious in your scrotum, go to your doctor and get it checked out. Don't be shy, and don't wait. It's better to go in and find out that it's nothing than to wait until the cancer is so advanced that it's no longer curable.

The Prostate

T he prostate is an internal gland whose job is to make the seminal fluid, the material that carries and nourishes the sperm, and forms the bulk of what comes out of the penis when a man ejaculates (comes). The prostate sits just inside the pelvis, in front of the rectum, and behind the base of the penis. The urethra, or urinary tube, passes through the prostate on its way from the bladder into the penis.

The prostate is quite sensitive, and many men enjoy stimulation of their prostate during sex, by means of a finger, penis, or sex toy inserted into the rectum. The prostate is also subject to various ills that occur most commonly in men over 40 but may happen earlier.

Benign Prostatic Hypertrophy

John: *I've been having more and more trouble urinating. I have to stand and wait for a while until the stream starts, and when it does, it's awfully slow. In fact I am finding it easier to pee sitting down. And it never feels like I am emptying my bladder. Ten minutes after I pee, I feel like I have to go again. I'm up and down to the bathroom all night. When I was younger, this never happened to me; it seemed to start earlier this year, when I turned 62. Am I just getting older or what? Is there anything we can do about this? It's driving me crazy.*

Slow, weak, or hesitant urination is usually a symptom of a prostate problem. This is very common in men of John's age. Since the prostate surrounds the urethra, the urine must flow through the prostate on its way out of the body. Every man's prostate slowly enlarges with age. It never stops growing because testosterone makes it grow, and most of us never stop having testosterone in our bloodstream. In many men, with continued growth the prostate becomes large enough that it interferes with urination by clenching around the urethra. This is called *benign prostatic hypertrophy*. Eighty percent of all men develop BPH eventually.

With BPH, the urinary stream gradually becomes weaker and weaker. Urination begins to take more and more effort or straining. And the bladder cannot exert the pressure it takes to fully empty, so the man with BPH finds he needs to urinate again soon after he has finished going.

Dealing With BPH

There are several ways to encourage your prostate not to give you this trouble. First of all, acidic foods—especially coffee—tend to irritate the prostate and cause it to swell. I advise men in John's situation to cut down their coffee intake. I also encourage them to drink more plain water and to ejaculate regularly, to keep the system flushed out. But I also suggest that they stop all fluid consumption each evening a few hours before bedtime, in order to go to bed with the bladder relatively empty.

If prostate symptoms continue, my next advice is to take 160 milligrams of saw palmetto twice a day. This is a nonprescription herbal preparation made from the berries of a palm tree native to the southeastern United States. Saw palmetto appears to shrink an enlarged prostate and permit easier urine flow. A month's supply costs $15 to $30 depending on the brand. Side effects are usually few and may include headache, nausea, or dizziness. Studies are under way that may lead to approval for prescription use, which would permit insurance coverage for this medication.

When nonprescription measures are not enough, there are other treatments that can help. A type of drug called an *alpha blocker*, can temporarily "relax" or shrink the prostate enough to permit normal urination. Examples of such drugs include Hytrin (terazosin), and Cardura (doxazosin). You may have seen these medications advertised in magazines as prostate remedies. They tend to work within a few days after one starts taking them, but they are effective only if taken every day because they do not cause a permanent shrinkage of the prostate.

Alpha blockers were originally developed for the treatment of high blood pressure. Their effect on the prostate was discovered later, when men taking them for high blood pressure found that they were peeing more easily. These drugs can drop the blood pressure enough to cause light-headedness, but many people get over this side effect after a little while. A newer medicine, Flomax (tamsulosin), was developed specifically as a prostate remedy. It has the same effect on the prostate as the other alpha-blockers but is reported not to lower the blood pressure, so it should not cause light-headedness.

Another medication, Proscar (finasteride), blocks the conversion of testosterone in the prostate to dihydrotestosterone. Proscar deprives the prostate of this potent male hormone, causing the gland to slowly shrink. Proscar must be taken for months to have an effect, and for many people it does not make urination any easier, even when tests show that their prostate is smaller. It also may interfere with the detection of prostate cancer by blood testing. In my experience, alpha blockers work better than Proscar in relieving symptoms of an enlarged prostate.

When a man has BPH, often the prostate eventually grows so large that medications stop helping. Urination becomes a challenge. The stream starts slowly, urine dribbles out weakly, and the bladder does not empty completely. It soon reaches its capacity again, so the man with BPH must urinate frequently. Often he awakens many times during the night to urinate. He may have recurrent bladder infections, due to urine sitting in his bladder for long periods. The only solution at this point is the brute-force approach: to remove the core of the prostate, allowing the urine to flow through.

Such a procedure, called a *transurethral prostatectomy,* is a great solution to severe BPH symptoms. An instrument is inserted into the urethra, and once in the region of the prostate, a knife blade is released, shaving away the prostate from the inside. An overnight hospital stay is typical with this procedure.

Newer methods involving freezing, electrical burning, or lasers are becoming popular. They may have quicker recovery times. Whatever the method, my patients who have had a transurethral prostatectomy are generally very grateful to recover the ability to properly urinate. Unwanted side effects, such as incontinence (urinary leakage), are rare but can occur. However, after a transurethral prostatectomy a man no longer ejaculates because much of the prostate, where semen is made, is removed. All other sexual functions, including orgasm, continue to work just fine; it's only that no semen comes out when the man orgasms.

Prostate Cancer

BPH, as indicated by its name, is a benign (noncancerous) condition. But cancer of the prostate can have all the same symptoms of BPH. For that reason, if you have developed difficulty urinating, it's important that you see your doctor and get checked to see whether it's BPH, prostatitis (infection or inflammation of the prostate), or prostate cancer.

Examination of the prostate requires the doctor to perform a digital rectal exam—feeling the prostate through the rectal wall, with a gloved finger. Any irregularities in the contours or texture of the prostate may be a sign of cancer, and if these are found, the next step is an ultrasound of the prostate and usually a biopsy (removal of a sample of tissue for analysis).

In addition, there is a blood test, called the *prostate-specific antigen*, that can be helpful in the diagnosis of prostate cancer. The PSA test measures the blood levels of a protein that is made only by prostatic tissue. Every man normally has a certain amount of PSA in his blood, but an excessively high level can be a clue to cancer.

The PSA is a useful test when cancer is suspected, and the American Cancer Society recommends that all men over 50 have their PSA checked annually, to screen for prostate cancer. However, prostate infections or just benign enlargement can also elevate the PSA. A high PSA does not prove that a person has cancer. It does mean that additional tests are warranted to find the cause of the elevated PSA.

Recently a more refined test measuring the "free PSA" in the blood as opposed to the PSA that is bound to blood proteins has been introduced. If the total PSA is high, a high free PSA means cancer is less likely to be the culprit than if the free PSA is low.

Prostate cancer is very common. In fact, aside from skin cancer, it is the most common cancer a nonsmoking man is likely to get. One in ten men is ultimately diagnosed with prostate cancer, and there are over 300,000 new cases annually in the United States. It is important to keep in mind that many, perhaps most, prostate cancers grow very slowly and never cause a problem. The average man with prostate cancer dies of old age or other causes, before the cancer gets out of hand.

But some prostate cancers are very aggressive, spreading throughout the body and causing disease and premature death. Annually, more than 30,000 men in the United States die of this disease. The problem is, when a cancer is found in the prostate, it can be difficult to know whether it is a relatively harmless, slow-growing tumor or a more aggressive one. This has led some professionals to question whether it is proper to screen healthy, asymptomatic men for prostate cancer.

My opinion is that it's good to find out if you have prostate cancer, especially if you have symptoms or are younger than 75 years old. But how and whether prostate cancer should be treated depends on many factors, including your age, symptoms, and size and location of the cancer. Discuss your options with your doctor, and don't assume that all prostate cancer needs to be treated.

Dealing With Prostate Cancer

Treatment for prostate cancer is a significant undertaking. Once the cancer is confirmed by biopsy, you will undergo some tests (a bone scan and possibly a CT scan of the pelvis) to see whether the cancer has spread to the bones or to the lymph nodes around the prostate. If it has not spread, there are two main ways to get rid of it: remove the entire prostate with a major surgical procedure called a radical prostatectomy or treat it with radiation, either by beaming X rays into the prostate from outside or by implanting radioactive pellets (seeds) into the prostate, which will fry it from within.

There are various potential complications of treatment for prostate cancer. Your urologist will go over them with you in detail, but here are the most important ones.

With the surgery, there is a risk that the nerves that allow you to have an erection will be damaged or destroyed. Even with the use of advanced, "nerve-sparing" surgical techniques, erectile function is often never as good as it was before the surgery. In addition, the surgery can sometimes lead to incontinence, or involuntary urinary leakage. Finally, without a prostate, you will no longer ejaculate. Orgasm will feel just as pleasurable, but nothing will come out. It may seem like a trivial thing, but it bothers some men a lot that they don't produce any "come" when they come.

Radiation has fewer potential complications than surgery. However, some men still have erection problems or urinary problems after radiation therapy. In addition, radiation can damage the delicate rectal tissue next to the prostate, causing the equivalent of a burn. Rectal pain and bleeding can result, and it may take a while to heal.

It can be physically and psychologically traumatic to have prostate cancer, especially because there are so many uncertainties about the right treatment option: Do nothing?

Radiation? Surgery? And the aftereffects of treatment can be significant. Most urologists are more accustomed to helping straight men go through the experience of dealing with their prostate cancer, and these men's wives are involved in the process. Many of my middle-aged and older gay male patients have had to face prostate cancer, and they have sometimes complained of a lack of support from the treatment community and from the gay men's community. Fortunately, the urologists I work with are not homophobic, and they involve my patients' partners in discussions about treatment choices.

When a patient of mine is diagnosed with prostate cancer, I now give him the names of other gay men who have dealt with this condition. One of my patients is starting a support group for gay men in Seattle with prostate cancer, and I suspect such groups exist in other cities with significant gay populations. Another patient has found significant support via the Internet. If you find you have prostate cancer and there is no support group for gay men with prostate cancer in your home town, consider starting one. Your physician may be able to help you find other gay men with the same condition.

Prostatitis

Keep in mind that prostate infections, or prostatitis, can also give symptoms similar to those of BPH or prostate cancer: urinary hesitancy, frequency, weak stream. The difference is that with prostatitis the symptoms tend to come on relatively rapidly, over a few days or a week or so rather than over weeks to months, as with BPH. In addition, with prostatitis the prostate is usually swollen and sore. Men describe this as a deep ache that they feel in the rectum or up behind the scrotum. It is often worse with urinating or defecating, both of which put pressure on the prostate. Some men with prostatitis also have pain when they ejaculate, and they may notice blood in their semen.

Prostatitis is usually obvious by physical exam. When examined by finger, an inflamed prostate is softer or "boggier" than normal, and it is also very, very tender. If that doesn't clinch the diagnosis, then sometimes the doctor will massage the prostate, which causes some secretions to drip out of the end of the penis. This material can be checked for white blood cells under the microscope, and if they are found, prostatitis is confirmed.

Prostatitis is treated with oral antibiotics. It may take weeks or even a few months to cure prostatitis. Even then, it frequently recurs because antibiotics do not penetrate well into prostate tissue. Some health care providers feel that regular ejaculation helps to prevent or treat prostate infections by keeping the gland cleaned out. I can recall a patient telling me—with a grin on his face—that his urologist told him he should try to jack off daily.

If you do get prostatitis or any prostate problem, at least you can take comfort in the fact that it has nothing to do with your being gay. Prostate problems are just part of being a male. Gay men do not appear to be at any higher or lower risk of prostate problems than anyone else. Of course, if you looked at the pictures in the ads in medical journals or the patient-education pamphlets put out by drug companies and professional organizations, you would think that we are immune to prostate problems because gay couples are never depicted or addressed in this literature.

The Anus and Rectum

For all humans, the rectum (the last part of the large intestine) and anus (asshole, or butt hole, the opening out of the body "down there") have a very important function in our bodies. We use this part of our body regularly to eliminate solid waste, a process known medically as *defecation* or *passing a stool*—shitting, in the Anglo-Saxon terminology. This is a very important human function, as we learn when something goes wrong with our anus.

For many gay men the anus is also an organ of sexual function and pleasure. So for us it is even more important that we keep this part of our body working properly and from causing us trouble.

Many of us have a problem in thinking about our bottom, much less discussing it, even with a doctor. It is frequently the butt of jokes (no pun intended) and of slurs. Why is it an insult to call someone an asshole? It should be a compliment. The anus is a very useful, important, and (to many) pleasure-giving part of the body.

Our negative attitude about our butts probably comes from our childhoods, when we were potty-trained. We were taught that our anus was a dirty, nasty part of our body, that we were not to touch it except when necessary to clean it. There is no rational reason for this. It's just another part of the body. Treat it well. If you are good to your anus, it will reward you with years of trouble-free service.

General Anal Health: Constipation, Diarrhea, Regularity, Fiber

The anus forms the opening for the digestive tract out of the body. The part of the colon just above the anus is called the *rectum*. These are the parts of the lower digestive tract that have a dual role of waste elimination and sexual pleasure for many gay men.

As digested food moves through the colon, water is gradually absorbed from the fecal mass to produce a formed stool (piece of shit). The stool accumulates in the sigmoid colon, which is just before the rectum, near the end of the digestive tract. When it is time to evacuate the stool, the colon moves the fecal material into the rectum, which is richly endowed with nerve endings that allow it to feel a sensation of stretch or fullness. These resulting nerve impulses signal the person's brain that it is time to have a bowel movement.

Diarrhea occurs when an unformed, loose, or watery stool rather than a formed one, is evacuated, often urgently. Constipation means that the stool is too firm and dry, and bowel movements are difficult and infrequent, requiring much effort. "Regularity" is a euphemism for the relatively effortless passage of soft, formed stools, at convenient times.

The number one rule of keeping a healthy and happy anus and rectum is to eat lots and lots of fiber. Fiber, or roughage, is indigestible material, generally of plant origin, which passes through our intestinal tract unabsorbed. Most commonly it consists of the cellulose-type material that makes up the coats of seeds and grains and is also found in fruit and vegetables.

Our digestive tracts were designed to process a diet that is much higher in fiber than most of us eat. I picture our primitive ancestors chewing on leaves, coarse seeds, and roots all day, unless they were lucky enough to kill and eat an occasional animal. With the current Western diet, it is almost impossible to take in that much fiber. The result often is bowel irregularity: constipation and/or diarrhea.

If your fiber intake is high enough, you will regularly have a soft, bulky bowel movement that comes out easily, quickly, and cleanly, without straining. Depending on the person, it can be normal to have a bowel movement as infrequently as every several days or as frequently as two to three times a day.

Whatever the frequency, the stool should be formed, bulky, easily eliminated, and it should float. If you have to strain to expel a hard "sinker" that makes a *thud* when it hits the bottom of the toilet bowl (OK, I'm exaggerating a little), you are not getting enough fiber, and sooner or later you'll have anal, rectal, and colonic troubles because of it.

It is not difficult to increase the fiber content of what you eat. Avoid processed grains and flours, and stick to whole grains. Eat lots of fresh fruits and vegetables. Have your bowl of bran cereal or a bran muffin every morning.

But often dietary fiber is not enough. The solution for many people is to take a daily dose of a fiber supplement and to drink plenty of water. The most popular form of fiber supplement is psyllium seed husk, which is a high-density fiber that can absorb a large amount of water. This material is sold as a powder that you mix with a glass of water and drink. Popular brands include Metamucil, Konsyl, and various generic and bulk types are available. There is also a synthetic called Citrucel that may cause less gas than natural roughage.

A few spoonfuls of fiber concentrate daily, consumed with plenty of water, should give you a good, healthy, bulky, easily eliminated, floating stool. Contrary to popular belief, fiber is not a laxative nor is it addictive, and it is not just for your grandmother. It is for everyone.

Darius: *I'm a bottom, so I take Metamucil every day.*

I was amused by what Darius said, but it made perfect sense. He should be a spokesman for the product—though I don't think his testimonial would go over well on network television. The point is that Darius's preferred sexual activity is to get screwed anally. By taking a daily dose of fiber, his solid waste is eliminated cleanly and efficiently, in one big dump each morning. This keeps his anal canal clean for sex later on in the day.

Fiber therapy does have lots of other benefits. For one thing, it helps keep your colon clean with its sweeping action. It reduces your risk of hemorrhoids, which are swollen perianal veins that can be itchy or painful. It also reduces your risk of diverticulosis (pouches that form in the wall of the lower intestine, catching food and becoming inflamed).

Some types of fiber reduce your cholesterol level, perhaps by binding to cholesterol in your gut and eliminating it. Fiber may even cut down your risk of colon cancer by absorbing toxic substances rather than allowing them to sit in the colon and cause mutations that lead to cancerous growth.

The Anus as a Sexual Organ

Men have been having anal sex since time immemorial. Many gay men appreciate this form of sexual activity. The recipient, or "bottom," enjoys feeling his partner inside him. The anal area is very richly endowed with nerve endings, and the prostate, which is also very sensitive, is just inside and is easily stimulated by anal penetration. The active partner, or "top," enjoys the sensation of having his penis inside his partner's body.

It's important—with few exceptions—to use a condom and use it properly to prevent disease transmission during anal intercourse. It's also important that both partners communicate before and during anal sex. Screwing usually needs to start gently with foreplay, perhaps with a finger, to help the bottom relax his sphincter. Sudden penetration can cause pain, which can make the sphincter involuntarily tighten up, causing more pain.

A little preparation can help make anal sex a more enjoyable experience. Prior to sex the bottom should try to make sure that he is relatively clean inside by having a bowel movement if he needs to. Regular use of a fiber supplement helps take care of this. An enema (douching) can also help. There is nothing wrong with this practice as long as it does not become the only way one can have a bowel movement.

Some men do not like to get fucked, and some would like to but find they are too tight. Most people can learn to relax their anal sphincter enough to have satisfying anal intercourse. Start with objects smaller in diameter than a penis. A finger, for example—yours or a buddy's. Tapered candles or small rubber sex toys also work well. Practice clenching and relaxing your sphincter. Hint: "pushing" with the sphincter, as if you are trying to expel a bowel movement, will actually relax the sphincter.

If done properly, anal intercourse cannot cause serious trauma or damage, other than the rare tear or fissure. In fact, some men maintain that getting screwed regularly keeps them from developing hemorrhoids. In any case, I have never seen an anus that was seriously injured by a penis.

Other things besides penises can be inserted in the rectum for sexual pleasure: fingers or fists, for example. Fisting is not for everybody, but it has a dedicated band of practitioners who often describe it as a religious experience. An object as large and unyielding as a fist can theoretically cause a great deal of damage. However, if done carefully and without the influence of drugs, fisting is generally safe. Fisting accidents are known to occur, but I am impressed that I have not seen one in eight years of taking care of hundreds of gay men. It is a tribute to the care and communication with which fisting enthusiasts approach this activity. I suspect that fisting accidents are generally associated with drug-impaired judgment on the part of one or both participants.

Inanimate objects can also be used for anal play. But one must be careful about what one puts up his butt. Dildos are fine if they are reasonably sized (in other words, not too big). A good dildo should have a large "handle" so that it cannot get swallowed up inside the rectum. Unfortunately, there is no federal agency that regulates dildos, so some are sold that are tapered at both ends and can easily get lost inside a person. It is very embarrassing and expensive to have to go to the emergency room to have a lost dildo retrieved, but sometimes it is necessary.

Large objects inserted into the rectum—especially if they are rigid and/or breakable—can and do cause major internal damage. I see about one man a year who has torn the inside of his intestine by inserting an oversized dildo or some other large object such as a wine bottle. Usually the patient is terribly embarrassed, and sometimes even delays seeking medical attention for a few days, making the situation even more dangerous.

Perforation of the rectum by a foreign body leads to a life-threatening abdominal infection called peritonitis. Treatment of this type of injury requires hospitalization and emergency surgery with a colostomy. My advice is, if you have had big toys up your butt and you get abdominal or pelvic pain, fever, or anal bleeding—see your doctor immediately. Your life could be at stake. And please, don't play with breakable objects, such as light bulbs. If they break while they are inside you, you're in big trouble.

Butt Clinic Now in Session

For the remainder of this section, we will have a "butt clinic." In the words of patients, I will present the common anal problems that gay men bring me every day. One by one we'll discuss how to deal with them. If you should develop an anal symptom, perhaps these stories will give you a clue as to what is wrong, and what to do about it. You'll notice that part of my recommended treatment for most anal problems is to take a fiber supplement. Fiber helps the anus recover from or avoid many maladies.

You may want to examine yourself down there. Although you can't look at your anus directly, you can see it by squatting over a hand mirror. Try it. When a man comes to me with an anal problem, he usually has no clue what his anus looks like. It impresses me when he can say, "It looks like there is a lump at six o'clock." You too can squat over a mirror and impress your doctor.

Anal itching

Percy: *My hole itches, and it's driving me crazy. I'm not exactly comfortable scratching myself back there while I'm in front of my classroom of third-graders, and sometimes I just have to run to the rest room to do it. Some mornings I wake up and find I've scratched myself raw.*

There are several possible causes of Percy's problem, which is called anal itching, or pruritis ani. He could be allergic to something: a soap or a lubricant, for example. I advise him to use unscented, hypoallergenic soap such as Dove. If he has been getting screwed, I recommend that he use the plainest of water-based lubes without perfume or spermicide.

He might have pinworms, tiny parasites that live on the perianal skin. I would examine his anus and look for them, though I'd be surprised if I found any. They are mostly found in kids. But he's a schoolteacher, so who knows. Herpes or warts can cause itching, which is another reason I told Percy it was good he came to the doctor with his symptom. Fortunately, when I examined him, he didn't have either of these.

Certain foods can cause anal itching. It turned out that Percy's coffee consumption was way up, and he also had a new Mexican boyfriend who was cooking special, spicy meals for him almost every night. I suspected that Percy's spicy, acidic diet was irritating his sensitive anal skin. My recommendations: Cut down on the coffee and the spicy food; buy some 1% hydrocortisone cream over the counter, and apply it several times a day to cut down on the itching immediately; and (of course) start a daily dose of fiber to help keep the area clean. It worked. The next week Percy reported that his itching was nearly gone.

Anal warts (condylomata)

Will: *I've been having this scratchy feeling in my ass, and it's been bleeding a little when I wipe myself. I thought I had hemorrhoids, but my partner looked, and he saw all these little bumps around my asshole.*

Will's story is repeated in our section on sexually transmitted diseases because anal warts are a common problem for gay men. It is important to find them and treat them because they are caused by a virus, and are contagious. In addition, they can lead to anal cancer, especially in HIV-positive men. For this reason it is a good idea for a gay man to have an annual rectal exam, to look for warts, cancer, and other problems. I can't count how many times I've discovered anal warts on a guy who didn't know he had them.

Will had lots of warts, both on the outside of his anal opening and also on the inside. I discovered this by looking inside him with a short, rigid tube called an anoscope. Because of the extent of his warts, I referred him to a proctologist (rectal surgeon) for laser surgery. I reassured Will that the proctologist was comfortable with gay men, nonjudgmental about anal intercourse, and would make sure that his anus would be OK for sex after the surgery had had time to heal.

The same virus that causes anal warts can probably cause anal cancer. Gay men, especially those with HIV, have an increased risk of anal cancers and of precancerous conditions. Studies are underway to determine whether routine Pap smears (using a cotton swab to obtain cells from the anal surface for analysis in the lab) are helpful at detecting and preventing anal cancer. For now, an annual examination of the anal area is certainly recommended for any man who receives anal intercourse.

Anal pain: proctitis or abscess

Kevin: *I haven't had sex in a few weeks, but for the past few days my butt has has felt like I was fisted by Godzilla! It is so sore I can barely sit down, and I'm afraid to go to the bathroom because it'll hurt so much.*

Without examining him, I can tell that Kevin probably has an infection. He either has some form of proctitis or a rectal abscess. *Proctitis* literally means "inflammation of the anus." An abscess is a pocket of infection, like a boil. Both can cause the severe pain that Kevin is describing.

Herpes is a common cause of proctitis in gay men. Herpes is particularly bad the first time, and primary anal herpes is awful. If it happens to you, you'll never forget it. Especially if it is misdiagnosed by a doctor who does not know you are gay and does not think you might have anal herpes. So if you have recently had anal sex and you get symptoms like Kevin's, get to a doctor, and let the doctor know what you think it might be.

Sexually transmitted bacteria, like gonorrhea, can also cause a bad inflammation of the rectum. Since Kevin had not had sex in a few weeks, I thought this was less likely but not impossible.

When I examined Kevin, I found that one whole side of his anal sphincter was swollen, firm, red, and extremely tender to the touch. This confirmed a diagnosis of perianal abscess, a bacterial infection in the tissues of the anus and environs. I gave Kevin a prescription for antibiotics and pain medication. I had him come back a few days later, when the area had softened. At that time I injected it with a local anesthetic, then lanced it to allow the pus inside to drain.

Kevin came back a month later, reporting that he had brown leakage mixed with a little blood in his underwear. This time I found a little hole in the outside of his anal sphincter that apparently tracked through to the inside of his rectum, probably as a result of his previous infection. That situation is called an anal fistula. I referred Kevin to a surgeon to have it repaired.

Anal fissure

Ralph: *I have this pain near the top part of my asshole, and sometimes it bleeds a little there when I wipe myself. It's worse after the area is stretched by a big, hard BM or a dildo or a cock. It's very annoying. I've been avoiding getting laid because of it, and that's not good for my mood.*

When I looked at Ralph's sphincter, I saw a little red crack through the top part of the sphincter. The medical term for this is an *anal fissure*. It is basically a tear in the sphincter, which has a difficult time healing. Trauma reopens it.

I told Ralph that the first-line treatment was to try to get it to heal on its own. I recommended Metamucil (of course) to soften his stools and asked him to apply 1% hydrocortisone cream several times a day to encourage healing. I asked that he not use dildos or allow himself to be penetrated for the next two weeks.

When Ralph came back for followup, the fissure was better but had not yet healed. Frequently this happens, and the best way to get it to heal is to artificially relax the sphincter. There are two ways to do this. A surgeon can operate, using a general anesthetic, and cut the sphincter just enough to loosen it a little, which will let the fissure heal. Or I offered to prescribe Ralph a medication, nitroglycerine ointment, to apply twice a day to his butt hole for a week, in order to keep it in a bit more of a relaxed state.

Ralph chose the latter. He later reported that the ointment gave him a weird headache, which got better after the first day, but that it worked, and he did not have to have surgery. Many doctors are unaware that nitroglycerine ointment can help relax the anal sphincter and help anal fissures heal. If your doctor prescribes this medication for you, be warned. Some people find that it really burns, and some find the headache intolerable. But several of my patients swear by it. I have tried it and can report that it did not burn, and the headache was tolerable.

External hemorrhoid

Lovell: *I just flew back from a one-week business trip, and I wasn't real "regular" while I was on the trip. Now I have a lump on my anus, and it hurts, and I'm getting spots of blood on my underwear.*

I looked at Lovell's anus and saw a firm red lump just on and outside of the sphincter, as big as the end of my little finger: an external hemorrhoid. Hemorrhoids are the veins of the anal area. When a person is constipated and has to strain, the pressure causes these veins to fill up with blood, and sometimes the blood can clot in the vein. This causes back-pressure, swelling, and pain.

Hemorrhoids can be treated with our old friends: fiber (of course), to soften the stool, and hydrocortisone cream, to relieve local inflammation. But when a hemorrhoid has a clot in it, the fastest way to fix it is to have your doctor numb the skin over the clot, then slice it open and remove the clot. It will stop hurting as soon as the clot is removed, though it will bleed a little for the next few days while it's healing.

Rectal bleeding: internal hemorrhoid

Jorge: *I'm bleeding "back there". When I sit on the toilet, blood drips out. Sometimes, if I push, it squirts out. It doesn't hurt at all. It's pretty scary to squirt blood out of your butt! The only other thing is that I've been a little constipated lately, but that's common for me.*

Rectal bleeding is alarming when it happens, but most commonly the cause is not serious. Using an anoscope, I looked inside of Jorge's bottom and found internal hemorrhoids. These are basically the same as external hemorrhoids, but they tend to bleed more. They seldom hurt because they do not have nerve endings. I told Jorge to start taking a daily dose of a fiber supplement (of course) with lots of water. His stools became softer, and his bleeding stopped.

If the bleeding had continued, I would have suggested looking further inside for other possible causes, such as a tumor or polyp. If only hemorrhoids were found, he might consider surgery to have the hemorrhoids removed. I did tell Jorge that it was important that he had gotten the problem checked out because rectal bleeding can sometimes be a sign of a serious problem, such as cancer or colitis.

Sexuality

Sexuality is an essential part of being human. It can be an expression of love, affection, and intimacy. It can be an act of lust and passion It can be can be playful, in a world where adults don't play nearly enough. Sex can be a great release of tension. Sometimes it can even be a decent form of aerobic exercise. As gay men, whose sexual desires and activities have long been stigmatized and proscribed, our sexuality helps define who we are, whether we like that or not.

A gay man's sexual life focuses, obviously, on other men. Many men do have sexual attraction to and interaction with members of both sexes. Depending on the degree of same-sex versus opposite-sex orientation, a man may consider himself gay, bisexual, or straight. Gay sex—the kind I will be discussing here—is sex between and about men. Any man, whatever label he chooses for himself, can have gay sex.

Barriers to a Fulfilling Sex Life

When I ask a patient if he is having any sexual problems, the most common response is, "My main problem is not enough sex." Many men want to have fulfilling sex life, yet it seems that that's not easy to achieve. There are many aspects of our gay culture, many social games we play with each other, that keep many of us feeling lonely and isolated. Our society as a whole has hang-ups about sex that carry over into gay men's lives. We do have certain institutions (bars, clubs, baths) where gay men go seeking sex, but many men come away from these experiences feeling just as lonely and isolated as they did before.

Some gay men who socialize with other gay men in nonsexual settings—such as gay athletic teams, choruses, or political organizations—seem have an easier time meeting people for sexual relationships. For the more isolated gay men that I see in my office, I sometimes wonder if I should hire a matchmaker to introduce some of them to each other, but I guess that's outside of my job description.

Finding a prospective sexual partner is just the first step. The next is that the plumbing must all be in order. Sexual dysfunction is common, and it is definitely considered a medical problem. We all have the right to expect our bodies to work the way they are supposed to, and something is wrong if they don't.

Another important medical aspect of sexuality is the opportunity for transmission of various sexually transmitted diseases, including HIV. Fear of catching (or giving) something can really put a damper on someone's sex life, and we need to make "safer sex" such a routine habit that we don't have to think about it all the time.

Doctor-Patient Communication Is Essential

Every man is entitled to a satisfying sex life. (Isn't that written somewhere in the Constitution?) As a doctor, part of my job is to help people with their sexual problems, just as I help them with other medical problems. But I can't help unless my patients and I can discuss the subject frankly and openly. It is important for a patient and doctor to use terminology that both are comfortable with. The terminology must also clearly and unambiguously describe various sex acts.

Because most of us are at least a little uncomfortable discussing sex, we have various euphemisms, vague terms, and medical terms for sexual parts and acts. It is helpful to try to be more precise when discussing these things medically. For example, if you tell a doctor you are worried about being exposed to a sexually transmitted disease because you have had "oral sex three times in the last month," what does that mean? Did you give three blow jobs or get three blow jobs, or both, and was ejaculation involved? Was a condom used? Some of the time? Or if you say you have a rash "down there," where exactly is that? The groin? The penis? The anus? The foot?

The point is, it is important to be as explicit and precise as possible with your doctor when you talk about these things. Don't worry—it's almost impossible to shock a doctor with words. Most have seen and heard a lot of fairly extreme things. But do be sure that you and the doctor are clear on what you are talking about. The doctor may not understand some of the words you use, even if they are precise to you because many doctors do not know a lot of gay men's sexual slang.

For example, recently when I gave a lecture on gay men's health to a class of 175 medical students, I asked if anyone knew what "rimming" referred to. Not a single hand was raised. Now, maybe a few of the students knew that rimming is a gay men's term for oral-anal contact, and maybe they were too embarrassed to raise their hands, but I suspect most of the students had no idea.

When I am meeting with a patient in my office, I use whatever terminology the patient seems to prefer. For example, I am perfectly comfortable discussing with a man his difficulty in "getting fucked," and that phrase seems much more graceful than "receiving anal intercourse." Either will do. I do tend to hesitate to use the cruder-sounding Anglo-Saxon words unless I hear them from the patient first. When you have this sort of discussion with your doctor, you should find a vocabulary that you both are comfortable with.

For the purpose of this book, I will use a range of terminology to describe sex organs and acts. My goal is to communicate as unambiguously as possible. I will frequently use medical, Latin-sounding sex terms because people need to know these words for "polite" conversation. But some of this vocabulary is more awkward than the vernacular equivalent (for example, *perform fellatio on* versus *give a blow job to*), so I will use any term that seems appropriate for the context. Expect to see some words or phrases that may sound a bit pornographic. After all, we are grownups, we all know most of these words, so in this book, we'll use them.

What's Next

The following sections consist of a discussion of various topics relating to gay men's sexuality. I start with a section describing the most common ways that men can relate sexually with each other. Next is my highly opinionated discussion of safer sex, or how to avoid disease transmission while still having fun. Following that is a section on sexual dysfunction from a gay men's perspective. Finally there is an essay on patterns of gay men's sexual behavior. Included is a discussion of sexual compulsiveness, a disorder that lately is trendy for gay men to diagnose either in themselves or in others of whose behavior they disapprove.

Gay Men's Sexual Vocabulary

What constitutes a sex act? A wide of range intimate activities between men can be considered sex, from heavy petting, where he may just barely get his hands in your pants, to anal intercourse and beyond. In general, sex involves some sort of physical-genital stimulation that may or may not lead to orgasm (ejaculation, coming). This may be solo (masturbation, or jacking or jerking off) or with one partner or more than one partner. Additionally, for most gay men sexuality has a broader physical focus than on just the genitals.

This book is not meant to be a sex manual. There are good sex manuals available for gay men, though of course the best way to learn about the art of gay sex is firsthand, from a skilled practitioner-teacher.

What's important here is to describe some of the basic sexual activities available to gay men. This will facilitate the discussions of safer sex and of sexual dysfunction that come later in this section.

By listing these activities in a physician-written book about gay men's health, my intention is to give my wholehearted endorsement to each and every one of these ways that gay men can please each other. There is nothing inherently unhealthy or dangerous about any of these activities. On the contrary, each is a wonderful way that men can share intimacy.

Of course, such intimacy can also facilitate the transmission of infection from one man to another. All gay men should be familiar with the basics of safer sex, to reduce this possibility.

The following list is far from complete, just covering the most basic and popular gay men's sex acts. If your tastes are exotic, your favorite may not even be described here. If that is the case, good for you! Some of these may not be your particular cup of tea. Nothing wrong with that either. To each his own.

Deep kissing (French kissing): oral-oral stimulation, involving using one's tongue in the mouth of a partner.

Finger- or fist-fucking (digital-anal or manual-anal stimulation): insertion of one or more fingers—or the whole hand, wrist, or forearm—into the anus of a partner.

Frottage (femoral intercourse): one partner stimulating his penis between the thighs of the other partner.

Fucking (screwing, anal intercourse): mutual stimulation by insertion of one man's penis (cock, dick) into the anus (asshole) of another man.

Masturbation (jacking or jerking off): the act of stimulating a penis by hand. May be done solo or involve more than one person.

Rimming: oral-anal stimulation.

Sadomasochism (leather sex, rough sex): a broad variety of sex play, involving roles, bondage, pain, humiliation, and other activities, with the mutual consent of the parties involved.

Sucking (giving head, giving a blow job, fellatio, oral sex): the stimulation of one man's penis by another's mouth.

Toys: often refers to dildos inserted into the anus, but innumerable varieties of sexual devices are available.

Water sports: urinating onto or into a partner.

There is no disputing taste, and some men find certain of these activities much more appealing than others. For some, anal sex of any variety is just not in their repertoire, while for others it's just not sex unless fucking occurs. Many people are uncomfortable with leather sex, yet to some practitioners it is the most exquisite form of human interaction. Fist-fucking is appalling to some, intriguing to others, and a sacred ritual to its devotees. Before you criticize someone else's sexual tastes, remember that as gay men, our entire sexuality has often been denigrated, reviled, and even outlawed by the larger society. We should be the last to criticize sexual activities that we do not personally enjoy ourselves.

All of these sex acts are quite safe if performed responsibly and with proper protection. Some require more expertise than others. None should be performed while under the influence of drugs, which reduce one's inhibitions and lead to risky behavior and consequences that may be regretted later.

Sexual Dysfunction and Its Treatment

I n order to have healthy sexual function, a man must have adequate sexual desire (libido, "sexual energy," horniness), and adequate ability to perform sexually (I guess you could call it "studliness"). Those are the minimum requirements, of course. In this section we will discuss problems with general sexual desire and with genital sexual performance. Anal sexual function and dysfunction are covered in the separate section on anal health.

The medical profession tends to ignore gay men's sexuality except when addressing transmission of HIV and other sexually transmitted diseases. Many doctors are not accustomed to helping their gay male patients achieve optimal sexual function. Perhaps this is out of discomfort; perhaps it is because in many states it is still illegal (unbelievably) for two men to have sex with each other.

For example, the manufacturers of erection-enhancing medical devices and other treatments have only sought heterosexual volunteers for participation in their studies. We must assume that these devices and medications work for both gay and straight men, but it is nevertheless insulting that we are excluded from studies of medical treatments for sexual dysfunction.

Gay men therefore face barriers in seeking care for sexual dysfunction. Our sexuality is still not well-understood or accepted by many health care providers. It is important for a gay man to have sensitive health care practitioners who respect his sexuality. Ideally, a doctor must be comfortable in discussing a range of issues—such as anal intercourse, water sports, and fisting—without making a value judgment about these activities. Sexual dysfunction is an area where it is very useful for a gay man to have a supportive primary care doctor, one who can initiate the evaluation and treatment and make referrals to equally supportive specialists when indicated.

Problems With Sexual Desire

Adam: *I've lost interest in sex lately, and it's really bothering my partner. I don't know what to do about it, though frankly I don't mind having a break from sex right now. I guess it bothers me because it bothers him. For the first two years we were together, there was no problem. Now I'm afraid I'll lose him if this keeps up.*

Adam's situation is very common. To understand why he might be having his problem, several possible causes need to be explored.

Many physical and psychological factors can disrupt a man's sex drive. Any medical illness, for example, can take away interest in sex. Various medications—most notably antidepressants—can lower or wipe out the libido. Hormonal disorders, such as deficiency of testosterone or thyroid hormone, can do the same. Sexual desire also tends to diminish during periods of high stress. Lack of libido is a common symptom of clinical depression. Finally, relationship problems can definitely interfere with someone's desire to have sex.

Lack of libido is not only a health problem, but it also can be a part of some other problem, whether that problem is medical or emotional. So it is important to bring this problem to medical attention. It is often easy to pinpoint the cause, which is the first step to getting better.

If you suffer from a serious or chronic medical illness and/or are taking medication on an ongoing basis, that does not mean that your sexuality must be set aside. If you find your libido is down or gone, discuss this with your doctor. It may only take an adjustment of medication or perhaps a medical workup to be on the way to getting your sex drive back. However, in some cases, illness may interfere with sexual feelings. It can be normal not to feel sexual when one does not feel well. That does not mean one cannot experience other forms of intimacy.

Hormonal problems are easy to treat once they are properly diagnosed. I have been surprised by how many of my male patients have deficiencies in testosterone, the major male hormone. Replacement of this hormone can restore sexual desire and function.

Depression is a major cause of libido problems. Clinical depression is a serious disease and has its own section later in this book. It is very treatable. If you wonder whether you suffer from clinical depression, read the section. If the symptoms fit, you should definitely consult your health care provider.

Erectile Dysfunction: The Problem

Erectile dysfunction, or impotence, is what first comes to mind when we talk about problems involving male sexual performance. In the United States, according to recent estimates by the National Institutes of Health, between ten and 20 million men suffer from this problem.

Undoubtedly, more than a few of these millions of men are gay, though you would never know it by reading mainstream medical journals. You'll see ads in these journals for impotence therapies, but they would never dare feature male couples. Generally the treatments for impotence have only been studied in heterosexuals, and some even carry a disclaimer to that effect, though there is no reason they should not work equally well for gay men.

Impotence is traditionally defined as the inability to achieve or maintain an erection sufficiently firm to achieve penetration and satisfactory intercourse.

For a gay man, the definition needs to be broadened. Depending on one's sexual tastes and goals, "penetration" means anal penetration and hence presumes the availability of a partner that is capable of anal penetration without great difficulty. But impotence in a gay man could also mean lack of a sufficient erection for satisfying oral sex or mutual masturbation. If the man has a steady partner, it is very important to include the partner in the evaluation and treatment process for this problem.

Erectile dysfunction can have many causes. How does an erection (hard-on) occur in the first place? It seems rather magical and mysterious. The penis in repose is a floppy appendage, hanging limply down. With arousal it starts to enlarge, get hard, and stick straight out. It does these things because blood is pumping into it faster than it is flowing out. The blood fills the spongy, soft penile tissues and makes them rigid. This rigidity compresses the penile veins, slowing the flow of blood out of the penis and making the erection firmer.

Nerve impulses cause dilation of the arteries into the penis and hence allow an erection to happen. The stimulus for the process can be psychological (thinking about a hot man or seeing a sexy picture of one), physical (manual stimulation, for example), or both. Also, during the night the penis goes through intermittent cycles of erection that may or may not be connected with erotic dreams. Think of this as the penis practicing its act while we're asleep.

The delicate chain of events that leads to an erection can easily be broken. For example, anxiety about one's ability to perform can spoil the psychological part of the stimulus.

Disorders such as diabetes, which damages nerves, can block the nerve impulses. Surgery—for example, for prostate cancer—can also damage the nerves that facilitate erection. Hormonal imbalances, particularly a deficiency in testosterone or in thyroid hormone, can prevent one from getting a good erection. Circulation problems, especially in smokers or diabetics, can interfere with the blood flow necessary to engorge the penis. And many medications, particularly those used to treat high blood pressure or depression, can keep one's penis from getting hard when it's supposed to.

Sometimes the nature of the problem will give a clue as to the cause. For example, if a man can get a good, hard erection when he's masturbating alone but cannot get it up with a partner, the problem probably comes from the psyche. If a man cannot get an erection under any circumstances and does not even have spontaneous nighttime or early-morning erections, the problem is likely to be physical.

Recent life changes can also be relevant to erection problems. If Joe recently started on a new medication or is very anxious about a new boyfriend that he really wants to impress, these things might interfere with his ability to get hard. So if a patient sees me with an erection problem, I tend to ask him a lot of questions in order to help us figure out where the problem may be coming from.

In many cases—perhaps most—erections fail for a combination of reasons. Some of these reasons are physical, and some are psychological.

Treatment of Erectile Dysfunction

If an erection problem appears to be mostly psychological, psychotherapy from an experienced sex therapist can help. But if the cause appears at least partly physical, it is easiest to try medical solutions first.

There are several quite efficient ways to force an uncooperative penis to get hard. Even if the problem is one of performance anxiety, which is psychological, then by artificially enhancing the performance a few times, the anxiety can be reduced, and the erections will begin to improve on their own.

The medically accepted methods of coaxing an erection out of an unwilling penis include both pharmacological and physical approaches. In other words, a man with erectile dysfunction can either give his penis drugs that trick it into becoming erect, or he can help it get hard via physical means, such as vacuum pumping or a surgical implant. It is important to learn about all the potential options before making a decision about which one to try first.

One way to create an erection is with oral medications. An old drug, yohimbine, is taken as a pill and has a reputation for enhancing male sexual function. However, this claim has never been proven, so the American Urological Association does not recommend this product. A promising new oral medication, sildenafil (Viagra), dilates the arteries into the penis and appears to improve erections in most men. It begins to work within an hour after it is taken, and a dose seems to improve the ability of the man to have a good erection, at the appropriate time, for up to several days. A similar drug, phentolamine (Vasomax), may also be effective. A nonprescription herbal preparation, Ginkgo biloba extract, is said to improve circulation. It is reputed to also improve erections.

Other drugs—such as alprostadil (Caverject) or papaverine—given directly into the penis, dilate arteries and increase the flow of blood into the organ. In the past, these medications have always been given by injection, just before sex, using a tiny needle, and injecting directly into the side of the base of the penis. Ideally this produces an erection of appropriate firmness and longevity.

Although many men freak out at the the idea of sticking their willy with a needle, the injection itself is usually not painful. It does, however, produce a break in the skin, which may increase the risk of HIV transmission if one partner is negative and one is positive. Penile injections are usually first done under a doctor's supervision until the dose is properly adjusted. Too low a dose won't work. Too high a dose can result in priapism, a painful erection that won't go down and can lead to permanent damage of this important organ.

A new product, alprostadil urethral suppositories, sold under the brand name MUSE, administers a similar drug but without the need for injection. Instead, a tiny pellet of medication is inserted into the penis through the urethral opening just before sex. The man is advised to urinate just before inserting the pellet to facilitate insertion into the urethra. The drug is absorbed through the delicate urethral lining. As with the shots, the dose needs to be adjusted for each individual. The proper dose will produce an erection within five to ten minutes that lasts an hour or so. The advantage is that no injection is involved. However, it is more expensive than the shots, and some men may be just as squeamish at sticking something into their urethra as they would be at sticking a needle into the side of their penis.

These pharmacologic methods are particularly appealing to men who do not have a steady partner and do not want to reveal to their occasional partners that they are using "artificial" means to get hard. For example:

Dave: *I never tell my dates that I get a little medical help with erections. At the proper moment, I duck into the bathroom and give myself the injection. There is never any bleeding— the needle is so tiny—but I make sure the condom covers the injection site. I emerge from the bathroom with a nice hard-on, and no one has ever asked any questions. Except when we fin- ish early, and I've still got some time left on my one-hour erection. Once I was showering with a guy after sex, and he commented that I was still hard. I told him it was because he turned me on so much.*

If giving drugs to the penis is unappealing or unfeasible, there are mechanical methods of making it get hard without drugs.

For example, for years some gay men have been playing with vacuum pumps to engorge their penises, sometimes to monstrous size. More recently, enterprising medical-supply com- panies have discovered these toys, modified them slightly, renamed them "vacuum constric- tion devices," registered them as medical devices, and now sell them for hundreds of dollars more than the sex shops do.

Here's how a vacuum pump works: A Plexiglas cylinder is placed over the penis and con- nected to suction. Air is pumped out of the cylinder, creating a vacuum that draws blood into the penis until it is big and hard. Then an elastic band is slipped over the device and onto the base of the penis, constricting it to hold the blood in, and the cylinder is slipped off. The penis remains hard as long as the band is left in place.

The resulting erection is quite adequate for sex, though it tends to be poorly anchored because the internal part of the penis (below the constricting band) is not engorged. Because of all the apparatus involved, this method requires a partner who is both patient and under- standing. It obviously can't be done without the partner's knowledge. But some guys enjoy helping pump up their partner's penis to get it ready for action.

Less extreme—and much more popular—is the simple device known as a cock ring. (Yes, that seems to be the term urologists use.) This is simply a metal, leather, or rubber ring that goes around the base of the genitals, just tightly enough to impede the drainage of blood out of the penis but not tightly enough to prevent blood flow into the penis. Many men find that wearing a cock ring gives them a somewhat firmer, longer-lasting erection. Urologists rec- ommend them to men whose erections are not quite adequate. If you use a cock ring, just be sure it is the kind that can be removed easily even when the penis is hard. Otherwise you might find yourself in an emergency room with a doctor approaching you with a pair of bolt cutters.

All of the above methods work in most cases of erection problems, whatever the underlying reason. If the cause is mostly psychological, then getting a few good erections may be enough to restore confidence and return function toward normal. If the cause of the dysfunction is physical, the preferred remedy can be continued indefinitely.

For a few men, however, none of these methods works or is acceptable, and the only solution is a penile implant. This should be used only as a last resort. Penile implants, or prostheses, are either semirigid (malleable) or inflatable rods that are surgically inserted into the penis.

Obviously a penile prosthesis is a big deal, with greater costs and risks than the other ways of dealing with erection problems. I recommend very careful consideration before undergoing such an operation. The surgeon should explain the pros and cons of the two types of implants, the potential complications of the surgery, and what to expect during the healing process.

Also keep in mind that implantation of a penile prosthesis usually damages the erectile tissue so that other therapies, injections for example, will not be an option for the future. And an erect "bionic penis" is not the same consistency as one that has become erect by being pumped full of blood. It is basically a soft penis stretched around a hard supportive rod.

Before having your penis operated on, you should definitely ask to speak to other men who have had implants. Good luck in finding a gay man who has had one. I have none in my practice, though there must be a few around. Also, ask yourself if there is really no other alternative for your and your partners' sexual satisfaction. Be creative. What about a strap-on dildo or some other form of sexual expression that does not require your penis to be erect?

Other Types of Sexual Dysfunction

There are other aspects of male sexual function besides the process of erection that can go awry and interfere with sexual satisfaction. These include orgasmic or ejaculatory dysfunction. Not infrequently, a man will have an orgasm (come) too soon or take too long to come. My question to men with this complaint is, are you practicing on your own? Often enough? Sometimes just the excitement or anxiety generated by being sexual with someone after a long dry spell will result in premature ejaculation.

Usually one can gain some control over the timing of ejaculation by masturbating and developing a sense of control over one's own orgasm. When you feel like you are near coming, squeeze the head of your penis as hard as you can until the feeling subsides, then begin stroking again. Continue this process until you learn to control when you come. This need not be done solo; it can be done with a partner.

If the "squeeze technique" doesn't work, there are desensitizing creams sold for the treatment of premature ejaculation. If using the cream with a condom, make sure the cream is water-based, and of course, in order to work it needs to be applied inside the condom (unless you want to numb your buddy's butt or mouth).

Premature ejaculation can also be treated medically. Controlled studies have shown that certain antidepressants, for example Zoloft (sertraline), can improve the situation for men suffering from premature ejaculation to the point that they are able to have intercourse for a satisfactory length of time before orgasm.

Delayed ejaculation, another form of sexual dysfunction, can be a type of performance anxiety, and it can be treated with psychotherapeutic techniques. Additionally, some medications—in particular antidepressants—can cause delayed ejaculation. (This effect is used to advantage when these drugs are used to treat premature ejaculation.) If medication is causing delayed ejaculation, you and your doctor may be able to adjust the medication to reduce or eliminate the problem.

Other abnormalities of ejaculation can be quite alarming or disturbing to the person involved. One is called *hematospermia,* or bloody semen. Since the seminal fluid is made from blood and the prostate is rich in blood vessels, it is not surprising that occasionally one of these blood vessels will burst and spill some blood into the semen.

Sometimes bloody ejaculation occurs after receiving particularly vigorous anal sex, which may traumatize the prostate. Fortunately, this is almost never a sign of a significant problem, and it usually goes away by itself. If hematospermia persists or is accompanied by pain, it can be a sign of a prostate infection, in which case it will respond to treatment of the infection.

Lack of semen is another problem that can be psychologically distressing. In this case, the pleasurable sensations and muscle contractions of orgasm occur, but little or no fluid comes out. This can occur in various situations. A reduction in the amount of seminal fluid is common with age. I have noticed that the volume of semen also decreases in men with with chronic disease, such as HIV infection. The reason for this is not understood.

If there is absolutely no seminal fluid, it is often a sign of retrograde ejaculation, where the amount of semen produced is normal, but it is ejaculated up into the bladder during orgasm instead of out through the penis due to a fault in the internal valve in the urethra. The semen mixes with the urine in the bladder and is eliminated unnoticed with the next urination. There's really nothing dangerous about that, and usually nothing can be done about it, so don't let it worry you. Orgasms should still feel just as good.

Prostate surgery also usually eliminates the ability to ejaculate semen, but again, the capacity for orgasm should remain intact. There is nothing one can do about this, so my advice is to concentrate on how good it feels to come and not worry that there isn't any come anymore.

Safer Sex

Sexual contact can transmit unwanted infections from one person to another. There are many sexually transmitted diseases, which include not only HIV but a wide variety of other types of infection. These diseases are described in several other sections of this book. The point of safer sex is to be able to enjoy intimacy without giving or catching any of these nasty bugs.

There are many components to practicing sex safely, and there are various degrees of sexual safety. Certainly solo sex is the only way to be sexual and yet completely ensure that you won't give or get an STD. But for most people there's more to their sex life than masturbation. Physical intimacy with other men is at the core of being a gay man, and we can have this without endangering each other's health if we know how to be careful.

Patients often ask me how safe a given sexual activity is. Researchers have attempted to measure the risk of disease transmission with different sex practices, and people have made scales of the relative risk of these different activities. *Relative* is the key word here. There are activities that are more safe, and there are ones that are less safe. No one can tell you the exact chances of catching a given infection from a given act.

My recommendation is that you read the information in this section, study it, and then decide where your comfort level is, and stick to it. Draw the line between what you will do sexually and what you won't.

Having safer sex is a little like driving a car safely. If you are in the habit of driving at 100 miles per hour without a seat belt, you know you're going to get in trouble pretty fast. If you always wear a seat belt and stick to the speed limit, you're more apt to be OK. But accidents can happen to any driver, no matter how careful and skillful. The only way to avoid a misfortune would be to stay locked up in your room and never venture out, and who would want to do that?

Also, the majority of auto accidents occur under the influence of alcohol or drugs. So it is with safer sex that alcohol or drugs impair a man's judgment and get in the way of his being safe. No matter how much a person knows about protecting himself, if he has sex in an intoxicated state, he is likely to get into trouble. If you want to have sex safely, then do it soberly.

A Bit of Historical Background

At one time, gay men didn't really need to pay much attention to STD transmission. During the 1970s, at the height of gay men's sexual freedom, many men played sexually with many other men, without inhibition. The main responsibility for a sexually active gay man was to go to the clinic every few months and get checked and treated for syphilis and gonorrhea. Or if he had a drip or a sore, to avoid playing until he got it taken care of. Sure there were a few clouds on the horizon as hepatitis started causing serious illness or even death in some gay men, and herpes, an incurable STD, started making the rounds. But these did not seem to deter gay men from exploring their sexual freedom.

The real wake-up call came in the early 1980's, when gay men began falling ill and dying from complications of what became known as the Acquired Immune Deficiency Syndrome. At first, no one knew what caused AIDS. But even before HIV, the virus responsible for AIDS, was discovered, gay men had discovered for themselves the connection between "catching AIDS" and the exchange of body fluids. Hence the notion of "safer sex" arose in the gay men's communities in California and New York. Safer sex, originally defined as avoiding the exchange of body fluids, not only lowers your chances of catching or giving HIV but does the same for most other STDs.

Fucking Safely

The most important concept of safer sex is: Have as much fun as you like, but don't let your ejaculate (come) or pre-ejaculate (precome) get inside your partner. Especially inside his butt. And don't let his get inside of you.

The biggest rule of safer sex is, to be blunt: No fucking without a condom. A cock does not go up an ass without a condom on. Period. End of discussion. As the ads say: no glove, no love.

This is one of the very few aspects of safer sex that everyone agrees on. It is also agreed that anal sex can transmit HIV from the receiver to the inserter and vice versa.

This is not to say that anal intercourse need be risky. We have a right to enjoy anal sex if we like, and that's why God gave us condoms. Anyone who ever suggests that gay men should stop having anal sex in order to stop the spread of HIV is homophobic, plain and simple. No one would dare suggest that straight people cease indulging in vaginal intercourse in order to stop the heterosexual spread of HIV.

Condoms are the mainstay of hot, safer sex. These little rubber sleeves that roll over the erect penis and prevent the semen (come) from spilling onto/into a partner have been around for a long time, though they have traditionally been used by straight men to prevent pregnancy and STDs. Gay men have never had to worry about pregnancy, and in the past, when most STDs were easily treatable, we didn't worry too much about those, either. So condoms were something used by some straight men but not by gay men. Now, however, they are very helpful for gay men who want to play safely. They allow us to have the types of penetration that might otherwise spread disease, and now we realize how important that is.

There are various types of condoms. The standard kind—and the only ones that have been proven to work reliably—are made of latex rubber. These come in various sizes, shapes, and varieties (plain, lubricated, and flavored). They must be used with water-based lube only; oil-based lube will dissolve them.

Do not use "natural" condoms made of lamb intestine because HIV can leak through them. Don't bother with them at all. They are of no value for gay men.

There are also polyurethane condoms made of a plastic material. These are valuable for those folks who are allergic to latex rubber, and they can be used with oil-based lubes. However, they seem to have a high breakage rate, so they are less reliable than the latex rubber kind. Do not use them unless you have no other choice; they are probably better than nothing. Polyurethane condoms have recently been reformulated and are now thicker, but their reliability remains questionable in my mind.

There is also a receptive or "female" polyurethane condom called Reality. This consists of a polyurethane sac with a small, flexible ring at the closed end, and a larger ring at the open end. Many men have discovered that it is possible to use this type of condom anally. The device is inserted into the butt of the receptive partner prior to intercourse by using a finger to push it in until all but the larger ring is inside. The active partner then inserts his penis into the condom, which is already in the anus, and commences intercourse. Some gay men find this kind of condom quite comfortable.

But does it work? The company that makes the Reality condom is reluctant to test it for male anal sex, otherwise known as *sodomy* in those jurisdictions where it remains illegal. In heterosexual couples the Reality condom is fair at preventing pregnancy but poor at preventing disease transmission. Therefore, there is no reason to expect it to work well at preventing disease transmission during anal sex. My advice is not to rely on the receptive condom to protect you or your partner from any type of infection, especially if ejaculation occurs.

Even the best latex condoms are not 100% effective. Remember that women occasionally get pregnant despite their partner using a condom. If a sperm can leak through, so can an HIV particle, which is much smaller. Also, a condom must be used properly in order to work the way it is supposed to. Here are some basic rules of condom use:

Use a fresh condom. (Yes, they have expiration dates printed on the package.) Don't store condoms in a hot place, like the glove compartment of your car.

To apply the condom, roll it down over the penis as soon as it gets hard. If there is a foreskin, make sure it is retracted before applying the condom. Use only water-based lube, which can be used on the outside as well as the inside of the condom, if desired. Oil-based lubricant will damage the condom and make it leak. Unroll the condom all the way down to the base of the penis. You may want to be the one to put the condom on your own penis, but some couples also enjoy putting the condoms on each other's penises, as part of foreplay.

During sex, if it feels like the condom has torn, the insertive partner, or top, should withdraw immediately and replace the condom if necessary. In addition, he should try to avoid ejaculation while his penis is inside the receptive partner, or bottom, just in case the condom has torn or developed a leak. Afterwards, when pulling out, grab the base of the condom so that it is not left behind. Discard the condom after pulling out; do not reuse it. If you follow these rules, you are giving the condom its best chance to prevent disease transmission.

One more thing: When fucking, be careful what lubricant you use. Some lubes can injure your skin or mucous membranes:

Henry: *My new boyfriend is HIV-positive, and we wanted to be extra careful. So before we had sex for the first time I bought us a bottle of lube with nonoxynol-9—the spermicide that is supposed to kill HIV. We figured it would be extra insurance in case the condom broke. Well, when he screwed me it felt like fire, and for the next few days I had blood and mucus coming out of my ass. Not fun. Never again.*

For this reason I don't recommend that gay men use nonoxynol-9. It can be very irritating to some men's internal tissues, both inside the rectum and inside the urethra. And since it is considered a "cosmetic," it is not regulated by the government, so that the amount of nonoxynol-9 in a given brand of lube can vary wildly from one batch to the next. In studies in Africa, female prostitutes had a higher risk of catching HIV if they used nonoxynol-9. Stay away from it. Use a plain, water-based lube without perfume, spermicide, or any other unnecessary or potentially irritating ingredients.

Some of Us Still Fuck Unsafely

Many men—especially younger men who came out in the safer-sex era—would not consider fucking without a condom; they find the idea creepy. But the fact is that every day thousands of other gay men are having anal sex without condoms. Surveys of sexually active gay men in the United States have found that up to half or even more continue to screw without condoms at least on occasion. Since it seems that most HIV infection in gay men is transmitted this way, then if everyone who fucked used a rubber 100% of the time, the vast majority of HIV transmission in gay men would cease.

Why do some of us continue to have this type of unsafe sex? Some men say they do not like the feeling of a condom or have difficulty staying hard with one on. For some, a condom takes the spontaneity out of sex. Some men who are HIV-positive feel free to have unprotected sex with other HIV-positive men. It is likely that this is safe in terms of reinfection with HIV, but there is plenty of opportunity for the spread of other diseases, such as hepatitis or herpes, this way.

Some HIV-negative guys have a fatalistic notion that because they are gay, they are bound to catch HIV sooner or later, so why bother worrying about it? Many younger, HIV-negative gay men do not think that they are at risk of catching HIV if they only play with people their age; or they just haven't learned how to protect themselves or that they even need to.

There are gay community observers who believe that low self-esteem is the basis for many gay men's persistence in not protecting themselves or their partners from HIV. They maintain that if we as a community could improve our self-esteem level, feel like we had more to live for, and realize that we owe it to our community to stay healthy, then we would be more motivated to be safer sexually.

The Oral Sex Debate

What about oral sex? How safe is it? Can you catch or give HIV via a blow job? This is a very controversial subject among gay men and among public-health authorities. Everyone certainly agrees that anal intercourse is the easiest way for gay men to transmit HIV. Everyone also agrees that an occasional case of HIV transmission is probably due to oral sex because that is the only type of sex the person claims to have had.

But the chances of catching HIV orally are much less than the chances of catching it anally. This risk, people agree, is reduced further if ejaculation does not occur during oral sex. There is also agreement that the consistent use of condoms for oral sex should further reduce the risk of HIV transmission almost to zero.

I hear lots of stories about oral sex from my patients, and every man seems to have his own strong opinion about how risky it is. For example:

Mason: *I love giving head. In fact, it is the only kind of sex I really enjoy. You could call me an oral-sex slut. For instance, one afternoon I went down to the peep shows, and I wanted to see how many loads of come I could take. In four hours I scored 35! Over the years I have swallowed thousands—at peep shows, tearooms, rest areas, and parks. It's like a hobby with me, and I'm not giving it up. Besides, if oral sex can transmit HIV, how come I'm still negative?*

But I have also heard these stories:

Perry: *I went to New York to visit a friend who was in the last stages of AIDS. I was HIV-negative at the time. We slept in his bed together, and during the night I went down on him. He had some precome, but he did not ejaculate. Within a week I had fever, sore throat, and a rash—and I found out I had become infected with HIV, from that one exposure. I had not had any other sex in over a year, so where else could it have come from?*

Robert: *I don't mind using condoms for oral sex at all. I carry a few mint-flavored rubbers with me at all times. I was an Eagle Scout, and I still remember the motto "Be prepared." Some men think it's strange when I roll the rubber onto their dick before I suck them off, but I sure sleep better afterwards knowing I don't have to worry I might have caught something.*

So the verdict is: Yes, it is possible to contract HIV through unprotected oral sex. But no, it is not common, and it is not easy. Oral sex—even unprotected—is safer sex. Not *safe* sex but safer. In summary, to make oral sex safer yet, you can do the following:

■ Avoid giving head if you have any kind of mouth sores, recent dental work, gum disease, or other break in the lining of the oral cavity.

■ Avoid ejaculation during oral sex (but precome still presents some risk).

■ You may choose to use a condom for oral sex (though this is unappealing to many men).

Many gay men have come to terms with this issue by accepting the small risk involved with unprotected oral sex while religiously using condoms for anal sex. That reduces their risk of HIV considerably. The problem is, if you are that one unlucky person that catches HIV orally, you are just as HIV-positive as the guy who caught it anally. So each man must decide what his comfort level is with oral sex and act in accordance with that.

The Safety of Other Activities

Patients often ask me about the safety of other types of sexual expression. Most other activities are safer than oral or anal sex in terms of disease transmission. Masturbation, solo or mutual, is a very safe activity, as is frottage (body rubbing, or femoral intercourse, in which the penis is stimulated between the thighs of a partner). Kissing may transmit herpes and possibly hepatitis but not much else. It's never been demonstrated to my satisfaction that deep kissing can transmit HIV. Ejaculation on unbroken skin is not a risk, but be careful if there are open wounds or sores.

Urine is generally free of infectious bacteria or viruses, but water-sports players should probably heed the advice "on me, not in me" with urine as with semen. Rimming is not likely to transmit HIV, though it can transmit other germs such as hepatitis A virus, herpes viruses, and intestinal parasites. Fisting is unlikely to transmit infection but must be performed carefully and soberly, by skilled players, to avoid injury. Finger play in the anus is less traumatic than fisting and should not transmit disease if the skin is intact. Toys such as dildos or butt plugs are safe if they are not too big (to avoid trauma) and are not shared—or if they are, they should be covered with a condom.

Finding Safety in Relationships

Mutual monogamy, when both partners are free of infection, is theoretically very safe no matter what physical intimacies are exchanged. It is wonderful to be in a trusting relationship. But sometimes that trust is misguided. For example, this very distraught man came in to get his HIV test and had this story, which I have heard many times in several variations:

Nate: *I was madly in love with this guy, and we were going to be together forever. I had just tested negative for HIV, and he told me that he had also. We had wild, passionate, unsafe sex, night after night. Then he got sick, and we found out that he had AIDS. He had never actually been tested. He lied. So far I'm OK, but it's been six months, and I want another test. I'm going crazy with worry. Why did I trust him?*

When I see both members of a couple as patients, sometimes one will tell me, "We're monogamous, and we're both negative, so we don't use rubbers," while the other one will tell me, "He thinks we're monogamous, and we don't use protection, but it's OK because I use rubbers when I fool around with other people." This is a very risky situation, and such couples need to come to a better understanding so that one isn't deceiving the other. Even if the straying partner does not pick up HIV, he could bring home some other STD and inadvertently share it. Not only is he endangering his partner's health, but he is endangering the relationship by deceiving his partner.

I don't mean to breed cynicism or distrust by telling these stories. There are many gay male couples who are truly monogamous and who are honest with each other and who need not use any other type of precaution against sexually transmitted diseases. If that applies to you, then good for you.

Other committed male couples are not sexually monogamous and have various agreements permitting outside sex. Often in couples who are both HIV-negative, outside sex is permitted as long as it is "very safe," and the couple continues to have completely unprotected sex with each other. This practice, which is becoming known as *negotiated safety,* is more and more popular among couples whose relationships include permission for outside sex. But since no sex is 100% safe, this is a bit of a risky situation.

Serodiscordant couples—in which one man is HIV-negative and the other is HIV-positive—need to have an understanding about their sexual activity so that they can have a healthy sex life without the concern that the negative partner will become infected. Different couples deal with this situation in different ways. Some couples simply adhere to careful safer-sex practices. I favor this approach because it seems the least stressful—and the least risky. In other discordant couples, the positive partner will permit himself to be exposed to his lover's semen but not the other way around. And yes, some discordant couples ignore any protection. The negative partner assumes he will get infected at some point, so why worry about it? This is the cause of some of the new cases of HIV infection I see in my practice.

The Bottom Line

We can discuss all of these finer points of safer sex for pages and pages and hours and hours. But I like keeping things simple. So let's boil this down to three basic rules:

1. **Sober sex is safer sex.** It's impossible to be safe when you are messed up on drugs or alcohol.
2. **Oral sex is safer sex.** You can make it even safer by using a condom and avoiding ejaculation.
3. **Fucking with a condom is safer sex.** Use a rubber for all anal intercourse, every single time, whatever the situation. Fucking without protection is dangerous, and it should be considered bad manners, like eating ice cream with your fingers. That's why God gave us condoms—and spoons.

Patterns of Sexual Behavior

Gay men relate in many ways. Many gay men mate for life in monogamous pairs. Others are single or date or have a series of relationships that begin and later end. But human diversity is often much more complicated than that, and some men do not fit into a simple category of "coupled" or "single" for any length of time. There are innumerable patterns in which a gay man may relate lovingly and/or sexually to other men. There is no one right way, and there are very few wrong ones.

Gay men's sexual behavior runs over a huge spectrum, from celibacy to monogamy to promiscuity. Sexual behavior does not always correlate neatly with someone's relationship status. Sex can be an integral part of a loving, committed relationship between two men. But sex can have many other roles in a man's life. For example, a "single" man who is not in a loving relationship, can be celibate, monogamous with one sexual friend, or promiscuous. Likewise, a "coupled" man who is in a committed relationship with another man may be celibate sexually, monogamous with his husband, monogamous with another partner, or promiscuous.

Luigi: *Sex was never a big part of my life. My partner was the first man I had sex with. After he died, it never has really occurred to me to go looking for sex. If I meet another man and fall in love with him, then sure—but right now it's not something I'm interested in.*

Zak: *For the past couple of years I've been working as an escort. I have an ad in the paper, and men call and pay me to have sex with them. I enjoy the work. I'm in good shape, and I like sex, and I usually like my clients, and I'm told I'm talented at it. I know it's not something I'm going to spend my life doing, but for right now it's a good living. I was single when I started, but now I have a boyfriend. I told him about my work after we had a few dates. He's very understanding about it. In my mind, what I do with my clients is totally different from the relationship I have with my boyfriend.*

Marco: *I've known for a long time I was gay, but I'm only 19, and I haven't had sex yet. Most of my friends have. I'm just waiting for the right guy. My friends tease me, but I don't think there's anything wrong with waiting.*

Ryan: *I'm single, but I'm not a monk. I'm not into anonymous sex, and I'm usually dating someone. One person at a time. I tend to date a guy for a few months, then move on. Sometimes we have sex on the first date, sometimes not. I like the passion of just getting to know someone. I'd like to settle down with someone long-term, but I'm not sure I'm the marrying kind.*

Kai: *I guess you could say I have a husband and a boyfriend and also occasional tricks. My husband and I have been together for 18 years. We are devoted to each other and to our two daughters. We never had much of a sexual relationship, and we haven't had sex in years. My primary sex partner is the man I call my boyfriend. For several years we have been getting together one or two evenings a week, primarily for sex. Sometimes we go out for dinner or a movie, but that's it. We take care of a certain need for each other this way. When I travel on business I occasionally go to the baths, and the men I briefly play with there are what I call tricks. My husband seems to have less interest in sex than I do, and this arrangement works out fine for both of us.*

None of these patterns is inherently good or bad, healthy or unhealthy. The important thing is that sex be done safely and that each of us be comfortable with his own pattern of sexual behavior.

Identifying Harmful Patterns

When a man sees me for an annual checkup, we usually discuss his recent pattern of sexual activity. Sometimes he is unhappy or uncomfortable with his sexual habits. Often the complaint is not enough sex. But not infrequently it is the pattern of the sex that bothers a man. Here are two contrasting examples:

Glenn: *Last year I told you that I had been nearly celibate lately. That's changed recently. When I turned 50, for some reason I became more interested in sex. Maybe I needed to know that I was still attractive. Anyway, I found out that there are a lot of guys out there looking for a "daddy." I put an ad in the gay paper, and I also cruise a couple of computer bulletin boards. I get together with maybe three or four new guys a week, and I've been having a great time. I've also found a park where I go occasionally for anonymous sex, which can be a big turn-on* for me. *I think I'm being careful enough with what I do that I am not worried about HIV, though I'd like a test just to make sure.*

Dave: *I'm unhappy with my sexual behavior. Every few weeks I've been going to the park and having anonymous sex in the bushes. I don't know why I do it because afterwards I feel dirty, and I hate myself for it. I immediately go and have an HIV test; I've already had three tests this year, and it's only March. I keep promising myself I'll stop this anonymous sex stuff, and then the tension builds, and I find myself back in the bushes again. I want to stop, but I think I need help.*

Glenn has been having a lot more sex than Dave, but Glenn is happy with his sex life, while Dave feels he is doing something he doesn't really want to be doing. Dave could be described as sexually compulsive. Glen, who is more promiscuous, is sexually healthy because he has a pattern of sexual activity that he is happy with and that is harmful to no one. Promiscuity is not a dirty word.

In psychiatric terms, a compulsion is a behavior that a person persists in doing despite negative consequences and/or a desire to stop. Sexual compulsion is also called sex addiction. For some men sex can become an addiction, like alcoholism. Sex addiction has its own unique set of negative consequences, such as legal trouble, financial stresses, anxiety, poor self-esteem, and contraction of sexually transmitted diseases.

It is fashionable to speak of sexual compulsiveness as a disease that needs to be treated. Treatment can be helpful if the behavior is truly compulsive. If the behavior has negative consequences and the individual wants to stop but can't, then a therapist can help him achieve this goal. The warning signs of compulsive behavior are: The behavior is risky, or there are (potential or actual) negative consequences, and the person persists in the behavior despite a desire to stop.

Remember that promiscuity is not the same as sexual compulsiveness. Some gay theoreticians have proposed that monogamy should be the goal for every gay man, and they imply that promiscuity is an unhealthy, destructive, or even addictive behavior. But for many men, monogamy is not a healthy or natural pattern. Many gay men are happiest with a life of lots of sex with a number of partners. This is perfectly healthy. A given pattern of sexual behavior that is wonderful and gratifying for one man may be distasteful and upsetting for another man. What matters is how one feels about one's own sex life.

If your pattern of sexual behavior is bothersome or upsetting to you, help is available. Many counselors, psychologists, and sex therapists are skilled in helping people change behaviors with which they are uncomfortable. This may involve learning new ways to meet and relate to other men. Or it may involve becoming comfortable with one's current sex life. There is nothing inherently wrong with having multiple sex partners or anonymous sex, as long as it feels right and is done safely.

Sexually Transmitted Diseases

Sexual intimacy is a wonderful thing, one of the most pleasurable experiences a man can have. But with those intimate moments comes the opportunity for infections to spread from one person to another. No matter how careful you are, if you have sex with other people, then at some point you may catch a sexually transmitted disease. There is a whole platoon of bacteria, viruses, and parasites that are cunningly adapted to be transmitted during sex. They cause diseases ranging from annoying (crabs) to serious (syphilis, Shigella) to potentially fatal (hepatitis, HIV).

If You Develop an STD

STDs are common, and there is no shame in catching one. They are a part of life. If you develop something you think is an STD, don't panic. Instead get medical attention, and get it taken care of. In addition, you have a responsibility to notify recent sex partners so that they can be tested and, if necessary, treated as well. Sometimes this is embarrassing, but it is the ethical thing to do. There should be no blame involved.

Often guys react with anger, embarrassment, or revulsion when they catch an STD. They are mad at the man that they think they may have caught it from, or they think it is a sign from above, that sex is immoral, and now they are being punished. For example:

Allen: *For a year after my lover died, I was depressed and pretty isolated. When I started feeling a little better, I started feeling more sexual. Last weekend I went to the baths for the first time in a long time. I played with some hot men, and one of them gave me his phone number. But now I think I've caught crabs. I feel so dirty! I tore up that phone number. Isn't there a pill you can give me to take away my sex drive? I think I'd be better off if I never had sex again!*

It's very common for a man to have this kind of reaction when he catches something sexually. But life goes on, and after a while things go back to their proper perspective.

Sex is an important part of a healthy life, and we all should just do our best to be responsible about it. Sexually transmitted organisms have no morals. They are dumb (or pretty crafty, actually) beings that live on or in people's bodies and jump from one person to another during intimate contact.

Usually STDs are transmitted only by direct contact and not from inanimate surfaces such as toilet seats. However, shared sex toys can certainly transmit them.

STDs can be serious. If you catch one, it is important to deal with it as soon as possible because the longer you wait, the harder it may be to treat. In addition, having an untreated STD may put you at higher risk of catching HIV from someone because STDs can compromise your defenses against the entry of HIV into your system.

Usually the symptoms of the STD (genital sores, discharge, or anal pain, for example) are the first clues of a problem. But in more than half of cases, you may have an STD and have no symptoms, and blood work or other medical testing is necessary to make the diagnosis. So if a recent sex partner notifies you that he has been told he has an STD, you should take it seriously and get yourself checked. Try not to be angry at him. Instead, be grateful that he has been responsible and has told you.

Prevention Is the Best Treatment

There are cures for some STDs and treatments for others that can't be cured outright and even vaccines for a few. But the best way to keep from catching one is to try to avoid coming in contact with it.

Abstinence or mutual monogamy works great to prevent STDs, but it is not a reality for very many of us. In my practice, when a male couple professes publicly to be monogamous, frequently one or both partners will tell me about outside dalliances with a disclaimer like, "I'm very careful not to catch anything when I mess around." In such cases, sometimes the person does catch something, which can put quite a strain on the relationship. The moral here is that it's best to be honest with your partner from the start. If you and your partner can agree on guidelines for outside sex, then it is much easier to be levelheaded if one of you brings home an unwanted "pet."

You can reduce your risk of all sorts of STDs, not only HIV, if you practice a reasonable degree of safer sex. If a prospective sex partner wants you to have sex that you consider unsafe, stand your ground. Besides, if he wants to have less-than-safe sex with you, he has probably been doing the same thing with other people and may be catching who knows what in the process. Certainly make sure to use a condom for any anal penetration, and a condom adds safety to oral penetration as well (further discussed in the section titled "Safer Sex").

Remember that condoms are not 100% effective at preventing disease transmission. Even if you are quite careful, you still may catch something you'll need to have taken care of. With a single sexual experience, the chance of catching something is relatively low, especially if you protect yourself. The chances add up with each additional exposure. In addition, the more different sex partners you have, the higher your risk of catching an STD because you are more likely to run into someone who happens to be infected with something. But just one unsafe, unlucky contact can be all it takes to catch a sexually transmitted disease.

Getting Checked Out and Treated

If you go to a health care provider for screening or treatment for sexually transmitted diseases, what should you expect? First, you'll be asked some questions about your symptoms and your recent sexual history. Be prepared to tell the practitioner the gender of your recent sex partner(s), and be prepared for questions about how many partners you have had recently and what sorts of sexual activity you have had. This is relevant because gay men are more susceptible to certain STDs (e.g., hepatitis, HIV) and may have infections in places (anus, throat) where a straight man is less likely to.

It is your right not to answer any questions that make you uncomfortable, but remember that the point of the questions is to help figure out what you have caught, how you might have gotten it, whether you might have given it to others, and whether there might be other STDs lurking in your system. You and the doctor should use vocabulary that you both are comfortable with, whether it is clinical (*penis*) or vernacular (*dick*). The important thing is good communication.

The exam itself will focus on your oral, genital, and anal regions, depending on your symptoms and what kind(s) of exposures you have had. Swabs may be used to obtain samples from some or all of these areas. In addition, you may be asked to give a urine or blood specimen in order to help diagnose what is wrong.

Finally, in many cases you will be given treatment on the spot, even before tests come back. Often the diagnosis is obvious on the first visit, though the lab must later confirm it. It is better to begin treatment right away rather than wait the few days it takes for confirmation.

In many places, the local health department has a public sexually transmitted diseases clinic. This is usually run under the auspices of the city or county government or through the local public hospital; look in the phone book. The people who work at STD clinics tend to be particularly easygoing and nonjudgmental about sexually transmitted diseases. After all, they see people with these infections all day, and they are used to it. Their job is to get you better and to find and treat others who may have caught the same bug. Trust them.

Or, if you have a doctor you trust and are comfortable with, that is a great place to go if you suspect you might have an STD. Just don't wait. If you have a genital or anal discharge or a rash or a sore or warts or unusual genital or anal pain or burning and you've had sex in the past few weeks—*get checked out.*

If you are confirmed to have a sexually transmitted disease, you need to be aware that most STDs are required to be reported to local health departments, whose goal is to stop their spread. It is helpful to try to track down other links in the chain of transmission and identify and treat other people who may not be aware that they are infected. An epidemiologist may contact you and ask you the names of recent partners or ask you to inform them.

This may be unnerving to some gay men who might be (justifiably) afraid of gay witch-hunts. However, unless you are in the military, there is nothing to fear. Health departments do not keep lists of gay people. They are simply in the business of tracking down diseases that are a threat to public health to try to identify infected individuals and make sure they are treated.

In the following sections we'll talk about the common sexually transmitted diseases from a gay man's perspective. We'll discuss their symptoms and how they can be prevented and/or treated. HIV is a sexually transmitted disease, of course, but its unique features earn it its own sections in this book. There are a number of genital and anal conditions that are not transmitted sexually, and we'll discuss those in the sections devoted to the health of those parts of the body.

Bacterial STDs—Gonorrhea and Chlamydia

Bill: *I was in Chicago last week, and I met a man the night before I left. We went back to my hotel room, and I didn't have any condoms—but we just had oral sex. Now I've been home for a couple of days, and I noticed this morning that it really burned when I peed. And now this whitish-greenish stuff, kind of like come, is leaking out of my dick. I know something is really wrong.*

Bill has urethritis, and it's probably gonorrhea.

Urethritis means, literally, "inflammation of the urethra," the tube leading from the bladder, out through the penis—in other words, the tube that urine and semen come out of.

Certain bacteria like to live in the urethra, and they cause infections there. These bacteria include *Neisseria gonorrheae,* the cause of gonorrhea (the clap); *Chlamydia trachomatis;* and a bunch of less common ones such as *ureaplasma.* Chlamydia, incidentally, is the most common bacterial STD in the United States, with over 4 million cases occurring each year. Gay men do not seem to be at any more or less risk of giving each other these infections than anyone else, but they are quite prevalent in sexually active men of whatever orientation.

When your urethra is infected with one of these germs, it tends to hurt. When you pee it burns. Your body tries to get rid of the bugs in there, and it sends white blood cells to the area, forming pus that drips out of the end of your penis or at least stains your underwear. If untreated, the infection can cause scarring and narrowing of the urethra, leading to problems with urination. Gonorrhea can also spread into the bloodstream and cause serious disease with high fevers and swollen, painful joints.

These Bugs Have Other Hiding Places

The urethral bacteria can also live inside a man's throat. There they seldom cause symptoms, so a guy can carry the infection for months and not know it. If he gives someone oral sex without a condom, he can give that person urethritis.

These bacteria can also live in a man's butt. There, inside the anus, an infection often causes pain, cramps, or discharge. Sometimes it can be hard to culture the STD bug and prove that that's what it is because so many bacteria live in there anyway. For other reasons as well, an anal infection it may not be diagnosed as an STD. Some men who have received unprotected anal sex are embarrassed to tell a doctor because they've broken the biggest rule of safe sex. And some doctors are not really savvy about anal sex or don't even know the patient is gay or are shy about asking.

In any case, urethritis bugs are transmitted from the anus or throat to the urethral opening at the end of the penis and vice versa.

Confirming the Diagnosis

By swabbing the inside of the urethra (ouch!) or squeezing some of the discharge onto a swab (easier), the doctor can find out if you have gonorrhea, chlamydia, both, or neither. Some newer tests just use urine, which makes testing even easier.

Gonorrhea tends to make a heavy drip of thick, greenish material. Chlamydia causes a thinner discharge or none at all (just pain when you urinate). The other bugs, classified as "nonspecific urethritis," also cause a thinner discharge or just burning. If gonorrhea or chlamydia are in the throat or anus, they can be detected by doing the appropriate cultures or swab tests.

In many cases, an infected man has no symptoms at all, especially if the infection is in the throat but sometimes also if it is in the urethra or anus. Infection is discovered because the man has a partner who develops symptoms or because the man simply decided to have an STD screening performed.

Getting Treated

If you have evidence of one of these infections or a definite history of exposure, you shouldn't have to wait the few days it takes for the test results to come back. Your doctor should offer you treatment right away. The treatment takes care of all the common bacterial STDs, since the infection is often a combination anyway and the tests are not 100% accurate.

It's possible to treat these infections with just a few antibiotic pills that you take all at once. Cheaper, generic medications also work but must be taken for a week. It used to be that you had to have a shot of an antibiotic to treat urethritis. That's no longer necessary. Pills are now available that work just as well as the old shots.

After treatment the urethral discharge should stop in less than a day. But the pain can last several days because the delicate lining of the urethra has been irritated by the infection and needs to heal. Drinking plenty of plain water will help reduce urethral irritation. Any throat or anal symptoms may also last several days before they go away. Once the symptoms are gone, you can have sex again. Don't be alarmed if it burns the first few times you come. Just remember to use condoms!

Treatment for Bacterial STDs

Note: Any treatment should cover both gonorrhea and chlamydia, since they frequently coexist.

Gonorrhea:
- Ceftriaxone (Rocephin), 250 milligram (injected into muscle)
- Cefixime (Suprax), 400 milligram (1 pill, by mouth)

Chlamydia:
- Azithromycin (Zithromax), 1 gram (powder or tablets, by mouth)
- Doxycyline (generic), one pill twice a day for seven days

Both
- Ofloxacin (Floxin), one tablet twice a day for seven days

Stopping the Chain of Transmission

If you do discover you have a bacterial STD, any of your sex partners over the past two weeks has over a 50% chance of having the same bug somewhere. Therefore it's very important that you notify recent partners so that they can get checked out and treated, even if they don't have any symptoms. It really doesn't matter who gave it to whom; the point is to break the chain of infection. It would be great if there were vaccines for these things, but so far there are not, so all we can do is behave responsibly and treat them as soon as we can.

What about second-hand exposures? In this case it is less clear-cut. For example, this sort of scenario can occur:

Gerard: *Last week I went out with a guy from the office, and we had sex. To be specific, I went down on him. A couple of days later at work he told me that the health department had just called him and told him that he had been exposed the previous week to someone with gonorrhea. I feel fine, but should I be treated just in case?*

Gerard is a "contact of a contact," and I would not recommend he be treated. I would recommend that he come in for STD screening or at the very least just watch for any discharge or discomfort in his throat or in any other orifice that might have been exposed to his date's secretions.

When It's Not an STD

Sometimes the symptoms of urethritis can occur even if there is no infection, as the following example illustrates.

Sam: *I think I have an STD because it really burns when I pee, and I feel like I have to go all the time. I don't have a drip like I did when I had gonorrhea years ago, but it feels the same. The thing is, I haven't had sex with anyone in weeks!*

I swabbed Sam's urethra and sent the specimen to the lab to test for gonorrhea and chlamydia. But I also talked to him about his diet. Turns out he had started taking high doses of vitamin C a few weeks previously, and he also had been working overtime and drinking a lot more coffee than he used to. Both coffee and vitamin

Dietary Irritants of the Urinary Tract
Ascorbic acid (vitamin C)
Alcoholic beverages
Chocolate
Coffee
Fruits and fruit juices
Tea
Tomatoes

C are very acidic and can make your urine so acid that it burns when it comes out.

If Sam had been sexually active, I would have asked him about lubricants. Some lubes have additives such as fragrance or nonoxynol-9 that can get into the urethra and cause burning. Bladder infections, which are not sexually transmitted, can also cause burning with urination, so before Sam left the office I had him leave a urine sample to be sent for culture.

Sam's urethral swab as well as his urine culture proved to show no evidence of infection.

I gave him a handout about urinary irritants (see table) and advised him to cut down on his coffee, switch to a nonacidic form of vitamin C, and drink lots of plain water. He felt better after making the changes in his diet. The point is, not every case of urethritis is really an STD.

Syphilis

Syphilis is much less common now than it used to be, and boy are we lucky. Back in the days before antibiotics, it was incurable; it's probably what made King George, among many others, go mad. Now antibiotics make syphilis easy to treat, and since the advent of safer sex this infection has become much less common among gay men than it was a few decades ago.

Syphilis is caused by a tiny, wormlike bacterium, *Treponema pallidum,* that is introduced into the body through a break in the skin, usually in the genital or anal area. At first it just causes a small open sore (an ulcer or chancre) at the site.

Surprisingly, a chancre is usually painless. In fact, if a genital sore is painful, it's less likely to be syphilis. The chancre often heals by itself, and the person might think his problems are over, but they are really just beginning. By the time the chancre has healed, the syphilis germ has gotten into the blood stream and traveled throughout the body, often including the brain and spinal cord. At first it causes no symptoms, but later, if left untreated, it causes many kinds of symptoms, including rashes and various neurologic problems.

It's easy to detect syphilis by a simple blood test. If you are sexually active, you should have a syphilis test periodically, for example when you get an HIV test. Certainly you should be tested for syphilis if you come down with some other kind of STD. If you get syphilis, you may need some further testing to see how far the germ has spread. This may include a lumbar puncture (spinal tap) to obtain some of the fluid that bathes the brain and spinal cord, to see if the bacterium has infected the central nervous system.

Syphilis is easily treated with penicillin shots or with another antibiotic if you are allergic to penicillin. The treatments for gonorrhea and chlamydia (see the previous section) usually take care of any early syphilis and prevent it from taking hold. This may be one of the reasons why syphilis is fairly rare these days.

Herpes

T he sexual revolution of the 1970s taught us more about herpes than we ever wanted to know. There were even herpes support groups (for all I know, they may still exist). Ah, for the days when herpes was the worst STD we had to worry about!

The main bad thing about herpes is that it is an incurable STD, caused by a virus (the herpes simplex virus). The good thing about herpes is that it is usually more of an annoyance than a serious health problem.

A Typical Herpes Outbreak

Herpes is a rash that starts out as a patch of red skin, usually an inch or less across, which develops a cluster of small blisters on it. These can appear anywhere on the body but usually are on the genitals, anal area, or mouth.

The rash of herpes tends to burn or tingle, though rarely it can itch. The tingling often starts a few days before the blisters actually appear. Over a few days the blisters show up, then break open, and as time goes on they crust and heal.

The whole process—from tingling to blistering to healing—usually takes ten to 14 days in a healthy person. In HIV-infected folks herpes may not heal on its own.

Emotional Reactions to Having Herpes

Many people are extremely bummed out when they first find out that they have herpes. They feel unclean, damaged, ashamed. I tell them, "Welcome to the club! Over 30 million Americans have genital herpes, so if you are among them, then you are in good company." And even though herpes can't be cured, it is not hard to manage so that it has a minimal impact on your life.

The annoying thing about herpes is that it tends to recur in the same place, over and over. This is because the virus is lying dormant in the root of a nerve in the spinal cord, and at times it runs out along that nerve until it ends up at the skin, causing an outbreak. Such recurrences can occur frequently or rarely depending on the individual. In many people they are brought on by stress, either physical or emotional.

Types of Herpes

There are two strains of the herpes simplex virus. HSV-1 is the type that most frequently causes herpes on the lips. These nasty, crusting outbreaks are also known as *cold sores.* The origin of this nickname is debated. Perhaps it comes from the observation that the stress of having a cold can bring them on or perhaps from the fact that being out in the cold, skiing for example, can trigger them. Cold sores are not to be confused with canker sores, which are painful sores inside the mouth but are not known to be caused by any kind of virus.

HSV-2 is the virus that causes genital herpes. The difference isn't really important. As we all know, lips and genitals are often in contact with each other. So either virus can infect either end of our bodies, and the symptoms depend more on where the infection is than which strain of herpes it is.

Incidentally, the herpes virus family includes many other members besides HSV-1 and HSV-2. These relatives include varicella-zoster, the virus that causes chicken pox and shingles; Epstein-Barr virus, which causes mononucleosis; cytomegalovirus, which can cause severe infections in people with AIDS; and human herpes virus 8, which is associated with Kaposi's sarcoma. All of these "herpes cousins" have little to do medically with herpes simplex other than the name and some genetic sequences in common.

Treatment

Even though herpes isn't curable, it is treatable with an oral medication called acyclovir, and various newer drugs that are closely related. Acyclovir, if started at the first tingling of an outbreak, can make the outbreak a lot shorter and less painful. Regular daily dosing of acyclovir can prevent outbreaks. This is a useful strategy for those whose herpes recurs frequently.

People also use the amino acid lysine to prevent or treat herpes. It does seem to work for some people, but it has not been formally tested head-to-head with acyclovir. If your outbreaks are mild, you might try it for treatment or prevention of outbreaks. Efforts to develop a vaccine against herpes have not yet been successful.

With a scabbed, crusted, painful herpes lesion, people are tempted to put some sort of medication right on the area. But there is no kind of salve that helps herpes heal. Even an ointment containing acyclovir does little good. A newer, related medication, pencyclovir (Denavir), has a minor effect on shortening the duration of the outbreak. It's best to just keep herpes blisters clean and dry, and that way they'll heal on their own without getting infected.

The Experience of Herpes

Different people have different experiences with their herpes infection. To many people herpes is a familiar though unwelcome friend that pops up at inopportune times. Here are some examples of how herpes can manifest itself.

Bobby: *My anal herpes usually does not recur, no matter how stressful my life is. Except when I travel. Then it always recurs, and sitting on a plane is no fun when your asshole feels like it's on fire! Now I try to start on acyclovir before I leave on a trip, and I take it during the entire trip and for a week or two after to keep the outbreak from happening.*

Frank: *I only get a herpes outbreak every year or two, but it's so painful that I keep a supply of acyclovir on hand. The burning feeling starts on the left side of the head of my dick before I can see any rash, and that's what tells me it's coming. If I start the acyclovir soon enough, sometimes I don't even get the rash.*

Isaac: *I take acyclovir every day. I used to have ten to 12 herpes outbreaks a year, but now I don't have any, basically, as long as I take the acyclovir. If I stop, I get an outbreak within a few weeks.*

Primary Herpes

The first time a person gets herpes is often much worse than later recurrences. Because the immune system hasn't been exposed to the virus before, it is caught off guard, so a first-time infection (called *primary herpes*) may make a man quite ill. The rash can be very painful, and lymph nodes in the area are often swollen and tender. There may be high fevers, muscle aches, and an overall flulike feeling. If the herpes is oral, it may be difficult to eat because of the pain.

Primary anal herpes can be particularly awful, and doctors often have trouble figuring out what's wrong. The man with primary anal herpes can have so much pain that he can't have a bowel movement, and the infection may also interfere with the nerves that allow him to urinate. Primary anal herpes can make a person so ill that he requires hospitalization, to control the pain and to manage bowel and bladder problems. So if you have terrible anal pain, trouble urinating and defecating, and might have been exposed to herpes anally—let your doctor know. Otherwise the doctor might not suspect herpes, unless he or she is used to taking care of gay men.

Transmission of Herpes

Unfortunately, herpes is not hard to catch. Skin contact with some herpes lesions is all it takes. If you have herpes, the responsible thing is not to have sex while you are having an outbreak. If you must have sex during an outbreak, at least inform your partner of the situation and be very careful that he not come in contact with the infected area. Any skin contact can transmit herpes, so for example, if you touch someone's herpes rash with your finger, you could develop herpes on your finger. If you rubbed your eye with that finger, you could get it in your eye.

Even if everyone were very careful during times of herpes outbreaks, some transmission would still occur. This is because infectious herpes virus is occasionally shed from normal-appearing skin even when an outbreak is not occurring there. The chances of this happening are very small, though, and there is little one can do about it. It's part of life.

Venereal Warts

Venereal warts look like little bumps with a rough or "frilly" surface. They can occur on the genitals (penis and scrotum), around the outside of the anus, inside the anus, on the face or lips, and inside the mouth. If untreated they can sometimes grow to quite a large size.

Will: *I had this itchy feeling in my ass, and it bled a little when I wiped myself. I thought I had hemorrhoids, but my partner looked, and he saw all these little bumps around my asshole. They turned out to be warts.*

The Culprit

Venereal warts are caused by a virus, so they are contagious and are definitely transmitted sexually. The virus is spread by skin-to-skin contact with a wart. Venereal warts are not pretty, and besides, they can become cancerous, so they should be treated. Even after they are gone, the area where they were is still at risk of cancer in the future.

The incubation period—the time between exposure to the virus and the development of its visible signs—can be months to years. I have seen several cases where a person developed warts for the first time after not having sexual contact for years. This is because the wart virus can exist in normal-appearing skin for a long time before it triggers the development of a wart. Obviously this can be upsetting to the individual affected by this problem.

Treatment of Warts

There are several ways to treat venereal warts. They can be frozen with liquid nitrogen in the doctor's office. Or the doctor may paint them with a caustic substance called podophyllin, which is later washed off.

Some wart treatments can be done at home. A prescription version of podophyllin is now available that a person can use on his own. A newer medication called Aldara (imiquimod) comes as a cream that is applied repeatedly to venereal warts. It is reported to stimulate the immune system to attack and destroy warts to which it is applied.

In cases of severe warts, especially inside the anal canal, surgery may be required. Often this involves the use of a laser to vaporize the warts.

It usually takes several treatments before warts are totally gone. The virus is still present in the skin around the visible warts, and after the visible warts are treated, new ones can pop up. But after a while the immune system learns to attack the wart virus and prevents new warts. In fact, this immune effect can be so powerful that some people have been cured of warts by hypnotherapy or meditation.

What to Do in Case of Warts

If you have warts, treat them like any other STD. Notify recent or steady partners so that they can be checked. Be responsible and don't expose others to your warts; wait until they are treated and gone. If you are having sex with someone and notice warts, definitely avoid allowing your skin to come in contact with the warts.

If you have had anal warts—even if they have been treated—you should have an annual anal-rectal exam. This is both to look for recurrent warts and to screen for anal cancer. The same virus that causes anal warts can probably cause anal cancer. It is known that gay men, especially those with HIV, have an increased risk of anal cancers and of precancerous conditions. The use of anal Pap smears as cancer screenings is currently the subject of research studies. See the section on anal health for more details on this topic.

The ABCs of Hepatitis

Paul: *The first sign that something was wrong was that I lost my appetite. And after years of trying to quit smoking, I lost my taste for cigarettes. Just the smell made me nauseated. I had absolutely no energy. I was just dragging myself through the day. Also, my urine was real dark, though I didn't think much about it. The real tip-off was when my boyfriend told me the whites of my eyes were yellow. I don't know why I didn't notice that myself, but anyway, that's what got me to the doctor, and that's when I found out I had hepatitis.*

Introducing the Hepatitis Viruses; The Gay Connection

Hepatitis literally means "inflammation of the liver." Most commonly the term hepatitis refers to viral infection of the liver, though alcohol or drugs can also inflame the liver and cause noninfectious forms of hepatitis.

There are many viruses that can cause hepatitis. The most common forms of viral hepatitis in the United States—and the most important for the gay community—are hepatitis A, B, and C. Each type is caused by a totally different virus, and each is transmitted sexually among gay men. To some degree they are also transmitted socially (by nonsexual contact). Gay men are at increased risk of all three of these forms of hepatitis because we transmit them to each other during our sexual and/or social interactions.

All three of these hepatitis viruses can cause serious illness or even death, so they need to be treated with respect. In fact, hepatitis B is responsible for more deaths annually than any sexually transmitted disease other than HIV. Death can occur during the first phase of hepatitis, known as acute hepatitis. Or it can occur years later due to the long-term effects of the viral inflammation on the liver that can lead to scarring (cirrhosis) and ultimately liver failure, cancer of the liver, or both. Hepatitis C can also lead to liver failure, and it is now the most common condition leading to liver transplantation in the United States.

Many gay men are unaware of their risk for catching hepatitis, and unfortunately many doctors are unaware that their gay male patients should be warned about this problem. There are even vaccines for hepatitis A virus and hepatitis B virus, yet the majority of gay men do not know this and have not been immunized. These are in fact the only STDs for which vaccines exist.

The Symptoms of Hepatitis

Paul's story is typical of what happens when someone gets hepatitis. Fatigue, loss of appetite, and headache are very common when someone has hepatitis. These are all symptoms of a sick liver that is having trouble doing its job of processing proteins from the foods we eat and breaking down toxic substances that we ingest or that our bodies produce as a by-product of our life processes. The symptoms of hepatitis are symptoms of toxicity.

When the liver is sick it can't do its proper job to break down a substance called bilirubin, which is yellow-brown in color. When a person has hepatitis, bilirubin builds up in the skin and eyes, turning them yellow, a condition called jaundice. The bilirubin spills into the urine, turning it brown. Normally bilirubin is gotten rid of in the stool, making it brown, and this does not happen when a person gets hepatitis, so the stool becomes clay-colored or whitish instead.

All three types of hepatitis virus can cause these symptoms. However, hepatitis caused by each type of virus is different in its own way, so each will be discussed separately.

Summary of Viral Hepatitis

Type of hepatitis	A	B	C
Mode of transmission	food, sex, blood	sex, blood	sex, blood
Incubation period	2–8 weeks	4–12 weeks	2 weeks plus
Long-term outcome	complete recovery	recovery or chronic (cirrhosis, cancer)	chronic (cirrhosis, cancer)
Is there a vaccine?	yes	yes	no

Hepatitis A

Hepatitis A is caused by a virus that lives and multiplies in the liver and digestive tract and is excreted in the stool. Transmission of hepatitis A is described as "fecal-oral." Despite the way it sounds, this does not mean you literally have to eat shit or participate in rimming to get hepatitis A. Various forms of sexual or social contact can expose you to this virus. It takes a month, on average, to get sick with hepatitis symptoms once you are exposed to the hepatitis A virus, although it can be as little as two weeks or as long as two months.

Symptoms of hepatitis A are the ones described above for hepatitis in general: fatigue, nausea, headache, loss of appetite, yellowing of the skin and eyes, darkening of the urine, lightening of the stool. Fever, rash, and many other less common symptoms can also be part of hepatitis A. These symptoms may last only a week or two or can last for two months or more. Almost everyone infected with hepatitis A eventually recovers completely, unless they have liver disease already, in which case it can be very serious or even fatal. Once you have had hepatitis A you are immune for life and will never get it again.

Hepatitis A is very common. In the United States, one third of all adults have been infected at one time or another. In gay men, the rate of hepatitis A is even higher than it is in the general population.

Gay men can certainly catch hepatitis A sexually. For example, rimming would be a form of sexual activity that obviously could transmit the hepatitis A virus. But any sexual contact can expose you to traces of the other guy's stool. Licking his balls or sucking on a finger that has been near his anus—you can imagine it wouldn't be difficult. Also, hepatitis A virus has been found in saliva. Although no one has ever proven it can be transmitted by kissing, it makes sense that it could be. Your partner does not have to know he is ill in order to give you hepatitis A because someone who is newly infected can be shedding the virus for several weeks before he starts to feel sick.

Gay men also catch hepatitis A through social interactions that do not involve sex. The virus is spread easily when an infected person goes to the bathroom and does not wash his hands, then handles food. It happens a lot. That's why your mother told you to always wash your hands before leaving the bathroom, and that's why health departments have laws about hygiene for restaurant workers. But people still don't always wash their hands, so the virus gets transmitted. So you could catch it by sharing a beer with a friend, for example. A few years ago in Seattle, a bunch of gay men were exposed to hepatitis A from a Pride Day potluck. The virus is stable for months outside the body, so even leftover food in the fridge could harbor the virus.

Hepatitis A is common in less-developed countries that do not have good sewer systems. The virus gets into drinking water from sewage leaking into the water. You know you're not supposed to drink the water when you travel to third-world countries (see the section on travel advice), but sometimes some water sneaks in anyway, for example when you brush your teeth or eat a salad.

Now, say you hear on the news that a waiter at the restaurant where you ate last week has been found to have hepatitis A, and all patrons are advised to contact their doctors. If you find you have been exposed to hepatitis A but have not gotten sick from it yet, you should definitely see your doctor at once. You might be able to keep from getting sick by getting a shot of gamma globulin. This is a mixture of other people's antibodies that can fight the hepatitis A virus incubating in your system. If given within two weeks after exposure, it is 85% effective in preventing hepatitis A.

The best way to make sure you never get hepatitis A is to get the vaccine. This is a relatively new product. It is made of killed hepatitis A virus particles, so it will not give you an infection. The only side effect is some soreness at the site of the shot. It is safe for people with HIV, and I recommend it especially in that situation because hepatitis A infection is a big stress to the immune system, and it can be a big setback for someone with HIV. Two shots six to 12 months apart will protect you for life. In the United States each shot costs $60 to $75, but they are covered by some health plans. If you have never had hepatitis A, you should definitely get the vaccine if you can afford it.

If you do get sick with hepatitis A, there is no treatment proven to make you better. Your body has to take care of the infection itself. Just rest (you'll be tired enough; you won't have much choice); drink lots of water to stay hydrated and flush the toxins out of your system; avoid substances that are toxic to your liver, such as Tylenol, aspirin, other medications (ask your doctor), and alcohol; and wait to get better. An herbal preparation, milk thistle, may help your liver deal with the infection. Almost everyone makes a complete recovery from hepatitis A in a few weeks to a few months.

Hepatitis B

Hepatitis B multiplies in the liver as well, but it is shed into the bloodstream rather than the digestive tract and is transmitted by exposure to blood or other body fluids. It was first discovered in people who had received blood transfusions, and that led to the term *serum hepatitis.* If you had serum hepatitis years ago, it was probably hepatitis B. But hepatitis B is also easy to transmit sexually, and it is very common among gay men. Depending on your sexual history, as a gay man you have a 50% or greater chance of having been exposed at some time.

The reason hepatitis B is so common in our community is that a few men—perhaps one out of 16 gay men—are lifelong carriers of this virus. That is, they were infected a while ago and never got rid of it. In general they don't feel sick from it, and in fact many of them don't know it, but the virus is in their bloodstream, and they can easily give it to sexual partners. The virus can be found in high concentrations in the body fluids of hepatitis B carriers, and it has been said to be 100 times more infectious than HIV. Because of the patterns of sexual behavior among gay men, hepatitis B travels fast within our community and is much more common among gay men than other people in the United States.

Jamie: *I never knew anything about hepatitis. For sure I know I never was sick with hepatitis. But last month my new boyfriend came down with a bad case of hepatitis B, so I went to the doctor to see what I could do to keep from catching it. She did a blood test and told me that actually I was a carrier and that my boyfriend probably got it from me! I wonder how many people I've given it to over the years. Goodness knows how long I've had this virus.*

Hepatitis B is transmitted the same ways (sex or blood) that HIV is transmitted, but it is much easier to transmit because hepatitis B carriers tend to have much more hepatitis B virus in their bloodstream than HIV carriers have HIV. Basic safer-sex practices, which are pretty good at preventing HIV transmission, also prevent hepatitis B transmission.

Another tricky thing about hepatitis B is that you can be exposed and catch the virus and never know it. A blood test will show antibodies to this virus, indicating that you have been exposed and are now immune. Rarely, the blood test will show that you are a carrier.

So here's what happens if you get exposed to hepatitis B. A few months after exposure, you could get sick with all the symptoms of hepatitis (nausea, headache, loss of appetite, lack of energy, yellow skin and eyes). By the time you get sick, you have been infectious for several weeks and could have transmitted the virus to other sex partners. Or you might not get that sick from hepatitis B. You might just feel like you have a mild flu. Or you might not get sick at all. In any case, either your body will clear the infection and you'll be immune in the future, or you will become a carrier (which, fortunately, happens only rarely). As with hepatitis A, there is no specific treatment for acute hepatitis B. Just rest, drink fluids, avoid liver-toxic drugs (such as alcohol and Tylenol), and trust that you will get better.

Hepatitis B can be very serious. In fact, some people die from acute hepatitis B (the illness you get when first exposed). Carriers have what is called *chronic hepatitis B* because they never get rid of the infection. Years of infection leads to more and more scarring of the liver. Although the liver is a very resilient organ and has a great capacity to regenerate, eventually the amount of scarring is more than it can handle, and it will fail. In addition, cancer of the liver can develop after years of chronic infection.

If you have chronic hepatitis B, your doctor can do some tests to see how active the virus is in your system. It is possible to treat chronic hepatitis B, and some people have gotten rid of the virus with treatment. So far the only proven way to treat chronic hepatitis B is with a four- to six-month series of injections with a drug called alpha interferon. This treatment is effective in only 50% of cases or fewer. Other medications, taken orally, are very promising. These include lamivudine (also known as 3TC and used for treatment of HIV) and famciclovir (also used for treatment of herpes virus infections). These and several other antivirals are in the testing stages.

Hepatitis B is not a lot of fun, and it is much better to prevent it than to deal with it once you have it. Fortunately there is a vaccine for this virus. Unfortunately, only a small minority of gay men are aware of the vaccine. And many doctors do not know that their patient is gay or that this vaccine is useful for gay men. So it is up to you to be proactive. If you have never been tested, get tested for hepatitis B. Even if you've had only a handful of sex partners in your lifetime, there is a reasonable chance you have already been exposed and are immune or—hopefully not—a carrier.

If you find you have never been exposed to hepatitis B, get the vaccine. It is a series of three shots given over a six-month period and is very safe. It works for over 90% of people and will make you immune to hepatitis B for life. The total series costs between $125 to $150 in the United States. Many insurance plans cover it.

Incidentally, gay men can take a lot of the credit for the development of the hepatitis B vaccine. Originally, the vaccine was made from the blood of people who were carriers of hepatitis B and had lots of virus in their bloodstream. Their blood was collected, and the virus was purified and killed to make the vaccine. Most of these volunteer blood donors for the hepatitis B vaccine were gay men. The experimental vaccine was then tested in other, uninfected gay men. These studies proved that the vaccine worked, and it was approved by the FDA.

When the hepatitis B vaccine was first marketed, the favor was not returned to the gay community. The vaccine was not promoted to gay men. It should have been offered at a discount in return for our help in developing it. The medical community was not advised that gay men were at risk for hepatitis B and should be immunized. It took years before this situation was remedied. Even now, only a tiny percentage of gay men in their 20s have had the vaccine or are even aware that it would be useful for them. Eventually things will be better because now all young children in the United States are supposed to receive this vaccine.

Hepatitis C

Hepatitis C is one of the newer forms of viral hepatitis to be discovered. Like hepatitis B, it is transmitted by exchange of blood or by sexual contact. Starting in 1990, blood for transfusion has been screened for hepatitis C, but prior to that, many cases of this infection were transmitted by transfusion.

Between 1 and 2% of the U.S. population is infected with the hepatitis C virus. Once infected, the majority of individuals never get rid of this virus. Hepatitis C is the most common cause of chronic viral hepatitis in the United States, and like hepatitis B, it may lead to cirrhosis and to cancer of the liver after many years of infection.

It used to be thought that hepatitis C was found mostly in injection drug users and in people who had had transfusions. But now that there are better blood tests for hepatitis C, it is being found in many gay men. The medical literature says little about how common hepatitis C is among gay men. In my practice, I find hepatitis C fairly commonly in gay men—especially those whose blood tests indicate a problem with the liver.

Basically, hepatitis C virus is transmitted the same ways as HIV and as the hepatitis B virus. Safer sex should be reasonable protection against hepatitis C. Sexual transmission of hepatitis C is more difficult than for hepatitis B or HIV, but it definitely does occur.

Most people do not become ill when they contract hepatitis C, or they might just feel like they have a mild flu. They might have some achiness, some nausea, or other vague symptoms but no jaundice. However, in most cases this is the beginning of a long-term infection that may lead to serious problems years later. Usually the person is not aware they are ill until blood tests reveal abnormal liver functions.

There are tests your doctor can do to tell if you have hepatitis C and how active the virus is in your system. I recommend a test for hepatitis C only if a screening blood test shows a liver problem. If there is no evidence of any problem with your liver, then no treatment would be recommended for hepatitis C even if you had it, so why bother finding out.

If the hepatitis C virus is in your system and is causing damage, there is a treatment (interferon) that can cure your body of the virus, but it is not very effective. It works in approximately one out of every five people who try it. Better treatments are being researched. For now, the best way to deal with hepatitis C is to try to be sexually safe and not catch it in the first place. Unfortunately, there is no vaccine for hepatitis C on the horizon.

Intestinal STDs

We all get diarrhea or gas at times, usually caused by a virus or by eating some food that disagrees with us. But if you have diarrhea that lasts more than a few days, it is very important to get checked to make sure it is not a sign of an infection that should be treated. This is especially true if you have been sexually active.

Gay men frequently catch intestinal infections from each other during sex. Rimming (oral-anal contact) is the easiest way a man can catch another man's intestinal bugs. But any intimate contact poses that risk. We're always touching ourselves, and we don't wash our hands often enough, leading to stool contamination on our skin. So you can catch intestinal bugs from another guy even without rimming.

Many intestinal infections are therefore much more common among gay men than other people because we give them to each other sexually. These infections can be caused by bacteria or by protozoa, which are microscopic life-forms that are a little larger and more complex than bacteria.

Protozoal Intestinal Infections

Roger: *Something is wrong. I feel bloated all the time, and I'm farting a lot, and it smells really bad. Usually I'm not like this. I feel like I can't go out in public!*

Roger has Giardia, an intestinal infection caused by a protozoan. Giardia usually causes bloating, cramps, and gas. Another protozoan, amoeba, causes cramps as well, but more in the way of diarrhea than gas. There are other protozoa, such as Blastocystis, which may cause similar symptoms.

Protozoal-type parasites are very common among gay men. For a while they went by the semiobnoxious name *gay bowel syndrome,* but there is nothing gay about these bugs, and thankfully the term is no longer used. All protozoa can be treated with the right antibiotics.

Bacterial Intestinal Infections

Jason: *This is the worst diarrhea I have ever had. I have terrible cramps, and it comes out just like brown water. Sometimes there is blood or mucus in it too. I am having high fevers each night, and my appetite is shot.*

Jason turned out to have shigellosis, an intestinal infection caused by the bacterium shigella. Other bacterial causes of sexually transmitted colitis include salmonella, campylobacter, and E. coli.

These bacterial infections of the intestines tend to cause severe diarrhea with painful cramps and sometimes fever. There may be other dramatic symptoms, such as blood, mucus, or pus in the diarrhea. A person with one of these infections can easily get dehydrated and end up in the hospital for a few days. Fortunately these infections are easy to treat with antibiotics, such as Cipro (ciprofloxacin) or various older generic erythromycins or tetracyclines, depending on the offending bug.

Getting Checked Out and Treated

Proper diagnosis of these intestinal infections requires that a stool sample be submitted to the lab for microscopic examination and for culture. In a day or two the result should be back, and you're on your way to being treated and getting over the problem.

As with other STDs, it is your responsibility to notify any recent partners so that they can get checked and treated as well. The incubation period for bacterial intestinal infections is in the range of a few days, while for protozoal infections it can be up to a few weeks, or occasionally longer.

Scabies and Lice

I nsects or mites can live on people's skin and can be transmitted by contact just like other infections. There are two main kinds of sexually transmitted infestations: scabies and lice. You might think of these bugs as causing more of an infestation than a true infection, but that doesn't make them any less annoying.

People who get these critters on their skin just itch and itch and itch. If it's any comfort, scabies and lice are ancient companions of our species and live only on humans. They are elegantly adapted to feed off our skin and blood, and they take advantage of our tendency to touch one another, jumping from one unwitting host to the next.

Scabies (the word is both singular and plural) is caused by a tiny mite, *Sarcoptes scabiei,* that is barely visible to the naked eye and spends its life burrowing under the skin. Lice, or crabs, are a family of larger insects that live on the skin surface and lay eggs at the base of hair shafts. These nasties are transmitted by intimate contact (sexual or not) or social contact (shaking hands) or even indirect contact (via bedding, clothes, or the bench or towel in the locker room). Remember, they only live on people, so you can't blame your dog, cat, or ferret if you come down with them.

Scabies

Scabies is highly contagious but, fortunately, readily curable. It produces about the itchiest rash you can get. Most commonly the rash is in between the fingers, on the hands or wrists, around the waist, or on the buttocks and the head of the penis; but actually it can be anywhere. The rash starts with tiny water blisters that are infuriatingly itchy, so they are scratched raw almost immediately, and many people never notice the original blisters. People with scabies complain about nighttime itching the most. It keeps them awake. They come to the doctor with tiny scabs wherever the rash has been.

HIV-infected people can develop severe cases of scabies that make large, crusty sores and don't look like regular scabies. This is called "crusted" or "Norwegian" scabies, and it can be mistaken for other skin disorders, such as psoriasis. If you are HIV-positive and get a very itchy rash, it's important that you get checked for scabies.

Here's how you get a rash from scabies: The average person infested with scabies has ten to 12 mites living in their skin in various places. Each mite burrows under the skin, traveling up to one fourth of an inch daily for up to two months. It lays its eggs under the skin as it goes. The eggs are very irritating and allergenic, so they cause the itchy blisters. When the eggs hatch, new mites crawl out to lay more eggs.

You can catch scabies from contact with an infested person or from their clothing or bedding. The mites can survive on their own for several days, so wash those sheets and towels in hot water as soon as your guests leave.

Once you have scabies, it takes a while for the allergic reaction to develop and cause itching, so the incubation period (time from exposure to when you notice symptoms) can be one to two months. Many times I have seen someone with scabies who swears it can't be because, Where could they have gotten it? Who knows, but there it is, and it must be dealt with.

Unfortunately, many doctors don't suspect scabies at first. Frequently the person gets treated for all sorts of other things and is given medicine for itching but not for scabies. Sometimes they end up going to a dermatologist before the true cause of the rash is discovered. It is possible to prove a person has scabies by finding an unopened blister, scraping it open, and looking at the material under the microscope. With luck a live mite or some eggs will be found.

But it's hard to find the mites, and so even if they aren't found, it's worth treatment if the rash even seems remotely like scabies. Treatment involves putting on a lotion or cream, containing an insecticide, such as lindane (Kwell), crotamiton (Eurax), or permethrin (Elimite). You put this stuff all over your body, from head to toe, including under the fingernails where you might have scratched up some eggs. Do it in the evening, leave it on overnight, then shower it off.

At the same time, change your bedding, wash your sheets in hot water, and wash any dirty clothes before you wear them again. Nonwashable items should be dry cleaned or stored in plastic bags for two weeks, until the mites die.

After treatment for scabies, the itching may take a few days to wear off. You can use calamine lotion, Benadryl lotion, or Benadryl capsules (all available without a prescription) to help with the itching. If itching is severe enough and these measures don't help, your doctor may prescribe a strong cortisone-type cream to help calm things down. Those eggs are still under the skin and may still be causing irritation, but with luck they are dead.

As long as you don't get any new rash in the weeks after treatment, you're probably cured. If you start getting new bumps, however, the scabies are back. Some cases of scabies do not completely respond to one or the other of the treatments, so if one treatment does not seem to have worked, you might try the other product. The oral drug ivermectin appears to be very effective against scabies, and only one dose is needed, so it may become the treatment of choice for this problem.

If you've been intimate with anyone in the few weeks before coming down with scabies, it's worth letting them know. But lots of the time it's hard to figure out where the scabies came from. Don't worry about it—just treat the nasty critters!

Lice

Lice are bigger than scabies mites. They are wingless insects that require humans for survival; they live only on our species. They are such a part of human culture that their names have become part of our daily vocabulary. We call someone we don't like a "louse." And remember the funny-looking kid in third grade that got teased about having cooties? That's another word for lice.

While scabies mites are almost microscopic, you can easily see lice and their eggs with the naked eye. There are two main kinds of lice: pubic lice (crabs, *Phthiris pubis*) and head or body lice (*Phthiris humanus*) .

The pubic kind can infest a hairy man's body hair or beard and head lice can as well. Lice look like tiny brown dots or freckles on the skin, but they can be picked off, and if you put the brown dot on a piece of white tissue, you can see its little legs waving around. It looks like a teeny crab, hence the nickname.

Unlike scabies mites, lice prefer hairy areas, and they lay their eggs at the bases of the hair shafts. The eggs, or nits, look like tiny white pearls attached to the hair shaft, and can be picked off (hence the term *nit-picking*).

Lice are very contagious. If you have sex with someone who is infested, you have about a 95% chance of catching them. They are also spread by nonsexual body contact or by sharing clothes or bedding. Head or body lice can survive for a week without food (human blood), though crab lice survive only two days.

Like scabies, lice cause severe itching. Each louse attaches itself to the skin and bites into a tiny capillary. It feeds on the blood it sucks from the capillary. As it feeds, the louse injects its digestive juices and waste products into the skin, which is very irritating, so you can see why that would itch.

Lice also lay up to ten eggs a day. The eggs hatch in seven to ten days, and the baby lice start to feed and cause itching, so the incubation period may only be a week or two. However, especially with a small infestation, it may take a while to figure out what is causing that itching So, as with scabies, the incubation period can be a couple of months or more.

Lice are treated with medicated creams or shampoos. Lindane shampoo requires a prescription in the United States but not in Canada. It is lathered over all hairy areas of the body for five minutes, then shampooed off. Products containing permethrin (Nix) or pyrethrins with piperonyl butoxide (Rid) are also available without a prescription, but it appears that some cases of lice are becoming resistant to them. The oral drug ivermectin may be effective, but it has not been carefully studied for this purpose yet.

After treating for crabs, body lice, or head lice, you should comb the eggs out of the hair in the area with a proverbial fine-toothed comb that is sold with the medication. Some people prefer to shave the hair off, especially in the pubic area—though shaving there can cause its own brand of itching. It sure gets rid of the eggs, though. The itching can persist for several days after treatment, and sometimes a second treatment is needed after a week or so, to kill off additional critters that have hatched.

If you later find nits (eggs) on the hairs, it may mean you are still infected. But if all the nits are at least one-half inch from the base of the hair, they are probably just dead shells because the louse deposits the egg right at the base of the hair.

Some Final Advice

Getting scabies, crabs, or head or body lice is part of being a sexually active adult. It's no big deal, healthwise, and is usually more of an annoyance than anything else. The important thing is to recognize the problem and immediately deal with it. If we all did that, the problem would be eliminated because these critters live nowhere but on human beings. But that's wishful thinking. These ancient companions of ours will probably always be with us, jumping from one unsuspecting person to another. So when it's your turn, break the chain and get rid of them before you pass them on to someone else.

HIV Basics

The human immunodeficiency virus, which causes acquired immune deficiency syndrome, has become a part of every gay man's life. This is true even for those of us not personally infected with the virus. All of us are living with HIV and AIDS in one way or another.

Many of us do have this virus in our bodies and deal with its presence every day. Those of us who are not infected with HIV still live with the knowledge that the virus infects many of our acquaintances, friends, and lovers.

Society at large continues to view AIDS as a "gay disease" in this country. People blame us for the AIDS epidemic. Those religious or political leaders who do not want us to have civil rights as gay people or who feel that our sexual behavior is wrong cite AIDS as an example of the results of our "unhealthy" behavior. Of course that is untrue. HIV is just a virus that happened to find fertile soil in our community, just as it has found fertile soil in heterosexual societies in large parts of Africa and Asia, where the vast majority of HIV infections in the world occur.

The Impact of AIDS: Sex, Death, Burnout

HIV has irrevocably changed the ways that we, as gay men, relate sexually to each other. Sex is now associated in many men's minds with the fear of catching a potentially fatal disease. Many of us have adapted our sexual habits in order to prevent transmission of HIV. Unless an effective vaccine is developed, we will always have to be careful during sex not to give or get HIV. The days of unprotected, unrestricted sex are over for the foreseeable future. Many gay men are justifiably resentful of that, yet there is little choice, considering what is at stake.

Alexander: *I always use condoms, and I get them free, courtesy of the Northwest AIDS Foundation. They distribute them in little safe-sex kits—a cardboard envelope, like a big matchbook, with a condom and a little container of lube inside. The outside of the kit has four photos of men's butts, and in large letters it says NORTHWEST AIDS FOUNDATION. The other night, in the middle of fucking, I looked over at the empty envelope on the nightstand and there was that word, AIDS, staring right at me. It kind of put a damper on things.*

So AIDS intrudes into our sex lives, and when we are having sex we may be reminded of the risk of illness and death.

There have been far too many deaths. We have lost hundreds of thousands of precious lives in this battle. The premature death of any gay man—whether a political leader, a homeless person, an entertainment figure, an auto mechanic, an athlete—is a tragic loss to our community and to all of society.

We have a right to be angry at these losses. We should be angry that we have had to put so much time, energy, and money into fighting this virus. We could have been doing so many other worthwhile things. It's no wonder that AIDS is creating fatigue and burnout in our community. After nearly 20 years of living with the epidemic, many of us are tired. We need a break, but the reality is that HIV and AIDS will always be with us in some form.

Yet life does go on. While acknowledging the presence of the epidemic we must all continue to live our lives one day at a time. None of us—HIV-positive or negative—can spend all of our time dealing with this virus. We cannot let it rule our lives.

We Can Be Proud

Some good has come from the epidemic. To our credit, gay men have been in the forefront of the battle against AIDS, and have been leaders in providing support for those who are infected with HIV. During the 1980s, when the U.S. Government had an unstated policy of ignoring the AIDS epidemic, gay men and our friends were founding AIDS service organizations, providing services to people with AIDS, raising money for AIDS research, inventing the concept of safer sex, and educating each other. Many prominent HIV doctors and researchers have been gay men.

Threats to our community over the years have usually made us stronger. From the police brutality that led to the Stonewall riots to the antigay political campaigns pioneered by Anita

Bryant to the current AIDS epidemic—the presence of a common enemy has united us. In the years since Stonewall, the gay community has continued to become more and more cohesive and more insistent on our right to be treated with equal respect. The HIV epidemic is just one more enemy that we have had to deal with, and despite its agonies it has strengthened and helped unite us.

The Epidemic Is Changing

Fortunately, we are overcoming the epidemic through prevention and treatment. The number of deaths from AIDS has started to decline dramatically in the United States. New treatments are helping people with HIV stay healthy.

Although the annual number of new HIV infections in the United States is fairly stable, it appears that fewer of them may be among gay men. Still, recent rising rates of gonorrhea among gay men are a worrisome hint that some of us are taking more risks sexually. We must not become complacent and allow a "second wave," an increase in new HIV infections, to occur in our communities.

Even with a steady rate of new HIV infections, the number of people actually living with HIV is increasing because the death rate has gone down so much. For example, in the Seattle metropolitan area, where I live and practice, it is estimated that approximately 500 people annually become infected with HIV. This has not changed throughout the 1990s. Before AIDS could be treated very well, through the early '90s, our region also had approximately 500 AIDS deaths annually. So the actual number of people with AIDS stayed fairly constant from year to year. Five hundred new infections, 500 deaths.

But now with the new treatments keeping people with HIV healthy and alive, the AIDS death rate in the Seattle region has dropped to 150 or fewer per year. Five hundred new infections and 150 deaths annually. This means that the number of people living with HIV is actually increasing steadily. It's great that fewer people are dying. It's not so great that more and more are becoming HIV-positive when we know how to prevent it.

Why All Gay Men Should Read This Section

It is the responsibility of every gay man, HIV-positive or not, to know the basics about HIV and AIDS. The epidemic effects us all.

The following sections present an overview of HIV and AIDS. There are many books on HIV/AIDS that cover the subject in great detail. In this book, which covers all aspects of gay men's health, I present only the most essential information on HIV and AIDS. You might call it "HIV 101: The beginner's course."

In the following sections I will present a variety of information about HIV infection. I will describe the virus and what HIV infection does to a person's immune system. I'll go over the basic tests we use to tell if someone is infected with this virus and how we measure the progress of HIV infection. I'll discuss some of the manifestations of HIV infection, ranging from the symptoms caused by first becoming infected with the virus, to the illnesses that can occur much later, when someone's immune system has been damaged by the infection. I'll give some advice to help you decide when it's a good idea to consult your doctor and when it's OK to ride things out for a bit. We'll talk about the best ways to stay healthy in spite of having this virus—both by having a healthy lifestyle and by choosing the best medical treatment to fight the virus.

The easiest way an individual gay man can start to combat HIV is to keep the virus out of his body. Treating an established case of HIV infection is a lot of work and has a huge impact on the life of the infected person. Most people who are being treated for HIV would say that it would have been a heck of a lot easier not to get infected in the first place. Once infected with HIV, there is no going back. Not getting infected means being careful about how one has sex because sex is how we give HIV to each other.

Safer sex is not a straightforward issue. It means different things to different people. What is important for each gay man is to consider the risks of various types of sexual activity, find a comfort level, and stick to it. A whole portion of this book in the section titled "Sexuality" is devoted to safer sex. Read it, study it, decide what feels right for you—then go out and live it.

Our understanding of HIV/AIDS and its treatment is changing rapidly. Every day seems to bring another new advance. The material here is up-to-date as of the time it was written, but parts will certainly be out-of-date by the time it is published. So read it with that in mind, and remember that it's just a starting point to help you begin to understand this tiny virus that has had such a big impact.

What Is HIV and How Does It Cause AIDS?

HIV is a virus that infects certain types of white blood cells that comprise an important part of the immune system. HIV also infects other types of cells in the body. The virus consists of a piece of genetic material, RNA, surrounded by a coat of protein. When the virus infects a cell, it releases its RNA into the cell. The genetic instructions encoded in the RNA are then used to turn the cell into a little HIV factory, making hundreds of new virus particles. Eventually the cell dies in the process.

This is a gross oversimplification, of course. The whole explanation of how HIV damages the immune system is very complicated. The details are poorly understood and are the subject of much research. But this model is a good way to visualize how HIV does its dirty work.

The main type of immune system cell that is damaged by HIV infection is called the *CD4* or *T4* cell, often nicknamed "T cell." Healthy people without HIV generally have between 600 and 1,200 CD4 cells per milliliter of blood. Healthy people with HIV, on average, have a somewhat lower count. This number may remain stable for years after HIV infection begins. But eventually, over time, the CD4 count of an HIV-infected person begins to drop.

When a person's CD4 count drops below a certain point, he becomes susceptible to unusual infections, called opportunistic infections, which normally would be prevented by healthy CD4 defenses. Anyone with a CD4 count under 500 is susceptible to at least a few of these, and if the CD4 count is below 200, many different, serious infections are possible. So the CD4 count is a good way to measure the health of an HIV-infected person's immune system. The higher the number of CD4 cells, the more robust the immune system is. A CD4 count under 200 indicates a severe immune deficiency. This is why a low CD4 count has become one of the definitions of AIDS.

A Lifelong Infection That Can Be Transmitted

HIV is unique among viruses in that it actually attacks the cells of the immune system. In doing so, it interferes with the person's ability to get rid of the HIV infection. In addition, HIV is able to permanently infect some cells without killing them. So once a person is infected with HIV, he is likely to remain infected for the rest of his life.

This is part of why HIV is so sneaky. Many people who have it feel perfectly healthy. Yet they have a lifelong viral infection that can be transmitted to others by intimate contact. HIV is found in various body fluids, the most important for gay men being blood, semen, and pre-ejaculatory fluid, or precome. Transmission of HIV can occur when one person has internal exposure to one of these fluids from another person. This principle is the basis for safer sex. HIV can rarely be found in other fluids—such as tears, sweat, or saliva—but there is very little evidence that any of these fluids has ever transmitted the virus.

In Untreated Folks HIV Infection is Usually Active, Not Dormant

Since many HIV-positive people remain healthy for many years, with reasonably good immune function, it used to be thought that the virus was lying dormant in those people. Now we know better because we are able to measure the amount of HIV in an infected person's bloodstream. We have found that all HIV-positive people—even those who seem completely healthy—harbor thousands of HIV virus particles in every drop of their blood.

It is now known that in an HIV-infected person billions of new virus particles are made every day, and about as many are destroyed. The stress of dealing with this huge amount of viral infection is undoubtedly part of the reason that the immune system eventually weakens. Ongoing, untreated HIV infection can cause general symptoms of illness such as fatigue, night sweats, and weight loss suffered by many HIV-infected people.

The test that measures the amount of HIV in the blood is called a *viral load test,* or a *quantitative HIV RNA test.* This test is now used to see how well a person is combating his HIV infection. The lower the number, the better off the person is. People with viral loads over 100,000 have a very high risk of becoming ill with AIDS in the near future. The lower the viral load, the lower the risk of becoming ill, but everyone with a viral load over 5,000 has at least some risk of this happening in the future.

Medications that prevent HIV from multiplying can lower the viral load. There are many such medications available now, and some of them are quite effective. When used in combinations of two, three, or more, they are sometimes able to reduce the viral load below 20 or 50 copies per milliliter of blood. In that case the viral load test is no longer able to detect HIV, and we say that the viral load is "undetectable." In these people, HIV replication may be completely suppressed by the medication. But dormant HIV remains in some cells, ready to take off and multiply again if given a chance.

People tend to have their highest viral load early on in HIV infection and again in the latter stages of AIDS. They seem to be more infectious to others at these times. A person with a very low viral load is probably less infectious. However, even if an HIV-positive man's viral load has become undetectable with treatment, he is not cured of HIV. If he misses even a few doses of medication, the viral load will often begin to rise. Even while he faithfully takes every dose, he still may have small amounts of infectious HIV in his blood and in his semen that potentially can be transmitted to others. So safer-sex precautions should always be maintained—even by men who have achieved an undetectable viral load with treatment.

Getting Tested for HIV

E arly in the AIDS epidemic, HIV testing was controversial. If there wasn't anything that could be done about HIV infection, why take the test? Why find out about an untreatable infection that seemed to lead inevitably to illness and death? Why bring on the stress, worry, and helplessness of that knowledge?

But now there are good treatments for HIV. To stay healthy, every sexually active gay man should be tested regularly. There is so much that can be done to combat the virus, to prevent it from damaging the immune system, and to ward off secondary infections. But these treatments are only available to those who know they are HIV-positive. All too often men find out they are HIV-positive only when they become ill with an opportunistic infection, and by then their immune system has been severely damaged.

A man who tests positive may also choose to tighten up his safer-sex standards to more carefully avoid infecting others. Many people set new priorities and make changes in their life once they find out they are HIV-infected. A positive test can serve as a wake-up call, a reminder that life is short. None of those things can happen unless the person discovers he is infected with the virus.

Many gay men have never been tested. Some just don't feel they're at risk; maybe they've had only a few partners, or maybe they think none of their partners could possibly have been HIV-positive, or maybe they're sure they've been having the safest of safe sex. But nothing is 100%, so why not just find out and be certain?

Other men have not been tested because they are afraid they will not be able to deal with a positive test result, whether or not this is likely for them. They may be afraid that a positive result will take away their hope or that it will be a self-fulfilling prophecy and that they'll immediately get sick with AIDS complications. For example:

Lou: *I haven't had unsafe sex in over ten years. I've never been tested, but I've done fine, and I figure the longer I go without getting sick, the better the chances are that I'm negative. Somehow it feels like if I don't get tested, then I'll be OK.*

This is flawed reasoning, sometimes called "magical thinking"—the idea that taking the test will make a person have HIV. The fact is, either the virus is present or it's not, period. The test just finds out the information. A man like Lou might be sitting on a time bomb, as Roberto discovered:

Roberto: *I always assumed I was HIV-positive, but I figured if I took care of myself it would never be a problem. I never got tested, never even had a doctor. I felt fine. About six months ago I started losing weight and having fevers and coughing. I ignored it all. I told myself I just had the flu.*

Then one day I woke up and the vision in my left eye was gone. My neighbor dragged me to the hospital. It turned out that my immune system had been trashed by HIV, and I had three major infections— pneumonia, retinitis, and esophagitis—all at the same time. I was in the hospital for three weeks and then in a nursing home, being fed intravenously, for another two months, before I was strong enough to go home. I'm back at work now, and my immune system is doing a little better, thanks to a three-drug antiviral cocktail that has reduced the virus in my blood to undetectable levels. I am taking 24 pills a day, but it's worth it to have my life back. The doctor says that I will never recover the vision in that one eye. It was a tough way to find out I had HIV. I shouldn't have waited so long. I'm just grateful I didn't die.

What Exactly Is an HIV Test?

How does one test for HIV infection? The standard test analyzes blood to look for an antibody against the virus. Antibodies are proteins made by our immune system in response to infection. When a person is infected with HIV, their body makes specific antibodies that grab onto the virus so that it can be attacked by the immune system. These antibodies can be detected by a blood test.

When a sample of blood is submitted to a lab for HIV testing, the lab first runs a simple test called ELISA, which looks for one common antibody against HIV. This test is inexpensive and shows positive for just about everyone who has HIV. But the ELISA test also picks up a few false positives, especially in people with liver disease, for example. So if the ELISA is positive, the lab then runs a test, called the *Western Blot,* that detects a whole array of different antibodies against various parts of the virus. If the Western blot is positive, HIV infection is confirmed.

Sometimes, especially early in HIV infection, the results are inconsistent. For example, the ELISA may be positive, and the Western blot may be negative or only partly positive ("indeterminate"). If a person is at risk of being positive, the test should be repeated after a wait of a month or two. Alternatively, a test called the HIV RNA PCR can be run. This test measures the actual virus rather than the antibodies against it. Early in HIV infection, before the person has made antibodies to HIV, it is possible to detect the virus using this test, even when the standard ELISA test is not yet positive.

HIV infection can now be diagnosed without obtaining a blood sample. Other body substances can be used. A procedure using oral secretions, OraSure™, is now available and appears to be just as accurate. It does cost a little more than the blood-based test. Urine testing for HIV is also under development.

Traditionally, HIV testing has only been available in a medical setting: at doctors' offices or public health clinics. Because of the sensitive nature of this test, the person being tested is counseled, and their consent is obtained, before the test is done. It is illegal in most states for a person to be tested for HIV without his consent.

Sometimes HIV test results are given by phone. But often the individual is asked to return to the office to obtain the result in person, especially if it seems there is a good chance the result will be positive or if the person feels he may have some difficulty dealing with the test results.

The FDA has recently approved kits for home testing for HIV. These have the advantage that no medical appointment is needed. Some people are reluctant to go to a doctor for an HIV test and would only test in the privacy of their home. The disadvantage is that the person may not receive the proper counseling about HIV infection and prevention, and if he tests HIV-positive, he may be less likely to get the proper follow-up.

Making the Decision to Test

When should a person be tested for HIV, and how often? There is no firm rule. Every man who has ever had sex with another man should probably be tested at least once. If he is sexually active, he should be tested every six to 12 months, unless he is in a relationship that is truly mutually monogamous with an HIV-negative partner. How frequently a man should test depends on the frequency and type of sexual activity he engages in, number of sexual partners he has had, and other factors. Each person can use his judgment about when next to test. For example:

Morgan: *I'm HIV-negative, and my partner is HIV-positive, and we have a very active sex life. We are very safe; we even use rubbers for oral sex. But I find my anxiety level starts to build up if I haven't been tested in a while, so I get tested every six months. It reassures me that we are doing things right. It also takes stress off my lover because he keeps worrying that some day he is going to infect me.*

Jim: *Being single at age 64, I still date occasionally, but sometimes I go a year or more without having sex with anyone besides my faithful right hand. When I see the doctor for my annual checkup, I get an HIV test if I have had sex since my last test. Otherwise I don't bother.*

J.R.: *My main sex outlet is at the baths and the park, and I usually have sex with several different guys each time I go. I don't like to use condoms, but I never let anyone get near my butt—I just don't like anal sex. So I think I'm being safe that way. Occasionally I pick up a drip or a rash or whatever, and I get it taken care of at the free public STD clinic. They test me for HIV every time, which is every few months or so, whether I need it or not.*

Dealing With HIV Test Results

Men tend to react to a negative HIV test with a great sense of relief. For example, if a sexually active gay man hasn't been tested in a while, he may start to worry whether he has picked up HIV. Once his blood has been sent off to the lab, his anxiety may actually increase because soon he'll find out the "verdict." If he finds he has tested negative, this news should be met with a renewed pledge to adhere to whichever safer sex guidelines he has chosen.

If the man has been having risky or outright unsafe sex and then tests negative, the negative test does not mean he is immune to HIV; it just means he's been lucky. Sooner or later the virus will catch up with him, unless he starts protecting himself. This man should promise himself to develop safer sexual habits.

Sometimes a negative test can be difficult to deal with, surprising as that may seem. For example, two men who have recently started dating may go for testing at the same time, possibly even before they start to be sexual with each other. If one tests negative and the other positive, it may put a great deal of stress on the new relationship. The positive one may resent the negative one or become fearful of infecting him, and there may be some sexual difficulties. The negative one may feel guilty or embarrassed that he is not infected. Frequently a budding relationship will end when the partners discover that they are of different HIV status.

Of course, dealing with a positive test is usually hard. Some men who test positive have always assumed they were infected, and the test result comes as no big surprise. In a way, they have already come to terms with being HIV-positive. For some of these people it can be a relief to have the information confirmed. No more wondering.

But for many men, even if they have expected a positive result, it is painful to see it in stark black and white. And for many others, the positive result comes as a surprise and shock that is very hard to accept.

Carey: *I grew up in a small Midwestern town. I started having sex when I was 15, and I didn't know anything about safe sex. But the only people I ever fooled around with were some of my high school buddies and the soccer coach. When I left home this year to go to college in Seattle, the nurse at the student health service offered to test me for HIV, so I said sure, why not. I was floored when the test came back positive. I went to a private doctor and made him repeat the test, and it was still positive. I never, ever thought that I would be one of those people who gets HIV. I guess I'll just have to deal with it.*

When a person learns he is HIV-positive, it is natural to feel angry, upset, afraid, hopeless, or all of the above. Many people go through a grieving process at the loss of their negative status that is similar to the grief one experiences with any other loss, such as the death of a friend. With time the pain of grief will fade away.

The most important thing is not to panic. Life is not over; it has just taken a different turn than you might have hoped for. HIV infection is very treatable now, and new advances are being made all the time.

Knowledge is power. If you find out you are HIV-positive, ask lots of questions of the person that tested you, even if you are too flustered to pay much attention to the answers. Ask for written information. Find out about local support groups and/or advocacy agencies for people with HIV. Read the sections on the subject in this book. If you don't have a doctor or if your doctor is not experienced in HIV care, find one who is. That out-of-control feeling will fade away when you start addressing and fighting your HIV infection.

Some people benefit from professional counseling during the first few months of coping with the knowledge of their HIV status. If you think you may need help, ask for referrals from your doctor or the person who tested you.

It can be helpful if you have a buddy or confidant you can share the news with—a shoulder to cry on. It might be particularly helpful if that person is HIV-positive himself because he's been there, and he can help reassure you that you have a future. But be careful who you tell at first. Once you tell someone, you can never take the information back. Give the news some time to sink in, let your head clear a little, before you start telling everyone about your situation.

As gay men, we have all been through the coming-out process about our sexual orientation. For most of us this is a gradual, ongoing process in which we reveal this aspect of ourselves to other people a few at a time. People with HIV experience a similar coming-out process, with similar fears. Will the person reject me when I tell them? Will they blame me for getting infected? Will they ask me embarrassing questions? The more important the person is to you, the more difficult it may be to tell them.

Brad: *When I told my mother I was gay and that I was also HIV-positive, at first she just stood there and didn't say anything. She looked dazed. The silence was painful. I didn't know whether she was going to burst into tears or run out of the room or what. Then she put her arms around me and put her head on my shoulder and hugged me as tight as she could, and we both started sobbing. I have never felt so close to her.*

Primary HIV Infection

Christopher: *I was 32 years old, healthy, ran five days a week before work—never sick a day in my life. I partied a little on weekends, but I usually didn't let it get out of hand. One morning I woke up feeling achy all over, and by that night I was sick as a dog. I was vomiting, and my belly was cramping, and I had watery diarrhea. My head was pounding, and my body felt like it had been run over by a truck. My roommate took my temperature, and it was 102. That really scared me, so he took me to the emergency room.*

They hooked me up to an IV and gave me some fluid. They drew a bunch of blood for tests. The doctor examined me from head to toe. He asked me about my lifestyle and if I had been around anyone who was sick. He asked me if I had been tested for HIV, and I said, "Yes, a month ago, and it was negative."

After a couple of hours, the doctor came back into the room and told me the tests had all come out fine. He said I probably had a "stomach flu" and I should be better in a few days. He prescribed some pills for the diarrhea, told me to take Tylenol for the aches and fever, and advised me to drink lots of fluid so I wouldn't get dehydrated.

I went home, went to bed, and did everything he said. My roommate waited on me, brought me soup, juice, and tea. The vomiting went away, but nothing else got better. I kept having diarrhea, feeling achy, and having high fevers.

Three days later I went back to the emergency room. This time there was a different doctor, but nothing else was different. They gave me an IV, did a bunch of blood tests, and told me I had some kind of virus that would get better on its own, soon.

But it didn't. A few days later I was feeling no better, and now I was developing a rash, like measles, all over my body. And my throat started to feel sore—almost like I had swal-

lowed razor blades. I didn't want to go back to that emergency room again, but I knew I needed help. I didn't have my own doctor to go to, so my roommate offered to take me to his doctor.

The doctor examined me and asked me a lot of questions. He said it did look like I had a bad virus, and it could even be HIV. He told me that in my neck I had swollen lymph nodes, which often go along with a viral infection. He explained that when a person first gets infected with HIV, it can make them really sick with the kinds of symptoms I was having, but that it could also be mono or another kind of virus.

The doctor asked me about my sexual habits and whether I might have been exposed to HIV. I told him that I always used a rubber for anal sex, whether I was on top or bottom. I didn't use them for oral sex, but I never let a guy come in my mouth. I also told him that a few weeks before, I had gone out and drank more than usual and woke up the next morning in bed with a guy I didn't know. That had never happened to me before, and it shook me up a little, but I hadn't told anyone about it until this doctor asked.

Before I left the doctor's office, he took blood for more tests, including a test for mono and a test for HIV. He explained that he was going to do the standard HIV test, but that that test only looks for the antibody against the virus, and a person does not make this antibody until several weeks or a few months after they have been exposed. So he offered to do another test, the HIV RNA test, which looks for the virus itself. He said that even if I was just recently infected with HIV, the RNA test might show positive.

I left the doctor's office with prescriptions for the rash and the throat pain and was given an appointment for a week later to go over my test results. During that week, I started feeling better. The aches eased up, the rash disappeared, and the diarrhea stopped. I felt very weak, and I had lost ten pounds, but my appetite was coming back, and I started eating more. I decided maybe the doctors in the emergency room were right—maybe it was just a bad stomach flu, and now I was getting over it. I almost convinced myself not to go back to my friend's doctor for my test results, but my friend dragged me there.

When I returned to the doctor's office, he sat down with me and showed me my lab report. The mono test was negative, and the HIV antibody test was negative. But the HIV RNA test was positive, and it showed that there was HIV—lots of it—in my blood. He said I had probably been infected recently—maybe during that one night I didn't remember or maybe by unprotected oral sex—and that it was just too soon for the antibody to show up. So that's how I found out about my HIV infection—right after I got it.

It's been two years now, and so far so good. I made a complete recovery from all the nasty symptoms that HIV originally caused. The doctor referred me to a study, and the nurse practitioner there started me taking three different medications to stop the virus from multiplying. My HIV-RNA count soon dropped so low it couldn't be detected. It's stayed that way ever since, and I'm still taking the same three medications. I've gotten used to the idea that I'm going to have to live with this virus for a long time, and I am grateful that I feel 100% well.

The Spectrum of Primary HIV Infection

HIV can make a man very ill when it first infects him. When the virus enters a person's bloodstream for the first time, it is able to multiply freely because that person's immune system is not yet prepared to attack it. Viral counts in the blood can rise very high, to millions of virus particles per milliliter of blood. In many people, this results in serious illness similar to what happened to Christopher. This is called *acute HIV syndrome* or *HIV seroconversion illness.* Note that these are common symptoms that can occur with a variety of infections, not only HIV. Many other viral illnesses, such as mono or the flu, can be indistinguishable from primary HIV infection.

When someone first contracts HIV, after a few weeks he begins making antibodies that attack the virus. Viral counts in the blood drop to more tolerable levels, and the person begins to feel better. Energy returns, and the various symptoms of acute HIV infection—if there were any—begin to fade away.

Common Symptoms of Primary HIV Infection
☐ Diarrhea
☐ Fatigue
☐ Fever
☐ Headache
☐ Loss of appetite, weight loss
☐ Mouth sores
☐ Muscle and joint aches
☐ Nausea, vomiting
☐ Sore throat
☐ Swollen glands
☐ Rash

Not all people get ill like Christopher when first infected with HIV. In fact, up to 50% of new HIV infections cause no symptoms at all. That's why if you are sexually active outside of a monogamous relationship with an HIV-negative partner, it is a good idea to be tested for HIV every six to 12 months. If the test turns positive, it means that infection has occurred some time since the last test, and you can begin treatment promptly if you so choose.

Samson: *I'm pretty sexually active. I do use a rubber if the other person tells me he's positive, but otherwise I just assume they're negative, and then I don't use protection. I don't have sex with anyone who doesn't look healthy. I was in the habit of testing every year or so, and last year it came back positive. I guess it had to happen. The only reason I was surprised was that I never was sick that year, and I assumed I'd know it if I got infected. I guess the virus just snuck into my body without letting me know.*

Others with primary HIV infection may have been a little achy for a few days or had a mild sore throat and shrugged it off. Later they find they have become HIV-positive.

Many do become ill like Christopher or even worse. Sometimes a person becomes so sick from acute HIV infection that hospitalization is required. It seems that people who have the hardest time when they are first infected also go on to develop AIDS sooner than those who have a mild or unnoticed illness with their acute HIV infection.

If you are a sexually active, HIV-negative gay man and you develop a flulike illness that seems unusually severe or is accompanied by rash or some other odd symptom, it is very important to get checked out for acute HIV infection. It didn't used to make any difference because there was little that could be done. But now it is standard practice to slam the virus with a three-drug cocktail as soon as acute HIV infection is recognized.

Why do we like to give antiviral medication to people who are newly infected with HIV? Because it seems that HIV is most vulnerable to attack by drugs when it first enters the system. Also, if the infection is treated aggressively before it has a chance to take hold, much less damage may be done to the immune system, and the development of AIDS may be greatly delayed or possibly even prevented entirely.

The medical community is becoming more aware of the importance of recognizing and treating acute HIV infection. But many doctors remain fairly ignorant on the subject. If you are at risk and you think you might have just gotten infected with HIV, you should seek care promptly from a doctor or clinic with expertise in the area, and you should make known your concerns about what might be happening to you.

Prevention After Exposure

What about "morning after" treatment? We know that if a health care worker is exposed to HIV through a needle stick, infection can be prevented if the person starts immediately on anti-HIV therapy. It makes sense that this should also work for someone who is accidentally exposed to HIV sexually. Treatment should begin within a few hours—or a day, at most—after the exposure occurs.

In some cases, morning-after treatment seems very appropriate. For example, suppose you are HIV-positive and your partner is negative. You are screwing him with a condom in place, and after you come you pull out only to find that the condom is torn. It might make sense for him to immediately start a course of anti-HIV therapy in hopes of avoiding becoming infected. There is no proof it works, but it might.

Another situation would be in the case of rape. If you are negative and are forced to have nonconsensual, unsafe sex with someone who is HIV-positive or whose HIV status you do not know, antiretroviral therapy might be a good idea because it might keep you from getting infected.

It is not a good idea, however, to consider morning-after therapy as a substitute for having safer sex. No one knows how well it works, it is expensive, inconvenient, and potentially toxic. So do your best to avoid the need for morning-after therapy.

If you are HIV-negative and have a high risk exposure, you may decide to get treated or not. In either case, you should have a couple of follow-up HIV tests over the subsequent six months, and you should watch for the symptoms of seroconversion.

Staying Healthy

I f you are living with HIV in your system, you probably have an extra appreciation of how precious health is and how important it is to maintain your health. Before you were infected with this virus you might have been able to take your health for granted. Now you really cannot.

In this section I will be discussing the sort of lifestyle and habits that can help optimize your health when you are HIV-positive. The other part of staying healthy with HIV, which involves medical treatments, will be covered in the next section.

Most health advice for HIV-positive people is the same as it is for everyone, only it's that much more important if you're HIV-positive. So the advice in this section is really common sense. It applies to all of us—whether we have HIV or not. But the stakes are higher for those of us who are positive, and preventive care is crucial.

The media are full of discussions on what constitutes a "healthy" lifestyle. We are all constantly bombarded with recommendations about diet, exercise, and taking care of ourselves. Having HIV is one more motivation to do something about that.

Reduce Your Stress if Possible

Stress is a big issue for many people in our culture today. For those with HIV, stress is an even bigger issue. Just the knowledge of being HIV-positive is stressful. But it is usually just one of many stresses in the life of an HIV-infected person.

Stress causes immune suppression. It appears that the suppression isn't permanent but lasts only as long as the stress is present. It was shown many years ago that people who had more than a few major life stresses over a year's time were far more likely to become ill. This includes both "bad" stresses—like losing a job or the death of a parent—and "good" stresses—like falling in love or inheriting a fortune.

The immune system of an HIV-positive person is already working overtime to deal with the raging fire of HIV replication and trying to keep the virus from getting out of hand. External stressors have an impact on the immune system. So it's good to avoid further stress, as much as is possible. That's easier said than done because in our society, stress seems to be the norm. But it doesn't hurt to try to reduce your stress by saying no once in a while to some new project, activity, or responsibility. It also helps to have some regular time out from the pace of life—with meditation, prayer, massage, music, or whatever activity helps you relax and center yourself.

Spending time with friends is a good way to have some time out and reduce stress. In addition, many cities have support groups for people with HIV/AIDS, where you can meet with a group of people to share and unburden. There are many on-line bulletin boards and chat groups for people with HIV/AIDS, as well.

Get Enough Sleep

Sleep deprivation is a major stress that can cause medical problems. The average person requires seven to nine hours of sleep a night. Some people may require more, and others may require less. If your life schedule forces you to awaken before you feel ready or if you find you are frequently drowsy during the day, you may not be getting enough sleep. For many of us there just aren't enough hours in a day to do everything we want to do, so we steal some hours from the time we should be sleeping. If this has happened to you, try to restore those needed sleep hours to your daily schedule.

If you have trouble sleeping, read the section titled "Insomnia" later in this book. Sleep is important for your health, and it is worthwhile to put some energy into making sure you get enough. The suggestions in "Insomnia" may help. If they don't, consult your health care provider.

Avoid Abuse of Drugs

Alcohol, tobacco, and recreational substances can be a detriment to your health. Any drug may be safe in moderation, but moderation is often impossible with some drugs or for some people. Some studies have shown higher rates of progression to AIDS in people who smoke cigarettes, drink alcohol to excess, or use recreational drugs.

If you choose to use substances, try to be moderate. If it seems the drug is controlling you rather than vice versa, you need to seek help in cutting down or eliminating your use. Read the sections in this book on substance use and abuse, and if anything there applies to you or to someone you love, see if you can't do something to change it.

Make Time to Exercise

Exercise is a big plus for anyone's health. Too few people exercise regularly, and they are missing out on a lot of benefits. Everyone should have at least 20 minutes of relatively vigorous exercise each day, either all at once or in smaller chunks. This applies to people with HIV, even if they are suffering from fatigue or from HIV-related illnesses. It is always possible to do some sort of exercise, even if you have fatigue, and often the exercise will actually lessen the fatigue.

Exercise is good for the psyche as well as for the body. It cleans out those cobwebs from the brain, and it contributes to stress reduction. People who exercise regularly have better energy, better sleep, better sex lives, and better self-esteem. Try to make the time for some daily exercise. If you don't have a form of exercise that you like, read the exercise section in this book, and see if you can come up with something for yourself.

Avoid Infections

Any infection is a stress to the immune system, which is already stressed if it is dealing with HIV. Some commonsense habits can reduce one's risk of preventable infections.

Sexually transmitted diseases—including herpes, hepatitis, gonorrhea, syphilis, and intestinal parasites—can be avoided to a degree by using condoms when having sex. Some

HIV-positive men make the choice to have unprotected sex if their partner is also HIV-positive. The problem here is that they put themselves at risk of these other STDs. And they get them. They are usually very unhappy when they come to me with acute hepatitis, primary herpes, or rectal gonorrhea. None of these is a fun experience, and it's a high price to pay for the privilege of not using a condom. So safer sex remains important. In addition, hepatitis A and B may be prevented by immunization, and every sexually active gay man should have these shots if he has not already been exposed to these viruses.

There is also a vaccine called Pneumovax that is recommended for all HIV-positive people. Pneumovax provides some protection against a family of bacteria that can cause pneumonia and other respiratory infections.

Herpes recurrences are bad for the immune system. If you are HIV-positive and get frequent herpes outbreaks, it is probably wise to prevent them. The most effective way is to take a daily dose of acyclovir or one of its newer, more expensive relatives, like Valtrex (valacyclovir) or Famvir (famciclovir).

It has been recommended that HIV-positive people not clean cats' litter boxes. This is because cats often carry a parasite called toxoplasma, and cysts of this organism are excreted in cat feces. Toxoplasma can cause serious infections in the brain or eye of someone who is HIV-positive. However, it seems that most of these cases actually occur as a reactivation of a dormant toxo infection that was acquired in childhood. So my advice to HIV-positive folks is that it's fine to have a cat, and you can change their litter box yourself. You might want to use disposable rubber gloves when doing this, and be sure to wash your hands afterwards, and of course you should never handle cat feces with your bare hands. (But who in his right mind would do that, anyway? Not you or me. Maybe someone in a John Waters movie.)

Some people believe that all HIV-positive people should boil or filter their tap water before drinking it. This is to prevent infection with cryptosporidium or other intestinal parasites that may be found in tap water. If you choose to follow this practice, be sure you get a filter with a small enough pore size to filter out these parasites; it should be rated as 1 micron or less. With the newer treatments for HIV, it appears that people may be more able to resist infection with cryptosporidium, and I see fewer people filtering their water lately. This practice might be considered a bit more seriously if your CD4 count is under 200.

Similarly, it has been the habit of some people with HIV to avoid fresh fruits and vegetables unless they have been peeled or cooked. This is to prevent infection by any bacteria or parasites that may be on the outside of the fruit or vegetable. While this makes some sense, it is a hassle, and I am dubious as to whether the benefit is worth the trouble. Only a small proportion of HIV-positive people bother with this, though I support their effort to take the extra step to protect their health. You may certainly choose to follow this practice if it makes you feel more secure.

The same goes for sushi. Some HIV-positive men avoid sushi, fearing that they will catch a parasite from eating raw fish. In reality, sushi from a reputable restaurant should not carry any viable parasites.

On the other hand, undercooked meat, eggs, or poultry can carry harmful bacteria, such as salmonella or campylobacter, that can cause severe diarrhea. If you eat any of these foods, make sure that they are well cooked.

What About Nutrition?

People with HIV sometimes need to be a little more careful about their diet than other people. It's important to maintain good nutrition and hydration. Some HIV-positive people have trouble maintaining their weight, especially if they have secondary symptoms or infections. Such folks may need more calories than an HIV-negative person of the same size, weight, and activity level. The important thing is to eat a balanced diet while striving for the proper proportions from the various food groups.

The current recommendations for everyone are that grains and starches (bread, rice, pasta, cereal) should make up the majority of what you eat (six to 11 servings a day); vegetables and fruits should be the next most common component of your diet (three to five servings); meat, dairy, and beans the least common (two to three servings); with fats and oils used very sparingly. Eating a variety of foods within these guidelines will keep you from getting bored, and will make sure you get the proper array of vitamins and minerals in your food. If you find you are losing weight, try to increase the amount and/or calorie content of what you eat. The meat-dairy-bean component is the most fattening, so it makes sense to eat more of this type of food if you are trying to gain weight.

But some people with HIV who are healthy are also overweight. It is not that rare for me to see this in my practice. Because being thin is associated with illness in an HIV-positive person, for some there is a backlash the other way, resulting in a tendency to put on too much weight. One of my overweight patients calls this syndrome "ARF"—AIDS-related fatness. For such people it is perfectly OK to follow the usual weight-loss advice and cut down on calorie and fat intake while increasing exercise. Intentional weight loss is a reasonable goal for an overweight person who has HIV. To some people with HIV, being fat is like having money in the bank. But there is no proven health benefit for an HIV-positive person to be obese.

Maintaining hydration is important. Some medications used to treat HIV are more toxic if you are dehydrated. It's a good idea to drink at least eight glasses of water or other fluids daily. Juice is fine. Keep in mind that some fluids (e.g., milk, juice, Gator Aid) have calories and/or salts that may make them a more important part of your diet. Others, such as coffee or colas, may act as diuretics, causing you to urinate more than you drink, resulting in net dehydration rather than hydration—so be careful.

What about nutritional supplements? People who are having trouble maintaining their weight often supplement their diet with protein powders or other weight-gain products. These products are usually not nutritionally complete. They are only to be used in addition to a well-balanced diet. Otherwise, nutritional deficiencies may result. Beware of "immune-boosting" powders or supplements, which have no proven benefit in helping your CD4 cells, no matter what the package says.

I like to recommend Carnation Instant Breakfast, either as a meal or as a weight-gain supplement. It is inexpensive compared to other supplements. Reconstituted with whole milk, it provides excellent, balanced nutrition and plenty of calories. I am not a fan of the canned, synthetic nutritional supplements such as Ensure or Advera. They are a very expensive and unnecessarily high-tech way to obtain nutrition. Besides, they are not especially tasty. If real food isn't enough to keep you going, add a serving or two of Instant Breakfast to your day.

Finally, a daily multivitamin provides good insurance that your vitamin needs are covered, so some people take one for piece of mind, but if you are eating a balanced diet, it is not really necessary. The packs of many vitamin pills that people take every day are an expensive way to give yourself peace of mind, and that may be all they give you.

The Bottom Line

Now, having gone on and on about all the ways to give yourself a healthy lifestyle, let me step back and and say this: If you are HIV-positive and feel well; if your energy is good; if your weight is stable, your CD4 cells are doing well, and if you are happy—then your lifestyle is probably fine. I see plenty of HIV-positive patients whose lifestyles are far from perfect. They may smoke, drink, not exercise, stay out late, eat poorly. Yet they are happy and feeling well. If this applies to you, then more power to you. Sure, you might feel even better, and you will probably stay well longer if you make a few changes. But if you're not ready, then keep going the way you are for now. It's not that I approve of unhealthy habits. But none of us is perfect.

HIV Treatments

P eople with HIV infection often take a number of medications regularly, to protect or improve their health. Medications may be prescribed for various reasons. One category of medication, the antiretroviral, fights HIV directly and prevents it from multiplying. Another category of drug is known as prophylactic or preventive medication, used to ward off an infection before it happens or recurs. Yet other medications are symptomatic or palliative drugs. These are used to reduce symptoms such as pain, nausea, diarrhea, or anxiety. Finally, there is a large group of medications used for treatment of various secondary HIV-related infections or other problems.

In this section I will cover only the medications that are used to directly combat HIV in people infected with this virus. "Cocktails" of three or more of these drugs are enabling many HIV-positive people to stay healthy by successfully combating the virus. The drugs used for prevention and treatment of problems and for symptom management are generally needed only by those with more advanced HIV infection. The use of these drugs varies so much, on a case-by-case basis, that they are best discussed with an HIV-expert physician at the time that they are needed and are beyond the scope of this book.

If you are HIV-positive or someone you know is, then you may use this section as your reference catalog of anti-HIV medications. Keep in mind that this is an area of very active research, and new drugs are being developed and released all the time. Because of this, the information here will necessarily be a little out of date even before the book is printed. So think of it as a starting point. AIDS peer-education groups, Web sites, and AIDS-savvy physicians should have the very most up-to-date information.

There are so many anti-HIV drugs now and so many possible combinations that it is imperative to work with a physician who is knowledgeable in the area. Treating HIV has become an art. For most folks with HIV infection, it should be possible to come up with a drug combination that is effective, relatively free of side effects, and relatively convenient to take. But this often requires skill, knowledge, experience, and creativity on the part of the treating physician, coupled with good patient-physician communication.

A word about nomenclature: All medications have at least two names. They have a chemical, or generic name; they have a brand name; and many HIV drugs also have a nickname. AZT is a good example. The name AZT is its nickname. Its generic name is zidovudine. Its brand name is Retrovir. It's confusing for one drug to have two or three names, but that's the way it is.

A few words about cost: Drugs for HIV tend to be among the most expensive prescription medications around. Most of them are available only in brand-name versions. Generic drugs or off-brand versions, tend to be significantly less expensive than brand. However, most HIV drugs are so new that the companies that developed them still hold the patents, preventing the marketing of generic versions.

Because of these cost issues, HIV infection is a very expensive condition to treat. A typical combination of three anti-HIV drugs can cost in the range of $1,000 to $1,500 monthly. For the person with HIV, it can be a major task to find the funding to pay for such treatment.

Medications are often covered by health insurance if the insurance is available and if it covers medication at all. There are also state programs that specifically fund the cost of some HIV-related medications for those who lack coverage. For the poor or disabled there is Medicaid. An unfair aspect of this is that the medications are more easily accessible in some states than others, depending on the funding situations and insurance laws in each state. States with poorer funding are probably more than happy to have you move to a state with better funding.

Antiretroviral Medications—General Philosophy

Antiretroviral drugs slow down or stop HIV from multiplying, allowing the system to clear the virus from the bloodstream more rapidly, and permitting some recovery of the CD4 cells. They do not kill or destroy the virus nor are they a cure for HIV infection.

HIV is called a retrovirus. It is "retro" because its genetic material is RNA, which is "backwards" from the usual genetic material of living things, which is DNA. In addition to a piece of RNA, each HIV particle is composed of a number of proteins, which consist of

Common Antiretroviral cocktails

Pick one drug from each column. The best-tolerated drug is listed at the top of each column, the worst-tolerated at the bottom. Choice of drug is determined by many factors including: dosing schedule, side effects, prior treatment history, and personal preferences regarding certain medications.

Nucleoside 1	Nucleoside 2	Protease Inhibitor
D4T	3TC	ritonavir+saquinavir
AZT	DDI	indinavir
		nelfinavir
		ritonavir

Notes on use of NNRTIs: Nevirapine, efavirenz, or delavirdine may be used in place of a protease inhibitor and may be just as effective in someone who has never had anti-HIV treatment. Additionally, if someone is responding to a triple therapy but develops an intolerance to one of the three components, nevirapine, efavirenz, or possibly delavirdine can be substituted for that drug without loss of efficacy.

enzymes that help it do its work, as well as coat proteins that protect the interior of the virus.

In order to multiply, HIV must enter a human cell, typically a CD4 cell. Once the virus enters it takes off its coat, and its genetic material (RNA) is copied to make a piece of DNA in a process called reverse transcription. This DNA is then copied to make RNA again. Some of this RNA forms the genetic material of new HIV particles. Other RNA directs the cell to manufacture the various viral proteins. These proteins are originally produced as one long strand that is then snipped into pieces by an enzyme called protease to make the final, active protein molecules.

Researchers have studied the steps of HIV replication in order to come up ways to interrupt the process. Two steps so far have proved to be vulnerable: the reverse transcription, or copying of the viruses genetic material, and the snipping step by the protease enzyme.

Originally, when few drugs were available to treat HIV, doctors would prescribe just one at a time. Later it became more common to prescribe two because several two-drug combinations seemed to work better than any solo drug. We now know that one or two drugs are generally not an adequate way to treat HIV in the long run. There are a couple of reasons why this is so.

First of all, just one drug seldom works well enough to completely stop the virus from multiplying, and even if viral levels temporarily go down, they bounce back within a few months.

Second of all, if the virus is exposed to just one drug, resistant virus starts to multiply and take over, after which the drug is useless for that person. Resistance occurs because HIV mutates very rapidly as it grows, and if enough mutant viruses are around, chances are that one of them will be resistant to the drug being used. Then that viral strain will rapidly multiply.

If three or more HIV drugs are taken simultaneously, however, often no single virus is able to be resistant to them all at the same time. The result can be a profound or complete suppression of viral multiplication and improvement in symptoms and immune function. This type of treatment has become standard for people with HIV.

Catalog of Anti-HIV Drugs

Reverse Transcriptase Inhibitors: The Nucleoside and Nucleotide Drugs

The first vulnerable step in HIV replication is reverse transcription, the process of converting the viral RNA to a piece of DNA, just after the virus enters the cell. Reverse transcription normally does not occur in human cells at all, so the concept is that it should be possible to devise a drug that prevents reverse transcription and has little or no toxic effect on human cells. When this aspect of HIV's life cycle was first discovered, many existing drugs were tested for their ability to block this process, and one, AZT, showed activity in the test tube.

When AZT was first given to people with AIDS, in the late 1980s, it was used in relatively high doses. The drug had a lot of toxic effects, including anemia, headaches, nausea, and insomnia. However, it did seem to produce a temporary increase in the CD4 count for some people, and it seemed to make some live a little longer. It was far from a cure for AIDS, though. People with AIDS who took AZT still went on to become more ill and die. But AZT proved that it is possible to devise a medication that can interfere with reverse transcription and slow multiplication of HIV.

AZT is classified as a nucleoside (sometimes nicknamed a "nuke," although that does not mean it is radioactive). A nucleoside is a chemical mimic of one of the normal building blocks of DNA, the genetic material that the virus must make when it starts to infect a cell. This type of drug fools the virus into adding it to a growing DNA chain, jamming the works in the process, and terminating the chain early.

Several nucleosides that are effective against HIV infection have been developed since AZT was released. Each new drug seems to be more effective and less toxic than the last. The two newest, D4T and 3TC, are the least toxic and most effective yet. Others in the pipeline include abacavir and adefovir (Preveon), which is actually a nucleotide but works in a similar way to the nucleosides. In general, nucleosides cost approximately $300 for a month's supply.

AZT (zidovudine, Retrovir): The granddaddy of HIV drugs. Of little use on its own, it is an important part of combination therapy for many people. Although AZT has a stigma because it was used solo in the days when everybody died of AIDS, they did not die because of AZT but in spite of it. AZT is most commonly now used in combination with 3TC and a protease inhibitor. It is taken as one or two capsules, three times a day, or one tablet, twice a day. It may cause nausea, diarrhea, headache, or insomnia, among other things, but is better tolerated if taken with food. Anemia, or a deficiency of red blood cells, can also occur and needs to be monitored for.

DDC (zalcitabine, Hivid): A moderately effective drug, best used in combination with AZT, it has largely been superseded by 3TC and is seldom prescribed any more. Peripheral neuropathy—nerve damage that produces burning, tingling, aching, or numbness in the toes, feet, or hands—can be a problem. DDC is taken as one tablet, three times a day, without regard to meals.

DDI (didanosine, Videx): A potent drug that works well in combination with AZT or with D4T, DDI is unfortunately a very inconvenient medication to take because it is unstable in the presence of stomach acid. Because of this, it is sold as a mixture with a strong antacid, either as packets of powder or as tablets that can be dissolved in water or chewed up and chased down with a glass of water. DDI tastes bad and must be taken on an empty stomach, twice a day, although recent research suggests it can be taken once a day. Peripheral neuropathy (see above) can occur and diarrhea is common because of the antacid mixed with the drug. Because of the difficulties with taking DDI, it is not a very popular drug. The once-a-day dosing may increase its popularity.

D4T (stavudine, Zerit): This drug is similar in some ways to AZT. It is at least as effective, with easier dosing and fewer side effects and toxicities. I think of it as "AZT Lite." It should not be taken with AZT because the two drugs interfere with each other. It is very effective as part of a triple drug combination. D4T is generally taken as one capsule, twice a day, without regard to food. Peripheral neuropathy can occur but may respond to a reduction in the dose.

Preveon (adefovir): A nucleotide drug that is similar to the nucleosides. This has only modest antiviral activity, but apparently resistance is slow to develop, so it may become a valuable part of treatment cocktails. It also may have efficacy against other viruses, for example CMV and the hepatitis B virus. This drug can cause a deficiency of a substance called carnitine, and those taking this drug must also take a carnitine supplement. Preveon may also cause kidney or liver problems. It may be released by the end of 1998, but again it is not yet clear where it will find a role in HIV treatment.

3TC (lamivudine, Epivir): A very effective drug, but resistance develops quickly unless it is used in combination with other drugs. 3TC is very nontoxic, with no common side effects. It is usually given as one pill, twice a day, without regard to meals. It happens to be effective against hepatitis B virus as well, so it may be of benefit to chronic carriers of this virus, as are many HIV-infected folks. It is usually given in combination with AZT or with D4T. A pill named Combivir contains a standard dose of AZT and 3TC in one pill, making things a bit easier for those who are on that combination.

Ziagen (abacavir): This is a new nucleoside that is highly potent and is currently in the research phase of development. A rare but severe and potentially fatal allergic reaction can occur with this drug. Its role in treatment cocktails is not yet clear.

Reverse Transcriptase Inhibitors: The Nonnucleosides

A second class of drug, called *nonnucleoside reverse transcriptase inhibitors*, also known as *nonnucleosides* or *NNRTIs*, also interferes with reverse transcription. However, unlike the nukes, these medications do not work by being incorporated into the new DNA chain. Instead they grab the enzyme involved from behind and distort it so that it cannot continue making new DNA. NNRTIs are becoming an important part of treatment combinations. Some very promising drugs in this class have been released, and more are in the pipeline.

Delavirdine (Rescriptor): This NNRTI has not yet been shown to have a great benefit, but the proper combination studies have not been done. When used alone it initially blocks HIV replication quite well, but resistance occurs rapidly. The dosing is relatively inconvenient, requiring four pills three times a day. As with nevirapine, delavirdine can cause a rash. It currently is the least expensive anti-HIV drug.

Efavirenz (Sustiva): A very potent and promising drug, Sustiva can be given once a day without regard to meals, so it is convenient to take. Side effects may include nausea and dizziness. As with the other NNRTIs, rash can occur. Also as with the other NNRTIs, resistance to this drug occurs rapidly unless it is taken with one or two other anti-HIV drugs at the same time.

Nevirapine (Viramune): This was the first nonnucleoside reverse transcriptase inhibitor approved. It is a potent blocker of HIV replication, but resistance can develop rapidly if it is used alone, so it must be taken in combination with at least two other drugs. The dosing is just one pill, twice a day, without regard to meals. Most people tolerate nevirapine very well. Side effects can include some nausea, headache, and fatigue, which tend to go away after a few weeks. Nevirapine can also cause a rash, which can be serious. A two-week lead-in period of one pill a day is recommended before starting on a full dose. This reduces the chances of a rash. Nevirapine costs somewhat less than the nucleosides.

Protease Inhibitors

The big breakthrough in HIV therapy has come with the development of the class of drugs known as protease inhibitors. While the reverse transcriptase inhibitors block an early stage of HIV replication, the protease inhibitors block a late stage. This is the stage when the virus has made all of its proteins in one long string that then needs to be cut into pieces in order for the proteins to function properly.

Normally, a viral enzyme, the protease, comes along like a molecular scissors and snips this string into several pieces. This process results in smaller proteins that then go on to come together and create the structure of a new viral particle. Protease inhibitors jam these molecular scissors, preventing them from snipping the string into the proper segments, resulting in a long piece of useless "spaghetti." Protease inhibitors are very effective at stopping replication of HIV.

The problem with the protease inhibitors, as with all HIV drugs, is that the virus can become resistant to any given protease inhibitor if it is used alone. But the breakthrough with protease inhibitors is that if one of them is given in combination with other drugs (usually but not always two nucleosides), then frequently HIV replication can be completely halted and may remain completely blocked as long as the drugs are being given. In that situation, the viral load becomes immeasurably low, and the CD4 cells begin to recover. Usually the person also starts to feel better. Opportunistic problems may improve or even clear.

Protease inhibitors are challenging drugs to take. In most cases, a day's worth of a protease inhibitor consists of a minimum of six pills, and 18 or more pills per day are not uncommon. This does not include any of the other drugs the person may be taking. Also, each protease inhibitor has particular rules regarding when the person may or may not eat with respect to the medication dose. In some cases the drug must be taken with a full meal; in some with a light meal; and in some, on a completely empty stomach. If taken improperly, these medications will not be absorbed into the bloodstream, so they will not work. Also, it is very important not to miss any doses of a protease inhibitor because the virus will begin to grow during the gap in therapy, and this will promote the development of resistant virus.

Protease inhibitors may be inconvenient or have odd or unusual side effects. Ritonavir, for example, must be kept refrigerated, which is difficult for people who work odd hours or who travel. Indinavir can crystallize in the kidney, forming a blockage (kidney stone) that can be very painful. People on indinavir must drink large amounts of fluids to try to prevent this. Most protease inhibitors can cause diarrhea to a greater or lesser extent. They can cause dry skin, hair loss, and high cholesterol. They can change the distribution of fat in the body, with extra fat around the waist and loss of fat from elsewhere.

Protease inhibitors also interfere with the liver's ability to break down other medications or recreational drugs. This is especially true for ritonavir but to an extent is true for all protease inhibitors. Anyone who is taking one of these medications must make sure that his doctor and pharmacist are aware of everything else he is taking—including recreational drugs.

Despite all of their problems, protease inhibitors work so dramatically well that they are now taken by over 100,000 HIV-infected Americans, many of whom are enjoying continued or restored states of health as a result. Protease inhibitor therapy has helped change the face of AIDS, from a chronic, fatal illness to one that can be treated and managed, with the expectation that many HIV-infected people will be able to enjoy reasonably good health for an indefinite period of time. Because of this success, the drug companies are working hard to develop new versions of protease inhibitors that should have fewer side effects, interactions, and toxicities and (we hope) require taking fewer pills each day.

Indinavir (Crixivan): A very potent drug, indinavir is currently the most popular protease inhibitor because of its relative lack of side effects. The dosing schedule, however, is a challenge, with the standard regimen being two capsules, every eight hours, on an empty stomach (one hour before or two hours after a meal). A twice-a-day dosing schedule is being studied. Most people are able to schedule their meals and their meds such that this works out.

Indinavir can cause some nausea, and if this is the case it can be taken with a light snack. Some people on this medication develop a form of kidney stone, caused by crystallization of the drug in the kidney. This can produce severe pain in one flank, sometimes accompanied by cloudy, pink, or bloody urine, and it requires immediate medical attention. Crystallization of indinavir in the kidney can be avoided by drinking eight or more glasses of water or other beverage daily. Indinavir is the least expensive protease inhibitor, at approximately $400 monthly.

Nelfinavir (Viracept): This protease inhibitor seems to be as effective as ritonavir and indinavir, and it may have fewer side effects. It is taken as three tablets, three times a day, with some food. A twice-a-day dosing schedule is being studied. Unlike indinavir, with nelfinavir a strict every-eight-hours schedule is not necessary. Diarrhea can occur in people taking nelfinavir, but it is usually manageable with over-the-counter preparations such as loperamide (Imodium). The cost of nelfinavir is approximately $500 monthly.

Ritonavir (Norvir): This is a very effective protease inhibitor, but it can be quite difficult to take. The standard dose is six capsules, twice a day, with a big meal, to increase absorption and improve tolerance. Most commonly I prescribe a lower dose, in combination with saquinavir. Ritonavir capsules must be kept refrigerated. A liquid form is available, and is stable at room temperature for a month, but it has a very bad taste. A new, nonrefrigerated capsule is being developed.

Ritonavir can have significant side effects, including nausea, diarrhea, and a burning sensation of the skin, mouth, and windpipe. When starting ritonavir, these side effects can be diminished if the dose is started low and then built up over the first week or two of therapy. Ritonavir also interferes with the body's ability to break down many other prescription drugs and street drugs, which can lead to serious consequences, including death. A doctor or pharmacist needs to be aware of every drug you are taking, when you are on ritonavir. Full-dose ritonavir costs about $600 monthly.

Saquinavir (Invirase, Fortovase): Although very potent in the test tube, in people this has been the weakest protease inhibitor because it is poorly absorbed. A newer form, Fortovase, is better absorbed. Saquinavir is taken as three to six capsules, three times a day, with food. It can cause diarrhea that can be quite severe. This drug is best used in combination with ritonavir or nelfinavir, both of which significantly raise the level of saquinavir in the blood. In my practice, saquinavir is most often used in a low dose in combination with ritonavir. Depending on the dose, the cost of saquinavir is about $400 to $500 monthly.

HIV-Related Problems

All of us are subject to colds, coughs, stomach flus, the usual aches and pains of life. People with HIV get these things just as often as anyone else. But if you are HIV-positive or at risk but don't know your HIV status, these common symptoms could also be an early sign of a serious problem. It's important for you to have a good relationship with a primary care doctor who knows your medical situation. That way if you get a symptom that you're unsure of, it's easy to get it checked out.

In this section, we will discuss some of the common symptoms that can occur when someone is HIV-positive. Keep in mind that most of these symptoms can happen to anyone, HIV-positive or not. A gay man who knows he is HIV-negative can afford to ignore some of these sorts of things, at least for a while, and see if they'll get better on their own. A man who is positive or does not know his status should seek medical attention sooner.

For each symptom I will try to give some perspective on when to call or see your doctor and when it may be OK to wait. Most people have pretty good judgment about this. But when you're not sure, you might want to read the section on your symptom and see if you should wait or seek medical attention.

Changes in Vision

Any lasting change in vision warrants a visit to an ophthalmologist. If it is simply a matter of more difficulty focusing close up or far away, you probably just need new glasses. But if you see a spot out of one eye that won't go away or part of your field of vision in one eye is missing, you should seek evaluation immediately. It could be a sign of CMV retinitis, a sight-threatening infection that occurs in HIV-infected people with low CD4 counts (usually under 50 or so). So, especially if your count is low or you don't know your CD4 count or your HIV status, be alert to this sort of change in vision, and deal with it promptly.

Cough

A cough is often your body's response to an upper or lower respiratory infection, such as a cold, sinusitis, or bronchitis. Allergies or asthma can also cause a cough. Most smokers have a daily cough. A cough can be "dry" or it can bring up phlegm.

Most transient coughs can easily be dealt with by taking over-the-counter cough or cold remedies, which contain cough suppressants, decongestants, and/or antihistamines. Fever may be part of an infection that is causing a cough. If the fever lasts for more than a few days or if it is accompanied by shaking chills or if the phlegm is dark green, brown, or bloody— then it is likely that the cough is from a bacterial infection that should be treated. Often these symptoms are a clue to pneumonia.

Pneumocystis carinii pneumonia, the most common form of pneumonia in HIV-infected people, manifests as a persistent, dry cough, accompanied by fever and often by shortness of breath and weight loss. People who know they are HIV-positive and potentially at risk because of a low CD4 count generally take medication to prevent PCP. If you do not know your HIV status or CD4 count and you develop these symptoms, you should be evaluated for PCP.

Diarrhea

Everyone gets diarrhea at times, usually because of a virus passing through the body (stomach flu) or because of eating something that disagrees with the digestive system. These benign types of diarrhea are best addressed with medications from the store—such as loperamide (Imodium), Kaopectate, or Pepto-Bismol—and by drinking lots of fluids with some starchy, low-fat solid food, such as rice or toast.

When is diarrhea something to be concerned about? When it is extremely watery and in large quantity; when it is accompanied by abdominal pain, bloating, or excessive gas; when it is accompanied by fever; when there is blood, pus, or mucus mixed in with it; or when it persists more than 3-4 days. These types of diarrhea can occur in men with or without HIV infection. Often the diarrhea is caused by infection with a parasite or bacterium. In any of these cases, see your doctor to have the infection identified and treated.

Fatigue

Fatigue is another vague symptom that can stem from many things: hormonal disorders, stress, seasonal cycles, depression, sleep deprivation, or infection. If you develop fatigue that interferes with your daily activities and lasts a week or more, it could be a sign of an underlying problem. Again, any associated, concurrent symptoms may be a clue as to the cause of fatigue. In people with HIV, fatigue can be caused by a high viral load or an HIV-related infection or malignancy. Treatment with antiviral drugs to bring the viral counts down often can help fatigue if it is caused by high viral load.

Fevers

A fever is usually a sign that your body is fighting infection. Many types of illness can be accompanied by fever. Often the illness is a benign viral condition, such as a flu or cold. But if the fever persists for more than 48 hours or if it goes very high (say over 103 degrees), it should be looked into. A fever also makes any of the other symptoms described in this section, such as cough or headache, that much more worrisome.

Headache

Most people get headaches at one time or another. Common, benign headaches can be caused by stress, muscle tension, or by blood vessel constriction in the scalp (migraines). Seek care if you get an unusual or worrisome headache. Some clues would be: if you never get headaches and now you have a bad one; if you do get headaches but this one is different from or worse than any headache you've had before; a headache accompanied by neck stiffness or by extreme sensitivity to light; or a headache accompanied by high fever. Such headaches can be a sign of a problem in the central nervous system (brain and spinal cord and the fluid that bathes them). Possible problems there include infection, cancer, or bleeding. Sometimes the problem is elsewhere, and the headache is part of the overall illness. For example, people suffering from acute hepatitis A or B often have headaches.

Night Sweats

Sweating often accompanies a fever. However, some people with HIV develop drenching night sweats that require that they change their pajamas and sheets. Some people sleep on a bath towel to soak up the sweat. This is never normal. It can be a sign of a serious infection, such as pneumonia or tuberculosis, or a malignancy, such as lymphoma, or it may just be from HIV itself if the viral load is high. Night sweats that persist for more than a few days warrant a medical visit. If you don't know your HIV status and you develop night sweats, you should strongly consider getting tested. If you are HIV-positive, you and your doctor need to look for a cause for the sweats.

Purple Skin Lesions

It's good to be familiar with the geography of your skin, with the moles, freckles, and bumps that are normal for you. People frequently come to see me because they have discovered a skin lesion that they think might be Kaposi's sarcoma. KS is associated with a virus in the herpes family. In the setting of HIV infection, this virus may trigger the development of KS lesions anywhere on the body. They are general purple or dark pink. They are raised or at least can be felt with the finger. They tend to be one quarter of an inch across or more. They usually do not hurt, especially in the early stages. Treatment of KS may consist of cancer chemotherapy or radiation therapy. Effective anti-HIV therapy usually causes KS lesions to regress and disappear. Because of this, I seldom see cases of KS any more, though it used to be quite common among HIV-infected men.

A bruise is frequently mistaken for KS, but typically a bruise is not raised and cannot be felt with the finger, unlike KS. Color can also help distinguish the two. KS tends to be in the pink to purple range. Bruises have more shades of tan and greenish coloration as they age.

If the bruising is unexplained, it may itself be a clue to an HIV-related problem and needs to be looked into.

Sores That Don't Heal

Any sore in the mouth, genitals, or anus that lasts for more than a few days should be evaluated. Herpes, which has its own section in the STD section of this book, is a very common cause. Usually a herpes outbreak runs its course and heals on its own. In people with HIV, however, herpes can produce a sore that does not heal without treatment. Treatment for herpes entails taking an oral medication (acyclovir or one of its relatives). This will help the lesions heal faster, but it does not cure the person of herpes, which can recur later.

Syphilis can also produce a sore in the genital area that may heal very slowly. Syphilis is readily treated once it is diagnosed.

Open sores inside the mouth are often called *canker sores,* which are not caused by a virus but happen at random or under times of stress (often when the person is dealing with an infection elsewhere in the body). Some HIV-infected people develop an excessive number of canker sores that are slow to heal. Treatment of HIV can help. There are also some prescription treatments for these types of sores. One is thalidomide, a notorious drug that was banned in the 1960s because it caused birth defects. It is now available for treating weight loss and mouth sores in people with HIV. Another drug, prednisone, is a steroid anti-inflammatory medication that can help canker sores heal.

Swollen Lymph Nodes

Most people with HIV have enlarged lymph nodes to a greater or lesser degree. These are most often found in the neck, armpits, or groin. Normally they are rubbery, up to the size of a marble, are easily moved around under the skin, and don't hurt. They may swell up more at times of viral illnesses such as flu. A viral throat infection can cause the nodes on one or both sides of the neck to swell up and become tender. During the course of HIV infection, enlarged lymph nodes may shrink down on their own. That is not necessarily a good sign. It may mean that the nodes have "burnt out" from dealing with HIV and are withering away.

On the other hand, chronically enlarged lymph nodes can shrink down to normal when HIV is treated effectively with antivirals.

Swollen lymph nodes may be a clue to problems other than HIV itself. Such problems include lymphoma (cancer of the lymph nodes), tuberculosis, or other infections or cancers. Some clues to an abnormal lymph node or group of nodes include: nodes that grow bigger than the size of a marble, especially in one area; nodes that are hard like bone rather than rubbery; nodes that seem to be stuck down to the tissue underneath; or ones that become painful for no apparent reason. Any of these symptoms could indicate tumor or infection in the area, and evaluation by a professional is called for.

Unexplained Weight Loss

Many people consider themselves overweight and are constantly striving to lose weight by dieting and exercising. But it's cause for concern when someone starts to lose weight without changing his lifestyle. This can mean many things, including an uncontrolled infection, a tumor, depression, or a hormonal disorder, such as diabetes or a hyperactive thyroid gland. If you lose a little weight and it stabilizes, fine. But if you lose ten pounds or more without trying or if the weight loss is accompanied by other symptoms, such as cough, fever, or fatigue—see your doctor. The weight loss could be a sign of a serious problem.

Psychosocial Issues

Being in good health means much more than just having a body that is in working order. The mind and soul must be healthy as well. The body and the psyche are interconnected, obviously, and each influences the other to a great extent. As a physician, I often find myself confronted with the psychological issues of my patients. These issues are extremely common. In fact, millions of Americans have psychological problems of some sort, but only a small proportion seek professional help, whether from their primary doctor, a psychiatrist, psychologist, or other counselor.

We gay men have our own particular psychological issues. Of course our gayness, per se, is not a psychological problem to be treated. As gay men, we have come a long way from being labeled mentally ill solely because of our sexual orientation. When we are troubled and seek help, whether from a physician or a psychotherapist, we should expect that our emotional concerns and not our gayness will be the issue to be remedied.

However, our psychological health is certainly influenced by our being gay, in some ways positively and in some ways negatively. Some of the experiences that are unique to us include our sexuality; our relationships with friends, lovers, and family; and our stigmatized position in society. If we develop emotional problems, these important gay aspects of our lives need to be acknowledged. Otherwise therapy is difficult or impossible.

Wendell: *When I went to bible college, I had my first relationship with another man—my dorm roommate. The relationship was very stormy. My grades suffered. My academic advisor made me see a counselor because I was obviously in a lot of distress. The counselor was a minister in the church that ran the college. Of course I couldn't tell him the truth about my relationship. But I wanted to get something out of the counseling. So when I talked with the min-*

ister, I split my boyfriend into two people. One was my "roommate," and I talked about my trouble getting along with him. The other was my "girlfriend," and I talked about the romantic troubles I was having with "her." The counseling was a total waste of time because I couldn't be honest. I didn't really get my head together until I quit Bible college and moved to the city and really came out.

This section will discuss common mental health issues as they relate to gay men. The first section will address how to find an appropriate, gay-supportive therapist. The remaining parts of this section will discuss specific common psychological issues—including depression, anxiety, insomnia, and grief—from a gay man's perspective.

Choosing a Therapist

There are many types of professionals whose job it is to help people with emotional problems. If you are looking for a therapist, it helps to know what types of therapists are available, what their differences and similarities are, where to look, and how to find one who is gay-supportive.

Because of our unique psychosocial concerns as gay men, we are best served when we are helped by someone who respects and honors who we are. Keep in mind that a good psychotherapist will not be homophobic and in fact should be actively supportive of your gay identity. The psychotherapist will also recognize your particular support system in the context of your gay identity and will help you identify and take advantage of these supports as you progress in therapy.

Some gay men prefer to have a therapist who is also a gay man. There is nothing wrong with that if a good one is available. But try to be open minded. Many professionals who are not gay men are very supportive and effective therapists for gay male clients. Conversely, because a particular therapist is a gay man does not necessarily mean that he is a good therapist—or the right one for your needs.

Recent research indicates that gay men and lesbians may be much more likely to seek mental-health help than are other people. However, a significant proportion of gay men and lesbians report receiving poor or inappropriate treatment. Nearly half reported encountering a homophobic therapist. It's a jungle out there. Be careful!

If you have succeeded in finding a gay-supportive primary care physician, your best bet is to ask your doctor for some names of gay-supportive therapists. Some physicians will offer to provide brief, goal-oriented psychotherapy themselves, but that is not particularly cost-effective, and you may be better served by going to a person whose full-time job is mental health.

Types of Psychotherapists

Several types of qualified professionals provide psychotherapy:

Psychiatrists are M.D.s, and hence they are licensed to prescribe medication. Some psychiatrists also provide counseling or "talk therapy," but they are becoming a minority. Psychiatrists are best for a person who has a fairly serious mental illness, often one for which medication is indicated. Psychiatrists tend to charge the highest fees.

Psychologists are not medical doctors but have a Ph.D.—a doctorate in psychology. They have been trained in the workings of the human mind, but are not licensed to prescribe medication. They deal well with behavioral and emotional problems. If the psychologist feels that medication may help, the psychologist will often make a referral to a psychiatric colleague specifically to assess for this and to prescribe if indicated.

Clinical social workers have a master of social work degree and provide counseling similar to psychologists. Their expertise tends to include "life problems" or coping difficulties, rather than more severe emotional problems. Their fees are lower than those of doctorate-level therapists.

Counselors usually have a master of arts degree in counseling. They function similarly to their social work counterparts.

A psychotherapist's credentials are less important than the therapist's actual skill at counseling. Your doctor should be able to give you names of gifted therapists, and these may include M.D.s, Ph.D.s, social workers, and counselors. The choice often depends on your insurance coverage, and perhaps whether or not you may need medication for your problem. Of course, it is important that your prospective therapist be gay-supportive.

Finding the Right One

In looking for a therapist, you should get two or three names and prepare to interview them all before deciding. Don't assume that a given therapist will work well for you, just because a friend thinks he's God. Even if Joe Doe is highly recommended, he and you just may not click. Try to make sure beforehand that all three candidates are gay-positive so you don't have to screen out the homophobes yourself.

Lately, many health insurance plans have started using a program called "managed mental health." This means that if you want psychotherapy, then instead of consulting your doctor for advice or referral, you have to call the 800 phone number of the managed mental health company that has a contract with your insurance company. You will speak to a referral specialist who will refer you to a mental health professional appropriate for your problem.

Do tell the referral specialist that you are gay and that you want a gay-positive therapist if you are comfortable with that. Be prepared for a stunned pause. These referral people are not used to that question. You may get the answer that all of their therapists are fine with gay clients—which just means you'll have to check things out for yourself when you show up for your first appointment.

Depression and Anxiety

O liver came in for a general checkup, and as is common, we began to chat about his general well-being. He was a healthy 30-year-old single gay man who worked as a computer programmer. I had not seen him in a few years and wondered why he had decided to have a checkup at this time.

Oliver: *I just haven't been feeling well lately, and I don't know why. My energy is terrible. It's all I can do to get out of bed in the morning, and when I get home at the end of the day, I just want to go to sleep. I've stopped going to the gym, and I don't go out with my friends anymore. My appetite is gone. I've lost ten pounds. I'm really worried I might have AIDS. But I tested negative last year, and I haven't had sex with anyone since then. I don't know. Something's wrong.*

Oliver and I continued talking, and I asked him some more questions. It turned out that other things were going on with him. He was having a lot of trouble getting to sleep, despite being so tired, and he found he was waking up frequently during the night. He was on probation at work because he found himself staring into space instead of concentrating on his job, and his productivity was way down. He was also making more mistakes at work. Oliver said he was pretty discouraged and actually was beginning to question what the point of his life was.

Oliver: *I haven't talked to anybody about this, but I've been having these weird conversations in my head. I've been pretty down on myself. I'm 30, I don't have a boyfriend, I have a stupid job—I'm just not sure there's any point in going on. I haven't thought about suicide, but I guess if I died tomorrow it wouldn't really matter to me. It sure wouldn't matter to anyone else.*

Diagnosis: Major Depression

Oliver was suffering from a serious case of depression, a very common disorder that affects a significant percentage of the U.S. population at any given time. Gay men are more likely than other men to experience an episode of depression at some time in their lives. Often the man who is depressed does not know what the problem is. He only knows that something has gone very wrong with his life.

Depression is far more than just feeling blue or sad. Those feelings are normal. No one is happy all the time. We each have moments when we feel down. It's part of life. But people who are suffering from depression feel blue most of the time. Often this seems normal to them because their thinking is distorted by the disease. So they may not be aware that they are truly depressed.

Symptoms of Depression

Depression has many other symptoms besides a blue or depressed mood. Some of these symptoms are psychological and some are physical. Because of the physical symptoms, many depressed people, Oliver for example, assume that they have a medical problem such as AIDS or cancer.

To be diagnosed with depression, psychiatrists say that a person must have several (though not all) of the following symptoms in addition to a depressed mood:

- Sleep problems, either insomnia or hypersomnia (sleeping too much)
- Lack of energy
- Lack of sex drive (libido)
- Appetite problems, either lack of appetite with weight loss or excessive appetite and craving for sweets with weight gain
- Feeling hopeless and/or helpless about one's situation
- Irritability, rapid mood swings, crying easily or excessively
- Thoughts about death and/or suicide
- Inability to concentrate or focus, i.e. on work tasks, reading a book or magazine, or watching a TV program

In addition, many depressed people also suffer from a general sense of anxiety, and they may have panic attacks. Generalized anxiety can be a separate problem, but often it is part of the syndrome of depression, and it responds to the same types of treatment.

Some people suffer from a milder form of depression, called dysthymia. In this case, people may have a depressed mood but only one or a few of the above symptoms. Dysthymia can be treated in the same ways as depression.

Depression is very common. At any given time, perhaps one in twenty-five Americans suffers from depression. Younger adults tend to be more prone to depression than their elders. As noted previously, gay men are more apt to have at least one episode of serious depression during their lifetime. However, at any given moment, a gay man is no more apt to be depressed than a similar straight man.

What Causes Depression?

Sometimes, the symptoms of depression are actually the result of a medical problem, such as an underactive thyroid gland, or anemia. For this reason, a physical exam and blood testing are in order for anyone who may be suffering from depression.

More commonly, depression is the result of other factors. These may include any of the following:

- Life stresses, both good and bad, including:
  starting a new relationship or ending an old one
  death of a partner or relative, or birth or adoption of a child
  being promoted or losing one's job
  moving to a new home or a new town
- Poor self-esteem; coming-out issues
- Diagnosis with a serious illness
- Inherited or biochemical factors that predispose a person to depression
- Gloomy weather and/or short days (producing "seasonal depression," which I see frequently in Seattle's dark, drizzly winters)
- Overuse of alcohol, tranquilizers, or illicit drugs

Modern society is full of stressors and even more so for gay men. Many of us have complicated, stressful lives. We belong to a stigmatized group. Many of us take prescription or illicit drugs. Many of use have to deal with medical stresses, such as HIV infection, in ourselves or our loved ones. No wonder depression is a very common problem for us.

Despite all of these potential causes of depression, sometimes the cause of a given episode of depression cannot be found. The person has become depressed, and no one knows why. So be it. That does not make him any less depressed, and the illness must still be dealt with.

Prevention and Treatment

How can a person prevent depression? It's important to try to keep the stresses down as much as is possible. Don't pretend to be superhuman. Make sure to take time off from work. Cultivate playtime, recreational activities, hobbies, a sex life. Have a spiritual aspect to your life. Try to have a small circle of supportive friends, two or three confidants to whom you can talk about anything. Work on taking pride in your gay identity.

Sometimes depression comes along as a reminder that we are not doing these things that we need to do in order to nurture our souls. But sometimes depression comes along when everything seems to be going just fine and there is no apparent reason for it.

Untreated, depression can last for months or even years. It can resolve by itself, but it tends to recur. Many depressed people feel that they could "snap out of it" if only they could work things out in their head. That's unrealistic. Depression is an illness. Just as people with AIDS or cancer cannot "snap out of" their illness, people suffering from depression cannot will themselves to recover.

Fortunately, treatment for depression is very effective. This is a good thing. Depression is a lethal illness, with thousands of deaths from suicide each year in the United States. In order for it to be treated, depression must first be diagnosed. But tragically, only one in three depressed people seeks medical care for his condition. Often the person is unaware that he is depressed or that a doctor can help him.

Despite this, depressed people do tend to see their doctors more than people who are not depressed, usually because of some minor ache or pain. Often neither the doctor nor the patient realizes that the problem is depression, and the patient is treated for his headache, backache, or whatever and may even be labeled a hypochondriac.

Psychotherapy

There are two main ways in which depression can be treated. The first is psychotherapy. The depressed person meets regularly with a mental-health professional (either a psychiatrist, psychologist, or counselor) and discusses his feelings and his life. The goal is to gain insight into what is making the person depressed and how to change it. In addition, some therapists practice *cognitive therapy,* in which the person is taught how to identify the thought processes that lead to negative thoughts and how to stop this chain of events and hence ward off these negative thoughts.

Antidepressant Medication

The other way to treat depression is with medication. There are many good antidepressant medications available. These are usually in the form of a pill that is taken one or more times daily. Antidepressants work by changing the balance of certain brain chemicals (neurotransmitters) that are involved in mood. They do not work right away but must be taken daily for a few weeks before they begin to help. Once an antidepressant starts to work, the various symptoms of depression gradually fade away and the person feels "normal" again.

Antidepressants are not habit forming, and no one gets high from them. The worst things that can happen from an antidepressant are either that it does not work or has side effects.

Many men develop some degree of sexual dysfunction while they are on antidepressants. Often they feel so much better that they are willing to accept this as a reasonable price to pay. However, this side effect need not be accepted. Often switching to a different antidepressant will relieve the problem.

If a given antidepressant just does not seem to be working, it is a good idea to try a different one. Each type of antidepressant medication is successful in 70 to 80% of the people who take it. If the first one that you and your doctor choose does not work, don't give up. The next one should do the trick.

In general, people who respond to antidepressants should take them for several months or longer. Otherwise the depression tends to recur. Some people find that they relapse whenever they try to go off antidepressants, so they stay on them indefinitely. Some people with seasonal depression take antidepressants only in the winter. A daily exposure to high-intensity light is also effective for seasonal depression. These lights can be rented, and insurance often pays the cost. However, many people find it more convenient to take a pill.

Combination Treatment

A combination of psychotherapy and medication is often the best treatment for an individual suffering from depression. When I see a patient like Oliver, I discuss both modes of treatment. It is my bias that someone as seriously depressed as Oliver should be treated with medication. But since he seems unhappy with specific aspects of his life, he may also benefit from psychotherapy. Working with a therapist may help him have insight into his condition, regain control over his life, and change the things he does not like about it.

Often a patient of mine is seeing a psychotherapist for some life issues but does not identify that he is suffering from depression. He may have responded partially to the psychotherapy sessions, but at a certain point the therapist calls me to say that the client has some physical symptoms of depression and does not seem to be making further progress in therapy. We discuss a trial of medication. At that point the medication usually works quite well in alleviating the remaining depressive symptoms, and the patient is able to resume his progress in psychotherapy.

The point is, that depression is common; it is particularly common in gay men; it is not caused by a flaw in character; it frequently goes unrecognized; it can be life-threatening; and it should be viewed as a medical problem for which good treatment is available. If you think you or someone you care about might be depressed, it's worth a consultation with a health care provider.

Insomnia

Arnie: *I've never had much trouble sleeping. But lately when I go to bed, I just lie there. In my head I go over and over everything that I did during the day and all the things I have to do the next day. I just can't turn off my mind. Eventually I fall asleep, but pretty soon it's morning, and the alarm goes off. So I've been really tired during the day. Over lunch I've been taking a catnap at my desk—just so I can get through the day.*

The ability to fall asleep easily at night is a blessing, one that we tend not to appreciate until something goes wrong. Then we really miss it. Although not a particularly gay male problem, insomnia deserves a discussion here. It relates to many other gay men's health issues, and it is one of the most common concerns my patients bring me.

Insomnia, defined as the inability to get a restful night's sleep, is a common problem affecting a significant proportion of adults in the United States. There are many patterns of insomnia. Some people have trouble falling asleep. Others find that they awaken frequently during the night, or that they awaken too early and cannot get back to sleep. Insomnia may be a brief problem that is resolved on its own. Or it may be a long-term pattern that has a significant impact on a person's life.

Insomnia can have major consequences for a person. A sleep-deprived man will have difficulty with work performance. He will tend to be irritable. He may have memory or concentration problems. He is at risk of accidents while driving.

Causes of the Problem

A disruption in one's daily routine is the most common culprit for insomnia. We all know about the phenomenon of jet lag, but any type of travel can disturb a person's sleep habits.

Other changes in routine—such as moving to a new home, starting school, or starting a new job—can cause a sleep problem. Fortunately, in these cases the cause is usually obvious, and sleep returns to normal once the person settles into their new routine.

An acute stress can also interfere with sleep. Suffering the death of a loved one, being laid off from work, having a fight with a boyfriend—any of these can disrupt a person's sleep pattern. Again, in these situations sleep usually returns to normal over time.

More persistent insomnia can be a symptom of a significant underlying problem. Depression is the most common. When a patient sees me for help with insomnia, the first thing I ask myself is, "Is this man depressed?" The majority are. Treating the depression will usually make the sleep problem go away. The previous section describes the symptoms of depression. If you have a sleep problem and also have symptoms of depression, you should seek help.

Use of alcohol or other drugs can also cause insomnia. Although alcohol makes a person drowsy, it also interferes with normal sleep. Alcoholics have very abnormal sleep patterns, and many spend the night passed out from alcohol rather than truly sleeping. As a result, in the morning they feel hungover rather than rested.

Medical problems can interfere with sleep. Uncontrolled pain, frequent urination, and shortness of breath are just a few examples of symptoms that can prevent a person from being able to sleep through the night. A health care provider may be able to treat these problems and improve the person's ability to get a full night's sleep.

Drugs That Can Interfere With Sleep

■ Caffeine

■ Alcohol

■ Decongestants

■ Prescription medications—especially steroids, stimulants, and certain antidepressants and anti-seizure medications

---

Dealing With Insomnia

If a sleep problem is caused by an underlying medical situation—such as depression, anxiety, pain, or frequent nighttime urination—it is best to work with your health care provider to try to improve the situation and allow the return of normal sleep.

But if that is not the case, there are a number of things that you can do in order to encourage restful sleep. These collectively are called *sleep hygiene*. They are habits to cultivate that promote normal sleep. If you try to incorporate these habits into your routine, you may save yourself from the consequences of long-term insomnia without even needing to see a doctor.

> **Don't nap.** Even if you are tired during the day, a nap will make it harder for you to sleep at night.
>
> **Go to bed and wake up at the same time each day.** Keep to a regular routine. If you can't fall asleep easily at your usual bedtime, then move your bedtime to a later time. No matter how late you fall asleep, get up at the same time each morning. Don't sleep in.
>
> **Use your bed only for sleep and sex.** Don't do homework, write letters, watch TV, or read in bed.
>
> **Don't lie awake in bed.** If you cannot fall asleep after 30 minutes, get up and do something else until you are ready to fall asleep.
>
> **Get some exercise regularly each day,** several hours before bedtime.
>
> **Go outdoors for thirty minutes or more each day,** preferably in the late afternoon. This can help set your biological clock.
>
> **Don't go to bed hungry.** Conversely, don't eat a big meal just before bedtime.
>
> **Don't drink alcohol to excess,** and avoid alcohol in the hour or two before sleep.
>
> **Drink caffeinated beverages (coffee, tea, cola) only in the morning,** and consume them in moderation if at all.
>
> **Optimize your sleeping environment.** Make sure it is quiet and dark. Use a face mask or earplugs if necessary to shut out light and noise.
>
> **Make an effort to relax before bedtime.** A warm bath or a few minutes of meditation can promote sleep. Herbal sleep aids, such as a cup of herb tea or a small amount of valerian, can be helpful.

It is worthwhile to try these lifestyle efforts before getting medical help for insomnia. Keep in mind that insomnia does not get better overnight (ha-ha), and it may take a few weeks for good sleep hygiene to work its magic. If it does not, a visit to your doctor may be in order.

Medical Treatment of Insomnia

Your health care provider will work with you to try to find the cause of your insomnia. He or she will ask you some questions, and perhaps perform an exam. The treatment will depend on the apparent cause of the problem.

If insomnia is due to a simple change in routine or some stressful life event, then sleeping medication may help. Sleeping pills do not cure insomnia; they only help a person fall asleep. If the pill is not taken the next night, the insomnia may still be there if the cause has not been addressed. In addition, sleeping pills tend to lose their effectiveness if taken for more than a few weeks. Therefore, they are most useful for insomnia related to a life event.

What about melatonin? This is a naturally occurring hormone that plays a role in the sleep process. It can be purchased as a "dietary supplement" in health food stores. People take it for sleep, and it works for some. It may be safe for short-term use, but keep in mind that melatonin is a powerful hormone. The doses sold are often too high, though, because this substance is not regulated by the FDA, there is no guarantee that the dose on the bottle is what is in the pill. In any case, do not take more than one milligram at night. No one knows the potential long-term consequences of taking melatonin. I would avoid taking it on an ongoing basis.

If insomnia is a symptom of depression, then the depression should be treated. Sometimes sleeping pills are helpful initially, until the treatment for depression begins to work and sleep normalizes.

If insomnia is related to some medical symptom—such as pain, shortness of breath, or frequent nighttime urination—then you and your physician can work on alleviating that problem to allow more uninterrupted sleep.

Sometimes the cause of insomnia is not apparent. In these cases a true sleep disorder may be involved. Examples include sleep apnea, when a person stops breathing during sleep and hence awakens, and "restless legs syndrome," involving involuntary kicking movements during the night. If you sleep with another person, he may be able to provide useful information. Has he noticed that you snore or stop breathing? Do you kick him?

If it appears that you have a sleep disorder, treatment is available. It may require further workup by a specialist, to help characterize the nature of the sleep disorder and to taylor the treatment to your particular problem. But the good news is, nearly all sleep problems can be treated.

Grief and Loss

al: *It's been a month since Barry died. The last year of his life was hell with him being so sick, but between work and taking care of him, I didn't have time to think very much. Now that he's gone the house is terribly quiet. Too quiet. I miss him painfully.*

Every day I cry when something happens that makes me think of him. When I watch TV I avoid the programs he liked because they just make me think about him, and I lose track of what's on the screen. I don't go out to eat at the restaurants we used to go to. It's too upsetting.

Our friends are trying to help. They've been trying to get me out to do things. I keep putting them off. When I do go out, I look at other couples and resent the fact that they still have each other when I've lost Barry.

I find myself angry at Barry for getting sick and dying, which is crazy because realistically I know it wasn't his fault. Then I flog myself for being angry at him.

Work is a good distraction, though my coworkers are keeping their distance. They've stopped asking me how I'm doing because I've told them not to. But after work I come home and just sit.

It'll take me a while before I can really function again. I know life goes on, and I know that Barry would want me to get a life now that he's gone, but it's going to take time.

What Is Grief?

The death of a partner, close friend, or family member is one of the most difficult losses a person can experience. Hal's reaction to Barry's death is very normal. The feelings of grief, loss, emptiness, hopelessness, even anger are painful and can last for weeks, months, or longer. Some people say they are never the same after losing the most important relationship in their life.

Grief is best thought of as a wound in the psyche. Like any wound, it takes time to heal, and as it heals it forms a scar. The pain of the wound, the healing time, and the size of the scar all depend on many factors. These include how important the relationship to the loved one was, how long it had lasted, how the loss occurred, and how the survivor deals with the grief afterwards.

A Variety of Losses Can Lead to Grieving

Without volunteering, gay men have become experts at dealing with grief and loss. The first phase of the AIDS epidemic taught our community a great deal about loss. For years many of us were in a perpetual state of mourning as our friends, lovers, and community leaders succumbed to the plague. The obituaries were the most interesting section of the gay newspapers in a tragic sort of way

Things are better now, and the obituaries take up less space in the papers, but the epidemic is far from over, and people continue to die from AIDS. Many men who survived the epidemic have suffered the loss of most or all of their closest friends, and some remain numb and shell-shocked from the experience, like Holocaust survivors. They are faced in middle age with the challenge of assembling an entire new support network. Many have told me that they just don't have the energy for this, and as a result they are isolated and lonely.

It is not only AIDS, of course, that claims the lives of gay men, and the process of grief is basically the same whether a person loses a loved one to AIDS, cancer, a heart attack, an accident, or suicide. Only the details are different. Profound grief can come from the loss not only of a partner but of a close friend or family member. I have seen men suffer painfully from the death of a buddy, parent, or sibling, and they are as deeply effected as men who have lost their lovers.

It is not only death that can cause a loss worth grieving. Many times I have seen men in mind-numbing grief over a relationship that has ended or at the loss of their career or their health or their youth. Much of the pain—and the stages of healing—are the same as if a loved one had died.

Manifestations of Normal Grief

The symptoms of grief are very similar to the symptoms of depression and may be indistinguishable. The grieving person may suffer lack of energy and motivation, difficulty concentrating, insomnia, social withdrawal, loss of appetite, weight loss, and loss of a sense of purpose in life. To an extent, all of this is a normal reaction to the pain of losing someone so important, and it does not mean the grieving person is suffering from a clinical depression.

It is also normal for the survivor to feel anger toward the person who has died: "How could you do that? How could you leave me?" These feelings then sometimes lead to guilt at feeling angry toward someone who is dead.

There is also such a thing as pathologic grief. This is a grief reaction that is more extreme and/or longer lasting than normal grieving. In this case, the grieving person may begin acting irrationally. He may stop eating, stop bathing, stop going to work, not answer the phone, not pay bills. He may tell friends that he wants to join his loved one who has died.

Pathologic grief is a very serious and potentially lethal situation. It demands professional intervention. More than once I have seen a bereaved man commit suicide while suffering from pathologic grief. If you or someone you know appear to be grieving pathologically, get help as soon as possible.

Help for Grief

Most people get through normal grief without professional help. Their friends and family provide support. Gradually the wounds heal. Survivors sometimes find comfort in spirituality, which they may rediscover during the grieving process.

Human cultures have institutionalized various rituals, such as funerals and memorial services, to help the survivors deal with the emotions surrounding grief. In my experience, these rituals can be very useful.

For example, the Jewish religion, with which I am most familiar, has some strict guidelines to be followed when someone dies. The body must be buried within 24 hours, which immediately gives a sense of finality to the death. This is followed by a prescribed series of rituals over the subsequent weeks and months, making the grieving process less of an unknown. Two of these have helped me when grieving the death of my mother many years ago. One which is called *shiva,* is basically a week of potlucks immediately following the death. Each evening friends and neighbors bring food and hold a brief service at the home of the bereaved family. The other, which is called the *unveiling,* is a graveside ceremony on the one-year anniversary of the death. At this time the tombstone is displayed for the first time, and a service is conducted that formally concludes the one-year period of mourning.

Unfortunately, most Americans tend not to observe such rituals, which would help guide them through and out of their time of grief. We gay people, in particular, could develop more elaborate grief rituals that fit with our culture. If we can create our own commitment ceremonies to celebrate our loving partnerships, then we can create beautiful bereavement rituals to celebrate the lives of our gay brothers who have died and to support those who grieve them. The AIDS quilt is an example of a wonderful, innovative bereavement ritual that has helped thousands of people memorialize and celebrate those they have lost.

I have been to some heartwarming memorial services for gay men who have died. But after that, there is nothing, except perhaps a quilt panel if the cause of death was AIDS. And all too often the obituary states, "There will be no memorial service." The survivors are left to flounder with their painful feelings.

Assistance From a Health Care Provider

Many men suffering from normal grief see their doctors for help with the pain. Sometimes they ask directly for help. Other times they ask indirectly. The premise for the visit is for some other complaint—often insomnia—or an ache or pain somewhere. But the real reason is that they are suffering from the pain of grief.

When I see someone who is grieving my first task is to try to figure out whether the grief reaction is normal or extreme or pathologic. Usually it is the former, and in that case my job is often just to reassure the person that he is going through a normal process. The painful feelings are natural when someone so important is gone from one's life.

Some of the more troubling symptoms of normal grief, such as anxiety or insomnia, may be treated with small amounts of a mild tranquilizer or sleeping pill, for a limited period of time. I do not believe that that sort of medication interferes with the natural healing of grief, and it can make the process a whole lot easier to get through.

Additionally because of the AIDS epidemic, in many locales there are therapists and clergy who are skilled at helping gay men get through the grieving process. There are also grief-and-loss support groups for survivors of people who have died from AIDS. Often these groups are welcoming to gay men who have lost loved ones to other causes. I make referrals to such groups frequently.

In the case of a pathologic grief reaction, the grieving person should be taken very seriously by his health care provider. He needs to be treated similarly to anyone else who is profoundly depressed. In such cases I make a referral to a skilled psychotherapist, and I enlist the support of close friends of the grieving man to check in on him frequently.

I prescribe antidepressant medication to individuals suffering from pathologic grief. In such cases I tell the person that his normal grief has turned into a serious, life-threatening problem but that it can be treated and that wanting to feel better is not disrespectful to the memory of his loved one who has died. I tell him that the best way he can honor the memory of his departed loved one is to take care of himself. Nevertheless, suicide can and does occur.

A Postscript to Hal's Story

Hal survived and overcame his grief, as he and I predicted he would. Of course loss and grief are painful. But they are part of life. Life is a series of beginnings and endings, hellos and good-byes. We can allow the good-byes to hurt and scar us, or we can grow stronger and wiser with the memory of loved ones whom we have lost.

I know that the hundreds of thousands of gay men who have died of AIDS would be very proud of the way we survivors have dealt with our losses. Not to say that the losses have not profoundly affected our community. Of course they have. But in a way, they have also strengthened our community. We honor those we have lost by not forgetting them and by continuing with our lives in a way we all can take pride in.

Life Issues

Men often seek help from their doctors in dealing with life issues. In the following sections we will discuss a number of important life events and circumstances and how they impact gay men. We will identify ways in which a gay man can deal with these events in a healthy way and still maintain psychological well-being.

Why are life issues included in a book of health advice? Because all of these issues relate, to some degree, to a person's health. As the personal physician for hundreds of gay men, I am impressed at how frequently my patients seek counsel from me about some event in their lives. Major life events can have a huge impact on our health.

Some of these topics are universal. We all must deal with coming out, and we all age, and we all must die. For some these events are traumatic. Others find resources, internal or external that can help them through these processes gracefully.

Throughout our lives as gay men we have particular legal needs that relate to our medical care and to the quality of our lives. I always mention these legal issues to my patients at some point. Often I am the first person to have done so.

Other topics apply only to certain gay men. Some of us have experienced the joy of being parents or are planning parenthood. Far from joyful is domestic violence, an unfortunate part of some gay relationships, and one that the medical profession is only lately trying to recognize and address.

Illness is a process that most of us experience at some time in our lives. The issues of how to deal with chronic medical problems, disability, and death have become very important to many gay men because of the AIDS epidemic. But many other medical situations aside from AIDS can affect our health and our lives. Chronic illness and disability are a part of many of our lives. We can learn to adapt to this, not letting the illness rule us, while optimizing our quality of life.

Self-esteem and Coming Out

Paul: *I came out at age 19, in college, but it took me years to really feel OK about being gay. At age 20 I came out to my parents, with the feeling that they might reject me. They didn't—they embraced me—but I continued to feel embarrassed and ashamed at my gayness. In my 20s I couldn't figure out what I wanted to do with my life, and it had to do with my poor self-esteem. I had done well in school, but as a gay man I saw my career options being pretty narrow. The only gay people I knew of were flight attendants, ballet dancers, waiters, or florists. Not that there is anything wrong with those professions, but none of them seemed like something I wanted to do.*

In my mid 20s I entered therapy. My therapist helped me a lot, and I realized that I wanted to be in a helping profession. By then I had met some gay people who were nurses, doctors, and social workers, and I ultimately decided to become a psychologist. I went back to school at age 27, and I knew from that moment that I had found my calling as a gay man. Now I am in private practice, and I have many gay men as clients. Being gay is a big part of my professional life, and yet every day I'm still coming out, and I'm still working on that self-esteem.

Self-esteem Is Part of Health

Self-esteem is a huge issue for gay men. We keep using the word *pride* in connection with *gay,* as if maybe some day it will really sink in. Sure, we've come a long way since Stonewall, but gay people are still stigmatized in Western society. We are one of the few groups that can legally be discriminated against in many parts of the United States and in many aspects of life.

Even those political leaders who profess to respect our rights will only go so far and often cave in to bigotry when it comes to support of equal standing for us in the military or legalization of our right to marry. Certain religious leaders continue to feel free to call us "sinners" and worse. No wonder then that many gay men have problems with self-esteem. If society repeatedly sends messages that you are inferior, a sinner, not "normal," it is natural that some of that sinks in.

Pride and Health Are Related

There now is evidence from studies of African-Americans that the stress caused by discrimination can lead to serious medical problems. A Harvard researcher has shown that blacks who accept unfair treatment or deny that they experience prejudice have higher blood pressure than those who face and challenge discrimination. High blood pressure leads to serious problems, including heart attack and stroke.

By analogy, gay people who accept the status quo, live in hiding, accept society's homophobia, and even possibly try to "change" or "become heterosexual" may be putting themselves at risk of medical problems. Those who own their gayness and take pride in it and challenge society's unfair and unequal treatment of gay men and other sexual minorities are doing their mental and physical health a favor. In other words, gay pride is good for your health.

Coming Out—Its Difficulties and Its Benefits

Because of the stigma attached to homosexuality, many gay men take some time to accept their sexual identity for themselves, and then they take more time to reveal their gay identity to others. Most of us are born into heterosexual families, and as we grow we begin to realize that we are different. And what are we going to do with that information? This "coming out of the closet" process may be fast or slow, and it really is a lifelong process. Even if a man thinks he is completely out of the closet, he has to come out all over again whenever he deals with someone who does not know him.

Some people—myself included—feel that coming out is a unique and valuable experience for gay men and other sexual-minority people and that the soul-searching and self-examination involved are part of what makes us especially sensitive, creative, and intuitive. It is our baptism of fire. Maybe that's just my gay chauvinism talking, but I truly believe it. Heterosexuals usually do not have the experience of discovering that they are something other than what is expected and coming to terms with that and accepting that and becoming proud of it.

Some people become very scarred by this baptism of fire or do not survive the ordeal. Teenagers who are gay or who are questioning their sexual orientation have a significant risk of contemplating, planning, attempting, and successfully completing suicide. There have been several studies indicating that the suicide risk for gay teens is three or more times greater than that of their nongay peers. Some of these studies have been criticized for flawed research methodology, but newer studies using more valid sampling techniques have come to the same conclusion. In addition, surveys of street youth reveal that a disproportionate number of them are gay kids who have run away from their rejecting families.

Coming out is frightening for anyone but especially for an adolescent who does not have a lot of life experience. It's a difficult decision. One can remain in the closet and keep a very important aspect of his life hidden from those around him. Or one can come out and be open, sharing this wonderful aspect of himself but risking rejection or condemnation in the process.

Coming out is not a one-step event; it is a lifelong, evolutionary process, and every gay man is at his own stage. Along the way, one's degree of closetedness influences his relationships with his family, his coworkers, and society at large. In my practice I see a wide range of closetedness among gay men. Some keep their gayness so secret that only a few people know about their sexual orientation. Other men's whole lives are about being gay, and they are as out of the closet as anyone can be. And there is a huge spectrum in between. It is easy for a very out gay man to put down one who is more closeted. But remember, it's an unsupportive culture we live in, and many men would have a lot at stake if they ventured out of the closet.

Nevertheless, closets are definitely health hazards. The air gets awfully stuffy in there. Being closeted is stressful, and stress of that sort is not healthy. It is not fun to live in fear of discovery. Closetedness can be bad for self-esteem because hiding implies that there is something shameful about a person just because he happens to be gay. Men who are having a protracted struggle with their coming-out process seem to be less happy and relaxed than people who are further out of the closet.

But coming out is not without its price. Revealing can be difficult and threatening. There is the chance of losing relationships with people who are important. Often when a gay man decides to step out of the closet, he does so with the knowledge that he may be rejected by people he loves.

Granted, many of my patients have very supportive parents, siblings, children, friends, and coworkers who appreciate them for who they are as gay men. But others have been shunned or disowned by their families of origin. I have patients who have not spoken with their parents in 20 years or more and don't even know whether they are still living. That is very sad. It's a great loss.

It's much easier to be openly gay if you live in a city with a liberal atmosphere. If you live in a small town or in a more conservative city, the stakes of coming out are much higher. Still, there are many rural gay men who are completely out of the closet and accepted by their local community.

In summary, the best way to build self-esteem and to be happy and healthy as a gay man is to be honest and open about who you are and to live your life in a way that makes you proud of yourself. It's very helpful to have positive gay role models. We gay men have far too few.

For many of my patients, having a gay doctor is a big boost for their own self-esteem. If their doctor is gay, well, then it must be OK to be gay. I also enjoy serving as a mentor for gay medical students and other health care professionals in training. It's important for those of use who are secure in our lives as gay men and in our careers to serve as role models for others. And we can't do this unless we are out of the closet.

Parenthood

Being gay is not incompatible with being a parent. Many gay or bisexual men have children from previous marriages or relationships. Gay men who are single or in a same-sex relationship also have various parenthood options. It takes more planning for gay men to become parents than it does for many heterosexual people. As a doctor, I am usually involved to some degree when my gay male patients become parents. For example:

Jaime and Victor: *We are applying to adopt our 5-year-old foster son. We wanted to try out parenthood first, so we applied to be foster parents. Billy had had a difficult background, and the agency was happy to place him with a stable couple. After a year, the three of us seem to make a good family, so we're planning to make it permanent.*

Jerome: *My sister is a heroin addict, and when she went to prison I applied to the court for custody of her baby girl. My sister has given me permission to adopt her, and I'm planning to adopt as a single parent. Emily can attend the day-care facility at the law firm where I work. I never expected to be a daddy, but I'm happy about it.*

David and Dave: *We decided to have our own biological children after we had been a couple for six years. A female friend of ours agreed to be a surrogate mother. Dave contributed the sperm, and she used a syringe for insemination, and it only took three tries. Now we have a beautiful daughter. We'd like a second child, by David, with the same mother, but the mother is not excited about doing it again, so we're looking for another surrogate mom. Dave's sister might be interested, which would be cool because then the kids would be biologically related to each other.*

Adoption

Prospective adoptive parents must pass a health screen. In this situation my patients come to me for a physical exam and various other tests that are required by the adoption agency. In my experience—granted that I work in a liberal part of the country—men who are HIV-positive have not been excluded from adopting.

Adoption by gay people is easier in some parts of the country than others. In Seattle, where I practice, adoption by a gay couple or single gay man is not a problem at all. In some other parts of the country, adoption may be difficult or impossible. It is specifically illegal for gay people to adopt in certain states. In fact, children have been taken away from their gay or lesbian biological parents because of the parents' sexual orientation.

If you are considering adoption, you will need to explore the legal environment in the area where you reside. Local gay advocacy organizations may be helpful, and some places have support and information resources for gay or lesbian people who are considering adoption.

Biological Parenthood

Gay men who are considering fathering a child biologically with a female friend or a surrogate mom should also have a medical evaluation. Here the main goal is to screen for infections that could be passed on to the mom and/or baby during the insemination process.

Specifically, before inseminating, the prospective father needs to be screened for HIV, syphilis, hepatitis B, and hepatitis C. Syphilis can be cured, but a man who is infected with HIV or with the hepatitis B or C viruses should not donate semen because there is a significant risk that the mother will become infected.

If all the tests are negative, it is a good idea to wait three months, avoiding any new sexual exposures, then retest again before inseminating. In addition, the prospective gay male parent should also be screened for any potentially serious genetic disorders for which he may be at risk—such as sickle-cell disease, cystic fibrosis, or Tay-Sachs syndrome—which could be passed on to the child.

Questions and Answers

Gay men sometimes ask me medical questions about parenthood, such as:

I am HIV-positive. Is there a safe way for me to become a father?

Yes, by adoption. Otherwise, even if you are on medication that appears to be completely suppressing your HIV infection, there is still a chance that your semen could infect the prospective mother with HIV. In Europe there are clinics that will "wash" the sperm of an HIV-infected man and use it for insemination, but in the United States no one I am aware of is willing to take that chance.

My partner and I do not want the responsibilities of parenthood, but a lesbian friend wants one or both of us to donate sperm so that she can have a child. What do you advise?

First, you will need to be clear about who will have what responsibilities for the prospective child. Do you want to be involved in its upbringing at all? Will you have any financial responsibility for it? It's important to consult an attorney and get an agreement written up to avoid conflicts later over custody and financial responsibility.

Second, the sperm donor needs a health screen, as described earlier in this section.

Third, the mechanics of insemination are quite straightforward. The mother needs to determine when during her monthly cycle she is fertile. At that time insemination can be done by intercourse, which is not the method of choice for most gay men or lesbians in this situation.

Most commonly, the man will masturbate and ejaculate into a jar, and then the woman can use a syringe to inseminate herself with the (fresh) semen. She'll know where to put it, and you don't have to be there. This is the preferred method of "alternative" insemination for gay men and lesbians. No doctor need be involved with the insemination, except to provide a sterile jar (urine specimen cups work well) and syringes.

Is there any way for two men to have a baby together? Can a sperm from each of us be used to fertilize one egg so that the baby really has two fathers?

No. An embryo develops from an egg that has been fertilized by a single sperm. Two sperm cannot fertilize one egg and form a viable embryo.

What about if we mix our sperm and give it to the mother for insemination?

Not recommended. This can lead to psychological, medical, and legal difficulties. Such a child and the child's parents will find it hard not to wonder who the biological father is. Medically, it's important to know who the father is so that family tendencies for various medical problems can be known. If mixed sperm are used for fertilization, and there is ever a custody conflict, a paternity test will need to be performed. The child can still have two daddies, but it's a good idea to know which one donated the sperm. (Donating is the easiest part of being a daddy! Raising the kid is the hard part.)

If the two of us have a child, biologically or by adoption, will it be hard for that child growing up? What are the chances the child will be gay or lesbian?

Studies have found that the children of same-sex couples are as well-adjusted as other children. Kids always tease each other about something or other, but kids of gay or lesbian parents tend to grow up being very resilient and proud of their parents. These kids have no more chance of turning out gay or lesbian than any other kids. After all, despite the fact that most gay people grew up with heterosexual parents, we still turned out to be gay.

Most important, with two dads, what will the child call each of us?

Many kids with two dads call one "Daddy" and one "Papa," or a variation on that theme. Some call them by their first names: "Frank" and "Joe," or "Daddy Frank" and "Daddy Joe." I have seen children raised by a couple that the kid calls "Frank" and "Uncle Joe," but that reflects a situation where the child considers only one member of the couple to be the father. Incidentally, a heterosexual couple I know, who have many gay friends with children, recently told me that their daughter has started to call both of her parents "Papa" because she decided she wants to have two daddies just like her friends. The world is changing.

Domestic Violence

dam, a healthy man in his 30s who had been coming to me for several years, paid a visit because of a few days of cough and low-grade fevers. As I applied my stethoscope to his back to listen to his lungs, I noticed a large bruise on the back of his upper arm. I asked Adam about it.

At first he tried to tell me he had fallen. I remarked that it was an odd place to fall on and went on with the exam. I noticed some faded bruises on Adam's trunk and made a mental note to ask him about them after the exam. Before I got the chance, Adam told me that no, he hadn't fallen, that actually his boyfriend, Kam, had grabbed him there. Adam told me his story.

Adam: *I've never talked about this to anyone. I don't know what to do. I love him, and I just don't understand. Before we lived together things were wonderful for us. Something changed about the time I moved into his apartment a year ago. I remember how startled I was the first time he yelled at me. It was about something trivial—I think I had opened a bill that was addressed to him. Then it happened more and more frequently.*

At first it would happen if I looked at other men when we were out. We might be driving down the street, and I'd look out the window, and he'd holler at me if he thought I was looking at a man on the sidewalk. Then when we got home he'd scream and yell and call me awful names—whore, scumbag, things like that.

He got very possessive. He stopped letting me answer our phone. If it rings and I reach for it, he'll grab my arm, slam it down, and say, "Expecting a call from your boyfriend?" When my friends call, he tells them I'm not home. I can't really leave the apartment any more on my own except to go to work or, today, to come here. If I am the least bit late getting home, I have to give a good excuse, and then sometimes he hits me anyway.

I don't remember when he first started beating on me, but at some point yelling wasn't enough. He punches me, grabs me, shakes me. Sometimes he hits my head against the wall.

He's thrown cans of food at me. I know enough to duck, but there are marks on the walls of our apartment. There's always some reason, something I've done, even if I can't figure out what it is. Sometimes he gets mad at me because I don't know what I did wrong.

If I start to cry, then he calms down, apologizes, says it will never happen again, comforts me, holds me, tells me he loves me—we end up have sex. He's very passionate after he's been angry, but the next day it's the same nightmare again.

I'm afraid to tell my friends, or my family. They all love Kam, and I was so proud when I introduced him to them. What can I do now? How can I make him stop?

The Pattern of Domestic Violence

Domestic violence can occur in any relationship, and it is not uncommon in domestic relationships between two men. Battering is a problem that many gay men are reluctant to acknowledge. The victim often believes it's his fault, and that if only he could change his behavior, the violence would stop. He may be embarrassed and ashamed and not know where to get help.

The batterer has the attitude that it is his right to control the behavior and feelings of his partner and that the violence is somehow justified because of this. He blames the violence on the behavior of his victim. Irrational jealousy and possessiveness are commonly part of the pattern. It is often unclear who is the batterer and who is the victim. In some couples, the battering is mutual. Substance abuse is usually involved in domestic violence, generally by the aggressor but often by the victim as well.

The violence usually begins subtly and escalates gradually. The abuse may be verbal, psychological, physical, sexual, or (usually) some combination. It may take some time for the victim to acknowledge to himself that he is being abused. Each episode tends to follow a cycle of anger, violence, and apology or bargaining, as in the case of Adam and Kam.

Note that domestic violence is not—I repeat, *not*—the same as sadomasochism. S/M is a healthy form of consensual sex play involving roles, power, and sometimes bondage, humiliation, or pain. But it is safe, sane, consensual, and often playful. It is not abusive—a totally different situation from domestic violence. Do not confuse them.

Unchecked domestic violence can lead to serious physical injury or even the death of either party. Victims of battering are frequently subject to depression, anxiety, substance abuse, or suicide.

Coming to Terms With Domestic Violence

It is difficult for anyone to acknowledge being part of a battering relationship. For gay men it may be particularly difficult. Our relationships are often a badge of our success in life as gay men. When a gay man admits that he is being abused by his partner, he must acknowledge that his relationship has failed big time. In addition, it is hard for any male to admit that he is being beat up repeatedly.

It is also hard for others to see how someone could stay within a battering relationship and allow the situation to continue. But the victim is controlled by fear, and it can be very difficult to leave. Furthermore, although there are many shelters for battered women, few communities offer support for male victims of battering, gay or straight. Where will the victim go, especially if he has been threatened with harm or death if he attempts to leave his batterer?

I am sure that I do not find out about many instances of domestic violence among my patients. Frankly, I don't routinely ask my patients unless I see bruises or other clues. I probably should. Patients seldom volunteer the information. Sometimes I find out when one or both of the members of the couple end up in jail. When I do find out, I do what I can to help the couple resolve the situation.

If you are in a battering relationship, it is OK to tell your doctor. There is no law that requires the doctor to report the story to your partner or to the authorities. But the doctor can work with you to help you figure out how to end the pattern of violence.

Escaping the Situation

Nothing you do can change a battering partner so that he stops his abuse. The only solution is to get out. This can be difficult if, as is often the case, the batterer controls the money, car keys, and other items necessary for escape. The batterer may also threaten to hunt you down and "get you" if you leave. This is not an idle threat. Women have been stalked, assaulted, and killed by ex-partners who had battered them, and the same is undoubtedly true of gay men.

But there is always a way out. One man saved up money by hiding it in the freezer until he had enough for a bus ticket out of town. Several of my patients have escaped from a battering situation, at least temporarily, by calling 911 during or right after an assault by their partner. Sometimes the wrong party gets arrested or both spend the night in jail but usually the police get the right man.

While the batterer is incarcerated, the victim should get a "no-contact" order preventing the batterer from returning to the scene of the crime. It is also a good idea to move away because a "no contact" order can easily be violated.

Unfortunately, jail terms for batterers are usually brief, and the victim tends to be there waiting when the batterer returns from jail, continuing the pattern.

Batterers can be helped. Patients of mine have learned to stop battering, usually by attending anger-management group therapy or via individual psychotherapy. Usually the motivation is the loss of a relationship or the threat of such a loss. Treatment is often court-ordered in lieu of jail time.

Some batterers are only violent when they are intoxicated, which is a sure sign of a substance-abuse problem. Getting clean and sober, with the aid of a substance-abuse treatment program, can help them end their violent behavior.

Prevention and Early Intervention

The very first step in combating domestic violence is acknowledging that it exists. As a community, we must stop denying that gay men can beat on each other. We protest when we are subject to violence from outside our community. We must also admit that we can be subject to violence from our friends and lovers. With that awareness we can take care of it early, before it goes too far. It is certainly possible. For example:

Walkker: *I don't know about this dating business. Recently I met a man who seemed really sweet, and he definitely showed a strong interest in me. I'm just out of a difficult relationship, and I told him I needed to take things really slow. Last Friday evening was our third date. We had gone out for dinner and had had a few drinks. We hadn't had sex yet, and after we kissed good night outside his door, he invited me in. I was starting to explain that I didn't feel quite ready for that when he went totally ballistic. He grabbed me and shook me and started ranting and raving, calling me names. I broke free and ran away. Since then he's left me the sweetest, most apologetic messages on my answering machine. He sent me flowers at work, but forget it. No one gets a second chance after treating me that way. There are other fish in the sea.*

See the pattern here? Anger, violence, then apology, bargaining. This is how the cycle of battering begins. Not a good omen for a long-term relationship. Walkker did the right thing to end it when he did. If someone close to you is violent with you for the first time, don't let there be a second time. It is their problem, not yours, so get out while you can. It only gets harder to leave as time goes on.

Aging

ook in the mirror. How old are you? Who do you see? The man you are now, or the one you were ten, 20, or 40 years ago? Every day we age imperceptibly, and gradually we become old. Sometimes our image of ourselves lags behind our chronological age. Then suddenly one day reality hits, and this can precipitate an emotional crisis. One response is to try to fight the aging process in ways that may not be physically or emotionally healthy. A better response is to accept the natural changes that come with age, and do it with grace.

The fact is that life is a one-way trip, and aging is part of the ride. Many men would like to complete their journey without getting older along the way, instead staying young forever like Peter Pan. The ideal for these people would be to have the wisdom of an old man, and the body of a young man.

But of course that is just a fantasy. The best we all can hope for is to age gracefully and yet remain youthful in all of the important ways—to retain our vigor, our vitality, our ability to love, laugh, and cry, our feeling that we are an important part of our culture. For a gay man the latter can be especially difficult.

Aging in the Gay Community

American culture—and American gay culture in particular—seems to over-value youth. Age is not particularly respected in our society, even though older people have much to offer. When we are young, often the only elderly people we know are our grandparents or other relatives. Certainly it is rare that we meet any gay elders when we are young. Perhaps this is part of why some gay men have so much trouble with getting older. We don't have enough good role models, enough older gay men we can look up to.

Why do gay men have so very few senior role models? In part, it is because of a fundamental difference between the current generations of gay men. The oldest gay men presently living have spent much of their adult lives in a culture that did not permit them to be openly gay. Far fewer gay elders are out of the closet compared to younger gay men. Sometimes we only discover that a prominent octogenarian artist, composer, or author was gay when his obituary mentions that he is survived by a male "companion."

In addition, our gay community as a whole could do better at recognizing and supporting our elders and in the process make it easier for all of us to grow old gracefully. Open any gay magazine or newspaper and you will see how highly valued youth is. Look at the photos in the display ads. Look at the articles about gay celebrities and achievers. You would almost have to conclude that gay men disappear from the face of the earth sometime during their 30s. Well, maybe their 40s—at the latest.

But they don't. Gay men live as long as anyone else, as I see every day in my work. I am fortunate to have been able to take over the oldest gay medical practice in Seattle, where my predecessor, a gay man, had been taking care of gay men since the 1960s. As a result, there are many senior gay men in my practice. My oldest gay male patient is in his 90s, and I take care of many gay men in their 50s, 60s, 70s, and 80s—in addition to many younger men.

Many gay men do not have this experience of meeting other gay men of all ages. We all tend to socialize with our peers. Because there is little socializing between gay men of different generations, many younger gay men seem unaware that gay elders exist. A valuable opportunity for role modeling is being lost. Because younger gay men don't have enough older role models, the natural tendency is to be apprehensive about growing older. Because older gay men came of age in a different, less supportive culture, they may have few peer role models. We naturally tend to fear what we don't know, so the lack of models of gay aging can make growing older a difficult prospect for all of us.

The Goal: Aging Gracefully

At work I see a different spectrum of the gay men's community than I see in the gay media. I see a community that includes men of all ages, all generations. I see many beautiful older gay men who are aging gracefully. Here are some examples:

George just turned 82. He walks two miles daily and swims three days a week. His blood pressure has been a little high lately, but when I gave him medication for it, his erections became weaker. George is single but has a 68-year-old fuck buddy, Daniel, who made him ask me about alternatives to the medication. Now George is working on his diet and increasing his exercise program in an attempt to control his blood pressure without medication. His erections are back to normal, and he and Daniel are satisfied with their sex life again.

Paul and John are in their early 60s and they look their age. In fact, they look like twin Santa Clauses, complete with big bellies and bushy white beards. They have known each other for 20 years, and love each other dearly, but work and family obligations have kept them from developing a deeper relationship. When they first met, each was married to a woman. Now both are widowed, and both are granddads. They have just moved in together to start their life as a couple. In celebration, they had a reunion of their children and grandchildren, and all agreed they were perfect for each other.

George, Paul, and John are happy men. They are not young, they are not pretending to be younger than they are, and they are comfortable with their lives as gay men.

On the other hand, I also see some men who are ungracefully fighting the aging process and becoming battle-scarred. The following is a composite portrait of a man who is struggling with growing older.

Ringo turned 50 this year. He has had a face-lift and a hair transplant and wants to know a good clinic where he can get liposuction. He has never had a long-term lover, and he is panicking that he will not be able to find one. He tells his dates that he is 39. He looks like a 50-year-old man who is trying to look younger. He continues to smoke and drink to excess and says he does not have time to exercise. He tans regularly because he feels it makes him more attractive. From his smoking and sunbathing his face had become leathery and wrinkled. Since the facelift it is leathery and smooth, like a mask or the skin of a burn victim. Ringo is not interested in my advice regarding smoking, drinking, and exercise because he says his work is too busy, and it would be stressful for him to change his lifestyle at this time. He takes medication for an ulcer and for high blood pressure. He is unhappy and doesn't understand why.

In these examples, who would you rather be? Who seems younger and who seems older? Who seems happier?

Some Advice

The point is, that people who remain vigorous and happy, who are comfortable with who they are, and who take care of themselves tend to age with grace. It is much healthier to deal with aging in that way than to deal with it by using medication, surgery, and cosmetics to combat the signs of age.

The next question is, how can you maintain your vigor as you grow older? How can you grow old gracefully? Here are some ways that are generally suggested by doctors and that seem to be working for those of my patients who are aging successfully.

Stay physically active. Develop good exercise habits when you are young. Find a time in your schedule for at least half an hour of vigorous exercise each day, and stick with it. It's never to late to start, so if you are older and are not in the habit of exercising, start now! Brisk walking is an easy exercise that doesn't require any special equipment or facility. Walk to and from work, or the grocery store, if possible, or take the stairs rather than the elevator at work, or take a brisk walk some time each day. Don't use bad weather as an excuse not to walk daily; that is why God made shopping malls. (I knew they had to be good for something.) If walking doesn't appeal to you, there are many other forms of exercise, of course. The important thing is to find one that suits you, to make the time for it in your routine, and to prioritize it. Look at the section on exercise for more ideas.

Don't smoke. Smokers age faster than nonsmokers, have many more illnesses, lose their stamina at a younger age, and die younger. There are very few smokers over 70 years old. Most of them have either died or quit—often because of smoking-related illnesses. If you smoke, and plan to live into your 70s, you might as well quit now. In addition to the emphysema, heart attacks, and lung cancer that smokers get, men who smoke are much more likely to have sexual dysfunction as they age. Furthermore, smokers have more wrinkles. When researchers showed people photos of smokers and nonsmokers of the same age and asked them to guess their age, the smokers appeared to be five to ten years older than the nonsmokers.

Try to maintain friendships with people who are vigorous and enjoy life. Some older men tell me they prefer the company of younger people because their friends just "act too old," whatever that means. Others have found a circle of similar-aged peers who are remaining active and enthusiastic, year after year. In some cities there are social support groups for older gay men. This is a great way to network and to maintain a circle of peers. New York

City has an advocacy agency called Senior Action in a Gay Environment. In my town, Seattle, we have a social organization for older gay people called Mature Friends. If there isn't a similar group where you live, maybe you'd like to start one.

Exercise your brain. Develop interests that continue to challenge you. Work, hobbies, projects, or volunteering all help give life meaning and purpose. Some of my older gay patients have found it particularly rewarding to volunteer for AIDS support organizations, but the possibilities are limitless.

A Few Words About Sexuality

Aging gracefully means accepting that some things do change with age. Interest in sex can decline, for example, as can a man's sexual ability. A man's sexual peak is in his teens, a fact that seems more and more unfair as one gets older. Although sex drive and ability may decline with age, you should expect to have satisfactory sexual function your whole life. Granted, at age 60 you might not be able to orgasm three times in one day like you did when you were 18. But daily orgasm is still possible for many, and there are lots of seniors who have sex (solo or accompanied) on a very regular basis—be it daily, weekly, or monthly. (Being older does not mean that one is immune to HIV infection, though. Gay men in their 60s and 70s can—and do—become infected if they are not careful. I have seen it.)

The key to maintaining sexual function is "use it or lose it." The older guys I see who are sexually active have been that way their whole lives. They may masturbate regularly, and/or they may have a regular partner or partners or go to a sex club. Whatever. The point is, you've got to keep up with it to keep getting it up. Besides, regular ejaculation cleans out the plumbing, and some urologists maintain that men who remain sexually active have fewer prostate problems as they get older. My patients with prostatitis are often amused by the urologists' advice that they should ejaculate more frequently.

The prostate does tend to grow with age. Since the prostate surrounds the urethra (the tube that carries urine from the bladder out through the penis), an enlarged prostate can put pressure on the urine flow and cause difficulties with the stream. The section on prostate health more fully explains this situation and what can be done about it.

That "Mature" Look

Of course our physical appearance inevitably changes with age. Hair gets gray or white or falls out on top (male pattern baldness, it's called). Hair can be dyed; baldness can be covered with a wig or "repaired" with hair transplantation. But as a bald-and-proud man myself, I'd like to suggest that it's easier to accept graying and balding as a part of life. I resent any implication that just because I'm balding, I'm not sexy. Actually, the fact that I'm losing my hair means that I've got a lot of testosterone, lots of male hormones.

To prove to yourself that bald is sexy, conjure up the image of a sexy bald daddy like Patrick Stewart or Sean Connery. I think most gay men would have to admit that these two guys are pretty attractive. Now imagine them with wigs. Would that make them any sexier? It's not whether a man has hair but how he presents himself that makes him attractive.

The same with gray or white hair. Ernest Hemingway, in his later years, had a thick head of white hair and a close-cropped white beard. I recently saw a news item describing an Ernest Hemingway look-alikes convention held in Key West, Fla., where Hemingway lived. The accompanying photo showed a room full of very sexy daddy types, all with white hair and trimmed white beards. It looked more like a scene from a local gay bar on Daddy's Night than some Hemingway event. No one could see these guys and say they didn't look hot.

Wrinkles are part of aging too. There is nothing wrong with having them. But there are ways to prevent more extreme cases of wrinkles:

Stay out of the sun. That bronze tan that makes you look so attractive when you're twenty will cover your face with wrinkles (and maybe skin cancers) when you're forty. There is nothing, I repeat nothing, healthy about tanning, and we need to change our concept of what is attractive so that tanning is not desirable.

Don't smoke. Smoking makes your skin lose its elasticity, and it wrinkles up.

Choose your parents well. People with more delicate skin tend to wrinkle more with age. People whose skin is naturally darker—for example, those of African, Asian, or Mediterranean ancestry—wrinkle less because their skin is more resistant to the effects of sun damage.

If you have wrinkles and don't like them, there is a medication, tretinoin (Retin-A or Renova) that can smooth them. This is available by prescription in the United States. Again, you have to ask yourself, "Is it worth it?" Cosmetic surgery can also reduce wrinkles, but this is a big step to be considered carefully. See the section on cosmetic surgery for a more detailed discussion.

One Last Bit of Advice

The older a man gets, the more important it is that he have a relationship with a primary physician. There are many changes that occur as we age, some normal and expected, some abnormal and serious. If problems are identified soon, they are easier to fix. Your health care provider can help advise you about good habits that will keep you feeling and looking vigorous as you get older. And if you really must have that face lift, tummy tuck, or hair transplant, your primary doc probably knows the best place to get one.

Dealing With Illness

hen you are healthy it is easy to take good health for granted. Health is usually defined in a negative way—as the absence of illness—and illness is what most of us want to avoid. We'd rather not spend our time and energy being distracted by pain or discomfort. We have more important things to do!

Even a little thing—like a headache or a sprained ankle or a cold—can be a big interference with your life. It is also a reminder of how precious your health is. The goal of preventive care is to stay healthy and avoid illness. Good health habits give a gay man his best chance to stay healthy. Such habits include regular exercise, proper diet, avoidance of cigarettes and of excesses in alcohol and recreational drug use, and taking care to have sex safely.

Illness Can Be Acute or Chronic

Most of us, whatever our habits, eventually develop medical problems that need to be dealt with. Some problems—such as the flu, a bladder infection or a broken arm—either get better by themselves or can be permanently "fixed" or cured. These are called *acute* conditions. But many other conditions—such as diabetes, multiple sclerosis, or HIV infection, to name just a few—cannot be cured. These are called *chronic* conditions. Although it may not be possible for them to be cured, they can be treated or "managed" to minimize their impact on one's life.

Acute Illness

Acute illnesses often run their course without any direct medical intervention. For example, a cold or a sprain or a rash will usually get better on its own, and home remedies or over-the-counter products may help. This is common knowledge and does not usually require a doctor's advice. Many self-help books are available with information on dealing with common acute illnesses.

Other acute illnesses, such as a heart attack or pneumonia, can be serious or life-threatening and require medical evaluation or treatment. Most people have very good judgment about when they need to see a doctor and when they can deal with a problem themselves. Sometimes a symptom is so overwhelming that it is obviously a medical emergency. If you develop crushing chest pain, I trust that you will call 911 and take an ambulance to the emergency room rather than trying to get through to your doctor for advice.

Chronic Illness

Chronic, or long-term, illnesses are a part of many people's lives. For many gay men, HIV infection is a chronic condition, one that must be lived with day in and day out. Many other chronic illnesses are common among the population of gay men that I take care of. Examples include heart conditions, prostate problems, diabetes, arthritis, hepatitis, and high blood pressure.

Chronic illness is a situation where it is very important to have a personal physician that you trust, to help treat you and advise you on how to deal with your condition. Often, you will not need to see a specialist. Your primary care physician is able to manage most medical problems. In some cases, as with HIV infection, it helps to have a primary care provider who is knowledgeable enough to treat you without needing to send you to a specialist. See the section titled "Finding Your Primary Care Provider" for further discussion of this.

As a doctor, it's very rewarding when I can help "cure" someone of a condition so that they no longer have to deal with it at all. But the reality is that many conditions simply cannot be cured. Given this situation, my job as a physician is then to help the person manage his chronic medical condition(s) in order to minimize the impact on his quality of life.

Being diagnosed with a chronic or incurable condition can be emotionally devastating at first. Having such a condition means that you must accept and adapt to having the condition indefinitely. It can take some adjustment, if you have always enjoyed good health, to find out that you have a medical condition that cannot be cured. That sort of news can make a person depressed, angry, sad, hopeless. It is a reminder that our bodies are imperfect and that we are mortal.

With time most people with a chronic condition adjust and move on with life. They accept that the illness is a new part of their reality, and they cope with it the way one copes with all the other givens of life. As time goes on it seems like less and less of a big deal. Many people find that humor helps them deal with a chronic or life-threatening illness. An ironic sense of humor about the ridiculousness of it all, is a common theme in memoirs of people coping with serious illness. (See Appendix.)

Some conditions can be life-threatening when they occur. Having a brush with death gives a person a new and different perspective on his life. Anyone who has been near death or who has been close to someone who has had this experience is forever changed.

Life With a Chronic Condition

Marty: *Until I was 47 I was never sick a day in my life. Then out of the blue I started getting chest pain, and I ended up in the hospital with a heart attack. It was a shock. I had thought I was invulnerable. What a reality check! At first I was really depressed. I kept going over and over in my head—Why was this happening to me, what had I done wrong?*

Eventually I accepted that I did indeed have this condition and that it had to be faced and dealt with. Now I've stopped smoking, and have begun a careful exercise program. I take three different medications a day to lower my cholesterol, keep my blood pressure down, and protect my heart from further damage. It took me a while, but I know that these things are necessary for me to protect my health. I know I have a heart condition, and I know how precious my health is. I'm just glad I'm still here. I call the experience my wake-up call.

Management of a chronic condition may involve taking medication regularly. It also usually involves lifestyle changes that may include a particular type of diet, regular physical activity such as exercises or stretches, and other behavioral efforts. These efforts are rewarded by a reduction in symptoms from the chronic disease, a reduction in worry about the impact of the disease on one's health, and a sense of empowerment in doing something positive to maintain one's health.

Everyone responds differently to advice about his health. Some problems—such as diabetes, high blood pressure, and elevated cholesterol—can be treated very well by lifestyle efforts—such as diet, exercise, and smoking cessation—without any medication. It's always healthier to cultivate good habits in the first place than to simply take a pill for whatever goes wrong. But most people find it very difficult to stop smoking or to start exercising regularly, and most find it easier to take a medication. (Though taking medication faithfully is a challenge in itself.)

The Case of HIV Infection

HIV infection is the most common chronic disease I see among the gay men I take care of. People with HIV infection have some particular issues to deal with. For example, for years HIV was seen as a uniformly fatal virus. A diagnosis of HIV infection was equivalent to a death sentence. People with HIV had to work on trying to maintain their health with the knowledge that they would probably die of AIDS.

Currently, many people infected with with HIV are enjoying renewed or continued good health as the result of taking combinations of anti-HIV medications. But there are many problems with these medications, including cost, side effects, the psychological burden of taking HIV medications, and the challenge of remembering to take the pills.

Rather than leaving pills in their original bottles, many people find it easier to by a multiple-compartment box, or Medi-Set, which contains a space for each dose of medication during the day. At the proper time, one takes the contents of one of the compartments. That way the person can make sure he takes every dose, which is very important for these medications. Some people purchase watches with alarms on them to remind them of when the next dose is due. Some people have a partner, lover, or coworker help them remember to take their medications. Whatever it takes.

These new treatments bring new stresses. For one thing, they do not work for everyone. Some people cannot be helped by any of the anti-HIV medications now available, and they are becoming ill from AIDS. They must face friends and family who do not understand why they are becoming ill when AIDS now has a reputation for being manageable and not serious.

Others are doing very well with the new medications. Many who were ill and disabled are now better and returning to work or school, sometimes after years away. They are dealing with starting their lives over again, redirecting their goals after preparing and expecting to die young. They also have the uncertainty of wondering how long the medications will continue working. No one knows.

HIV can be a stress for relationships. It can make dating difficult. For example:

Kensho: *I'm still single, but I came close last fall. I met a wonderful man. We took it slow—dinner, movies. On our fourth date he said he had to talk to me about something. He told me he was beginning to have strong feelings for me. He wanted me to know he was HIV-positive. I told him that I was negative but that it didn't make any difference to me what he was. But he didn't agree. He said he wanted to stop seeing me because he didn't want to fall in love with an HIV-negative man. He couldn't deal with it. I understood, but I wasn't happy. For a minute I wished I was positive.*

Serodiscordant couples—where one member has HIV and the other does not—have their own stresses. Some couples deal well with this difference, and it does not harm their relationship. In others, a difference in health status can cause the relationship to end.

For example, sometimes the two members of a couple can take on roles around HIV. One is the patient, the other the caregiver. In the old days when the illness was fatal, often the caregiver maintained this role until the death of his partner. Now that HIV/AIDS may no longer be fatal, many couples are severely stressed by these roles—often to the point of breaking up. Some examples:

Dan: *Dean almost died of pneumonia, and I was there for him. He pulled through, and for the next year I was his full-time nurse. We were expecting him to die. Then when the antiviral cocktail came out, he wanted to try. It worked great for him. He got better. His energy came back. He isn't sick any more, and he is going back to school. Meanwhile I did some soul-searching and realized we didn't have anything in common any more. The only reason I stayed with him was because he needed me. Now he doesn't, and it's time for me to move on.*

Pat: *Pete was really sick with AIDS. He had given up. I was his advocate to his doctor. He belonged to an HMO, and it was very hard to get them to treat him right. The attitude was, "He's going to die anyway." Well, not if I had anything to do with it. I called the drug companies and found out how to get him on protease inhibitors before they were approved. I went with him to every doctor visit and made sure he got the most aggressive treatment. He did very well. The drugs gave him back his life. After four years on disability, he went back to work. Problem is, when he got better he decided he didn't need me anymore, and he left. I'm angry, and I feel like he used me.*

Disability Benefits

A person can feel perfectly healthy and function perfectly well while having a chronic condition. But despite everyone's best efforts, chronic disease sometimes does lead to disability. Disability means just what it says: a person is unable to work due to a physical or mental problem. In other words, just having a certain medical condition or test result does not necessarily mean a person is disabled.

I frequently encounter patients who feel they are disabled because they have a positive HIV antibody test or because they have a CD4 (T cell) count under 200 (meeting the CDC definition of AIDS). But these blood-test results say nothing about one's ability to work. Neither does high blood sugar, high blood pressure, or high cholesterol. All of these are simply indications of an underlying medical condition that needs to be recognized and dealt with.

A person who is disabled may be entitled to certain benefits. These may come from the government or from private disability insurance companies or from the person's employer. Part of my job is to communicate with these agencies on my patients' behalf.

The U.S. Social Security Administration handles Social Security Disability payments. To be eligible the disabled person must have worked enough to qualify. Application entails filling out a detailed questionnaire about symptoms, the history of the illness, the impact of the illness on the person's life, and current daily activities.

To corroborate the disability claim, I forward copies of the person's medical record for review. If the medical record does not indicate that the person is truly disabled, the claim will be denied, though it can be appealed. If a patient of mine tells me that he is applying for disability, I feel it is my obligation to tell him honestly whether or not I think he is truly disabled and whether his application will be granted. My prediction is not always correct.

In addition to Social Security Disability, many people have private insurance or a disability benefit from their employer that pays them a monthly stipend if they become disabled. Claiming disability benefits from a private policy seems to be easier, and it seems to rely more on the doctor's word that the person is truly disabled. Again, I think it is fairest to be honest, so if a patient of mine wants to claim disability, I tell him whether or not I agree that he is disabled.

Medical records are an important part of the documentation that helps determine whether a person qualifies for disability. If you have symptoms that are interfering with your life and your ability to work, it is important that you let your doctor know about these symptoms, even if nothing can be done about them. The doctor should document them in your medical chart to form a paper trail if the question of disability arises later.

Disability need not last a lifetime. This is a time of change for people with HIV and AIDS. AIDS used to be a progressive condition that was inevitably fatal. Once a person qualified for AIDS-related disability, he tended to get sicker and sicker until he ultimately died.

But now, many people who were disabled by AIDS are doing so much better that they are entertaining thoughts of returning to work. The Social Security Administration makes allowance for people to return part-time and/or for a trial period without losing their benefits. This makes it easier for a person who has been disabled for several years to test the waters. But in addition, the Social Security Administration staff are not a bunch of dummies. They realize that many people with AIDS have gotten better lately, so they are reevaluating the status of many individuals who have been disabled for AIDS-related reasons. If you have been on disability for AIDS and are doing better now, you should be considering reentering the work force, even though the long-term situation remains unknown.

Death and Dying

Death is an inevitable event in every human life. Each of us is born, and each must die, and the important part is what we do with the time in between those two events. We expect to be allotted the proverbial "three score and ten" years, but numbers of gay men have died far short of that mark due to AIDS. Our community has had to deal with the premature deaths of many of our brothers in the past 15 years. Fortunately, that situation appears to be changing.

Modern American culture is not good at dealing with death. We tend to fear and deny it. Things were better in the past, when dying people were cared for at home by their loved ones, and death occurred in familiar surroundings. Today, most deaths in the United States occur in hospitals, often in a cold, sterile environment filled with technological devices. Many adults have never been present at the death of a loved one or seen a dead body, though they have seen lots of very unrealistic deaths in the movies. As a result, most people do not have a good idea of the reality of the process of death, so they are poorly prepared to deal with the impending death of a loved one or with their own future demise.

Fortunately, there is a trend lately for people to spend their last days at home or in a hospice or other facility where their comfort is paramount and where their loved ones can be with them. But this sort of scenario is still the exception.

Discussing a Terminal Prognosis With Your Doctor

Doctors are frequently uncomfortable discussing death with their patients or helping them have a better dying process. Medical training has to do with saving and preserving life, and death is viewed too often as a defeat, despite our knowledge that every person dies some time. Often the patient knows he is dying or at least is terminally ill, yet the doctor will not acknowledge that for fear of taking away the patient's hope.

I admit that some of this applies to me. I have some discomfort in discussing a patient's impending demise with him, and I sense a similar discomfort on the part of many of my patients. I'm working on that. I have learned that some terminally ill or dying patients seem to feel very comfortable in discussing what's ahead for them, and I find that very helpful and actually liberating.

If a life-threatening illness affects you or someone you love, I encourage you to have an honest discussion with the doctor about what lies ahead. Try to put the doctor at ease with the reassurance that knowing the truth will not take away hope. If your time may be limited, it can be helpful to know that so that you can plan and prioritize how you will use that time.

Do remember that doctors are not clairvoyant. Terminally ill people sometimes ask me, "How long do I have to live? A month? Six months? A year?" I tell them, "A day—if you don't look both ways before crossing the street. Beyond that, I can't give you a number." Doctors cannot predict the future, and unpredictable things happen daily in medicine. Don't think your doctor is holding back on you by not telling you exactly what day you will die.

What doctors can reasonably do is quote statistics, such as, "Of people with your stage of prostate cancer, only 10% live five years." That statement does not mean you do or do not have five years to live; it tells you what the odds are that you will be alive five years from now. There's a big difference. Or: "Of people with pneumocystis carinii pneumonia, ten to 20% do not recover and die of the pneumonia." Again, that tells you roughly what your chances are. But maybe those ten to 20% were the very sickest ones, and where do you fit on that spectrum—how severe a case do you have? Ask your doctor.

You Have Choices

Doctors can also discuss the possible future symptoms of the disease, what course it might take, and what treatment options there are. We can discuss the pros and cons of various treatments—the possible benefits, potential risks, and side effects. As the patient, you have the final say about your treatment, so it is good that you know as much as possible about your chances with various options.

When faced with a terminal prognosis, it's helpful to let the doctor know what your priorities are. If you are almost through writing the great American gay novel, you may want aggressive treatment, in an attempt to prolong your life just enough to finish your life's work, even if the treatment causes pain or discomfort.

Or if you don't feel you have any unfinished business and just want to hold court in your bed, surrounded by your four cats and three devoted ex-lovers, then perhaps all you want is medication to keep you comfortable and nothing more. No law says that a person must accept any medical treatment he does not want, so that even if there is a treatment for your problem, it is your right to decline it if you choose. Your doctor works for you and should be able to help you set up the last stage of your life the way you'd like it.

The Goal: A Good Death

What is a "good death"? Given that we all must die, a good death is a process that involves the minimum of pain, discomfort, and indignity—ideally, one in which the dying person has had the opportunity to speak with his loved ones and say his good-byes; and one that leaves pleasant memories as opposed to nightmares for the survivors. Even with the best intentions of all concerned, this is not always achieved, but it is a good goal. If you learn that you may be dying soon, your doctor can help ensure that the process goes the way you want it to. The important thing is communication.

What about hastening death in the case of terminal illness? This is a controversial subject, and it has been litigated in several courts in the United States in recent years. The voters of one state, Oregon, have made physician-assisted suicide legal under certain conditions. The practice has always occurred, quietly. It is important to distinguish between depression with hopelessness and suicidal wishes and a terminal condition with intolerable suffering and a rational wish to end life. Sometimes a health care provider or mental-health therapist can help sort this out.

Here again, open communication between you and your doctor is essential. Some doctors are opposed to assisted suicide under any circumstances, and some are more open to the idea. Perhaps the doctor is just not aware of the symptoms, and perhaps better symptom control can easily be accomplished. Any doctor should be able to pledge to control terminal pain and suffering to your complete satisfaction. If you or someone you love is terminally ill and there are intolerable symptoms, the doctor is failing and needs to do better.

Coping With a Terminal Illness

I t's not pleasant to find out that you—or a friend, lover, or family member—is serious-ly ill. Especially if it's the first time you've dealt with serious illness, it can be very scary and difficult. But it's also a very rewarding experience. The story of Michael, Tony, and Matt will illustrate how one man's illness may affect his relationship with people who are close to him.

Michael: *I hadn't heard from my old lover Tony in a while, and now I hear that he has pancreatic cancer and isn't expected to live more than a few months. What a shock. We haven't been lovers in years, but he's one of my dearest friends. I guess I assumed he'd always be there. I don't know what to do. I'd like to call him but I just don't know what to say. Any suggestions?*

It's natural to feel uncomfortable relating to someone who is seriously ill. But if you have an ill friend, you can give him a great gift by continuing to be his supportive companion dur-ing his illness.

Many patients of mine have told me that their illness really separated out their true buddies from their superficial friends. The true buddies are not afraid to be there "in sick-ness and in health," while the superficial friends disappear when a problem comes up. Being around a sick person isn't as much fun as being with a healthy one. It forces the healthy person to confront his own vulnerability and mortality. Often a man who thought he had lots of friends finds out when he becomes ill how few really loyal friends he has. It is not even unusual for a man to become ill and then have his lover leave him shortly afterwards.

Tony: *When my doctor first told me I had pancreatic cancer, I was shocked. At 55 I expect-ed to live another 20 years anyway. But my father and brother both died of pancreatic cancer in their fifties, and now it was my turn. I decided not to have heroics, like chemo, since they did-n't help my father or brother.*

I was afraid to tell Matt, my lover. I guess I felt like I was abandoning him by dying. But he was wonderful. He has a great attitude. He helped me figure out my priorities, like for instance quitting my job. He also called my closest friends and told them, so I didn't have to. That was a great load off my mind. Some of our friends were great, really rose to the occasion. Others we never heard from.

If someone important to you becomes ill, remember that everything is the same except that now the illness is part of that person's life. Just as the ill person has had to make an adjust-ment to the fact of his illness, so you also will have to go through a period of dealing with the fact that this person is now ill. Once you accept that, you can use your past relationship with that person as the basis for your future relationship in the context of his illness.

Michael: *I called Tony, and his partner Matt answered the phone. He said that Tony was still weak since getting home after his surgery, but he wasn't in a lot of pain. He put Tony on the phone, and we chatted for a minute. Tony sounded very happy to hear from me. He asked how my new job was going, and he didn't seem to want to talk about his own situation. He invit-ed me to visit tomorrow afternoon.*

Visiting an Ill Friend

Michael was anxious about the visit, so I gave him some more advice. When seeing a friend for the first time after he has become ill, be prepared that he might look different. He might have lost weight, and his hair might be thinner or gone, for example. Remember that these are superficial things and that inside is the same person you knew before.

Avoid commenting on the person's appearance, unless he brings it up. Don't lie to flatter him because it won't work. Don't say, "I know you've been sick, but you're looking great!" If you do, the response will probably be something like this: "No I don't. Let's get real—I look like shit. You look like life's agreeing with you, though."

Some other suggestions for visiting an ill friend:

Don't stay too long. It takes energy to play host.

Bringing flowers or a small gift is OK. Bringing food can be OK if the illness is not inter-fering with the person's appetite or ability to eat. If in doubt, check it out beforehand.

Chat about how things are going or about outside things, such as mutual friends or recent events in your life. The ill person may not want to talk about his illness, and it may be refreshing for him to hear about what's going on with you. Let him guide you on this.

Offer to read to him—the newspaper or a short story.

It's OK to tell jokes, to laugh. In fact, it's therapeutic. People who are ill see more serious, grim faces than they should.

Consider sitting there with your friend for a while, holding his hand and not saying anything. Ask, "Do you mind if I just sit here with you for a few minutes?"

If the person is in the hospital:

You might offer to bring in some of his favorite music to listen to.

Some hospitals now allow pets to visit. If your friend has a pet, you might offer to bring it in for a visit. On the other hand, if the pet is a goldfish or a parakeet, you might offer to feed it while your friend is in the hospital.

If your partner is ill and hospitalized, many hospitals will allow you to sleep in his room with him, and they may provide you a cot for this purpose.

Caregivers Need Relief

Matt: *Michael's visit went very well. In fact, I used the opportunity to go out to the store. I realized that I had not been out of the house in the three days since Tony came home from the hospital. Michael has volunteered to come over every Tuesday afternoon to spend time with Tony. It's a great relief for me.*

No matter how much we love someone, we need some time for ourselves as well. Taking care of a very ill person is more than a full-time job, and it doesn't leave any time for the caregiver to recharge his own batteries. Caregivers must have the time and space to take care of themselves as well. Otherwise, they are in danger of burning out and resenting the person they are taking care of.

Tony: *Matt's been getting crabby with me, and I know it's not my fault. It's just cabin fever. I called my doctor, and he arranged for me to be in a hospice program. The hospice nurse will come over once a week to make sure everything is going OK, and two mornings a week a young man, called a chore worker, will change and wash the bedding, clean me up, and clean up my room. Usually Matt does these things every day. This will be great because it gives Matt a break.*

The Last Stages

A few months later Michael called to let me know that Tony was in a coma and would probably be dying soon. Again, he was anxious about visiting him in that condition and wanted some guidance. I gave him the following tips:

If you visit someone who is unconscious:
- It is OK to talk to other people in the room about him, but assume that he can hear everything you say.
- It is definitely OK to talk to him, hold his hand, stroke his cheek or his head.
- You can play music for him if you know what he might like.
- You may want to read something to him.
- Don't try to feed him.

If you visit someone (conscious or unconscious) who is dying:
- All of the above are OK.
- You may want to say good-bye to him.
- You may want to tell him you love him and that you'll miss him.
- It is OK to cry.
- It is *not* OK to say "Don't go" or "I don't know what I'll do when you are gone." Give him permission to die.

Tony ended up dying a few weeks later. Michael and Matt were both with him when he died. Each man has since told me that being with Tony during his illness and death was one of the most powerful and beautiful experiences he has had.

Too many of us abandon our friends when they become ill. But it is a great privilege to be permitted to walk alongside someone during the course of a life-threatening illness, be it cancer or AIDS or something else. Don't be afraid. Go for it.

Medical-Legal Issues

Gay people have a special, inferior legal status in the United States. We do not automatically have all of the same rights as others. We may have come a long way in social acceptance. We are protected individually by nondiscrimination laws in a few places. But that's about it. Our unequal civil-rights status means that at times of illness or death, the law is often not on our side. By taking the proper steps in advance, we can make things work a bit easier for ourselves when a medical crisis occurs.

Legal Issues for Gay Couples

Gay couples in general have no legal standing in the United States. No matter how long two men have been together, they are strangers in the eyes of the law. That is, unless they draw up certain documents that make specific provisions for each other in the event of illness, disability, or death. The majority of gay couples do not think to do this until it is too late.

Larry: *Claude and I were together for 24 years. We owned a home together, and we filled it with Claude's paintings. All of our friends knew us as a couple. Our lives were completely shared. We never thought about putting any of it in writing. Our relationship was based on trust.*

Last year, out of the blue, Claude had a massive stroke. It left him in a permanent coma. Claude had always told me and his doctor that he "did not want to be a vegetable," but he left no papers to prove that. I found out that I could not make medical decisions for him because I wasn't his legal spouse.

While Claude was in intensive care, his family arrived in town and insisted he be kept on life support. He had not spoken with his parents in years, and that was the first time I had met them. Even so, they were his legal next of kin, and they had the right to make these decisions for him. Claude was in the hospital and then a nursing home for a month. They fed him through tubes until his doctors and I convinced his parents to let him die.

Claude did not leave a will. After he died his parents came into our home and started packing up things from the house to take back to Kansas. These were the mementos of our life together. It took a court order to get Claude's parents out, but meanwhile they took most of his art. My lawyer says I have no chance of contesting their claim to his savings and retirement accounts, and now they are suing me for half the value of the house we owned together. If I want to keep living there, I have to buy them out.

This story is not an exaggeration. It happens all the time. I have lived through dramas like it over and over with my patients. It breaks my heart, it makes me angry, and it can all be avoided. Easily.

Of course I am angry at the law, which ignores the spousal rights of gay couples. But I am just as angry at men like Claude, who let themselves and their partners down by not making preparations in advance. The system is unfair, but the unfairness can be avoided with some simple preparation in advance.

Essential Legal Documents

Every gay man should have a set of legal documents, easily obtained, that will ensure that his wishes are carried out in case of serious illness, disability, or death. These include a living will (or advance directive), a durable power of attorney for health care, a general power of attorney, and a last will and testament.

Claude, like the majority of gay men, had none of these. They are especially important for those men with HIV/AIDS, who know that they may face illness or death earlier than the rest of us. But a medical crisis can happen to anyone, at any age. By definition, no one expects a sudden medical catastrophe. Why intentionally make it worse by being unprepared?

Nobody likes to think about the eventuality of his own incapacity or death. Maybe that's why the majority of U.S. citizens die without a will. But put yourself in Claude's place, or

Larry's, and maybe that will help motivate you to make provisions in advance. After all, we all must die, whether or not we like to deal with that fact.

If you have not made your wishes known in advance and become incapacitated by illness or die, laws do exist that dictate who should take over your affairs. The problem is that these laws were not written with gay people in mind, and they are not on our side.

For instance, if you become incapacitated and you have not previously designated a spokesperson, the law says that your legal spouse is your nearest next of kin and should speak for you. If you have no spouse, then your parent, adult child, or sibling becomes the decision maker—in that order. If you die without a will, the law says that your possessions go to your closest (legal) relatives. If you have no relatives, your estate goes to the government.

These laws can cause a lot of problems for gay men who have not taken the proper steps. First off, many of us have a same-sex spouse whose status is not recognized by the law. Claude and Larry may have been a couple for 24 years, but in the eyes of the law their relationship did not exist. Our affectional partnerships—no matter how enduring—have no legal standing at all unless we draw up specific documents to that effect.

In addition, some of us are not on the best of terms with our families. We have created a "family of choice" that may have much more importance to us than our blood relations. Yet our blood relations are the only ones automatically recognized by the State.

I cannot emphasize strongly enough how important it is for each gay man to have the proper documents so that tragedies like that of Claude and Larry are not repeated. It is easy enough to do, and a lawyer is not absolutely required, though one is strongly recommended to ensure that the documents are drawn up properly.

The Living Will

Every gay man—in fact everyone in general—should have a document known as a living will. This document describes what you would want, in the event of a terminal condition or a condition of permanent coma. In a living will, you can state whether you would want life-prolonging medical treatments continued in such a case or whether you would want them stopped to allow the dying process to run its course.

By having a living will you can ensure that you are not hooked up to tubes or machines providing artificial life support when there is no hope of recovery. Once a person has witnessed a loved one spend their last days on life support with a tube in every orifice, he is usually not interested in this happening to himself, whenever the time may come.

The Advance Health Care Directive

It is also possible to create a document that is more general than a living will. An advance health care directive describes what type of treatments you might prefer if you were seriously ill but not terminal. Would you want only to be kept comfortable? Would you want to be admitted to the hospital for aggressive care? Or would you want your loved ones to decide in consultation with your doctor, taking your prognosis into account?

For example, some people with a chronic illness, such as AIDS, may choose at some point to forego any further active treatment. If you were in such a situation, dealing with an ongoing illness, and developed pneumonia or had a heart attack, you might wish to be kept comfortable at home rather than have the problem treated. Relatives could pressure you or your doctor to treat you despite your wishes, but an advance health care directive can help ensure that your wishes are carried out.

The Durable Power of Attorney for Health Care

Another document, the durable power of attorney for health care, designates a person to make medical decisions on your behalf, if you were incapacitated by illness. Normally, a competent person must consent before undergoing any medical treatment. But if you became so ill that you could not express your wishes, someone else would have to make the decision for you. If you had not designated anybody, the law requires that a legal spouse or family member make the decision.

You can designate anyone except your doctor to be your durable power of attorney for health care. All that is required is that the person know what your wishes would be in case of a serious illness.

It is good to have a frank discussion when you choose someone to be your durable power of attorney for health care to make sure they understand your philosophy and make the kind of treatment choices that you might make were you able. Are you the kind of person who would want aggressive care no matter what? Would you just want to be kept comfortable and kept at home? Or something in between?

If you have a partner, you don't have to automatically choose him to be your durable power of attorney for health care, as demonstrated by this man living with AIDS:

Sam: *No, I would never want my partner, Simon, to be my durable power of attorney for health care. He is such a dizzy queen; he absolutely came unglued when I had pneumonia last year. My girlfriend from work, Julie, really has her head together, and she and I have talked a lot about my illness and what might be coming up. She went through this with her brother, who died a few years ago, so she knows what's involved. She has agreed to be there for me. Simon understands, and I think he's relieved.*

The General Power of Attorney

Another document, the general power of attorney, gives a person the right to take over all of your affairs, in the event of your incapacity. This person can, for example, write checks on your account, to pay your bills when you are too ill to do so. Obviously this must be someone you trust a great deal. If you have a partner, he is usually the person to choose for this responsibility.

You Don't Really Need a Lawyer, But....

The exact wording of a living will, an advance health care directive, and of a power of attorney document may vary from state to state, depending on local laws. It is not necessary to see a lawyer to complete these documents, though one is highly recommended. A copy of the document appropriate for you state, with a signature and sometimes a notary's seal, is all that is needed. A set of the documents for the State of Washington is included at the end of this section.

Even though a lawyer is not necessary for drawing up these papers, I do advise all of my gay male patients to have a session with a lawyer. Especially if you are in a relationship, it's important to make the effort to make everything as kosher as possible. For heterosexuals, a marriage license instantly legitimizes the relationship in the eyes of the law, creating hundreds of spousal rights. For gay men, on the other hand, every relationship right needs to be created by a legal document.

For example, a lawyer can write up a "relationship agreement" that defines who owns what in case of a dissolution. He can go over your advance directives and make sure they say what you want them to say. And he can write up a document that says who you would and would not want to visit you in the hospital. I don't know whether such a document has the force of law, but I have seen them, and I know they impress hospitals enough to get the job done.

Where to Keep These Papers

Once you have completed your documents, please, please, please bring copies to your doctor! Originals are not required. Your medical record definitely is the best place to keep a copy of them—not your safety deposit box, not your lawyer's office, not your office safe. Most people tend to keep them in one of these places.

Think about it. If you were in a terrible accident or had a heart attack on the dance floor and were rushed to the hospital, no one would run to the bank and open up your safety deposit box to find out who your durable power of attorney for health care should be or whether you have a living will describing your life support preferences. But your doctor should be able to go straight to your medical chart and find out. Make sense?

Hospital Visitation

Mike: *My partner Spike was in an accident at work. His injuries were pretty serious, and he was in the hospital for two weeks, having a series of operations. It was the first time we had slept apart in four years. The hospital had a policy permitting a family member to stay overnight in the patient's room, but since I wasn't officially family, they wouldn't let me stay. The next day I brought in Spike's durable power of attorney for health care, which named me as his decision maker in case of coma or whatever. The head nurse acted like I was crazy. She told me Spike was perfectly able to make decisions for himself. But I told her that this piece of paper was the only way I could show that I was Spike's family, and I demanded to spend the night in his room. The hospital eventually let me stay.*

Hospital visitation rights are a difficult area for gay people. We've all heard stories of gay men who, when they are hospitalized, find that the hospital lets their parents but not their lover visit. Fortunately, this is happening less and less. Thanks to AIDS, many hospital personnel understand gay relationships much better now, and they seem to respect gay men's partners and friends.

Still, there is no standard legal document that will give a gay partner hospital visitation privileges. You could try to have your lawyer invent one for you, and I'm sure he'd be happy to do so. If you have trouble with visitation rights, you might take Mike's example and use a durable power of attorney for health care if you have one, even if your partner is not incapacitated. Or if you live in a place that recognizes same-sex domestic partnership, a domestic partnership certificate can help. Your doctor might be able to intercede if all else fails. It's another reason your doctor should know you are gay and be aware of your support system.

Last Will and Testament

When you die, documents such as power of attorney or domestic-partnership certificates become invalid because legally you have no rights as a dead person. In the eyes of the law you no longer exist. But a will ensures that your wishes are carried out after your death. The will stipulates what happens to your property after you are gone. It also specifies an executor who will manage your estate. And it can dictate what is to be done with your remains. If you have a partner and you die without a will, your partner has absolutely no rights, and the consequences could be very difficult for him.

Look at what Larry went through when Claude died without a will. A man like Larry stands to inherit nothing. He may even have to move out of the house where he has lived for years. The entire estate goes to the deceased's legal relatives, and if there are none, the State claims the property. How any of us can do this to the man we love is hard to imagine, but remember that over half of us die without wills, so it happens all the time. We don't like to remind ourselves that we all must die some day, so we put off dealing with it. Our survivors have to deal with it.

Wills can be written without the help of a lawyer, especially if they are simple. You can buy a blank will at a stationery store. However, wills can be contested, so homemade ones are a bad idea for most gay men. If you have any significant assets or have a partner or want to clearly stipulate what happens to your remains or want to ensure that your blood relatives do not contest your will, then you will need to consult a lawyer. Lawyers have some useful tricks—like the nifty phrase that says, "Anyone who contests this will is entitled to inherit no more than $1." I like that one.

Many lawyers are experienced with the needs of unmarried couples and/or gay men. Such a lawyer can help you draw up a full set of the legal documents described in this section. Even if you are young and in perfect health, believe me, you'll feel a great sense of accomplishment when you've gotten it done. My partner and I finally did ours a few years ago, so I know.

Washington Advance Health Care Directives
(Courtesy of the King County Medical Society)

Expression of Intent to Physicians and Caregivers: Approach to Serious Medical Problems

In most instances, when medical problems arise, you and your relatives discuss the situation with your physician and make the appropriate decisions. Occasionally, medical decisions need to be made when you are not able to communicate your wishes and/or your relatives cannot be reached to insure that your wishes are followed. Therefore, it is important to state in advance what you would want if you developed a potentially disabling or fatal illness.

In all circumstances, measures that by current medical standards provide comfort and alleviate pain will be taken.

Measures that are considered futile by current medical standards will not be provided.

Please indicate the statement that best expresses your wishes in the event of serious medical problems:

_____ A. I want all measures to insure my survival (including hospitalization, consultations, surgery, life-support systems and tube feedings).

_____ B. I want my physician to use his/her judgment in providing measures considered likely to return me to an acceptable state of health. (If no choice is indicated, this option will usually be followed.)

_____ C. I want only those measures that provide comfort and maintain dignity. In making this choice I accept that my death may come more quickly.

A. In following my instructions I prefer:

_____ To be admitted to a hospital if indicated.

_____ NOT to be admitted to a hospital.

B. In following my instructions I prefer:

_____ IV fluid and/or tube feeding to provide nutrition and water.

_____ No IV fluid and/or tube feeding to provide nutrition and water.

Signature

(Print name)   Date

Witness

(Print name)   Date

Physician's signature

(Print name)   Date

Washington Advance Health Care Directives
Directive to Physicians
(Living Will)

Directive made this _____ day of _____(month, year)

I, _____ being of sound mind, willfully, and voluntarily make known

my desire that my life shall not be artificially prolonged under the circumstances set forth below and do hereby declare that:

1. (You may choose to check, by initialing, either one of the following options or both in order to provide direction to your physician.)

> (a)_____ If I should be in an incurable or irreversible condition with no expectation of recovery, I do not want any treatment that will merely prolong my dying. Thus I want my treatment limited to medical and nursing measures that are intended to keep me comfortable, to relieve pain, and to maintain my dignity.

> (b)_____If I am in a coma that my doctors reasonably believe to be permanent or a persistent vegetative state, I do not want any life-prolonging treatment to be provided or continued, including artificially provided nutrition and/or hydration.

> (c) Additionally, I_____

> _____

> _____

> _____

2. In the absence of my ability to give directions regarding the use of life-sustaining procedures, it is my intention that this directive shall be honored by my family and physician(s) as the final expression of my legal right to refuse medical or surgical treatment and I accept the consequences from such refusal.

3. If I have been diagnosed as pregnant and that diagnosis is known to my physician, this directive shall have no force or effect during the course of my pregnancy.

4. I understand the full import of this directive, and I am emotionally and mentally competent to make this directive.

Signed: _____

_____
City, County, and State of Residence

The declarer has been personally known to me, and I believe him or her to be of sound mind.

Witness_____

Witness_____

Durable Power of Attorney for Health Care
(Designation of Agent for Health Care Decisions)

1. I, _____ (your name) as principal, designate and appoint the person listed below as my attorney-in-fact for health care decisions (hereafter, Agent).

Designee: Name_____

             Address_____

             City/State_____Telephone_____

2. Powers Related to Health Care Decisions

My agent for health care decisions shall have the following powers:

To make health care decisions on my behalf if I am unable to do so, including informed consent to health care providers. Included in this power is the authority to make decisions about life-prolonging medical procedures, such as (but not limited to) a respirator, placement or removal of tubes to provide nutrition or hydration, antibiotics, placement or removal of tubes to provide nutrition or hydration, antibiotics, and cardiopulmonary resuscitation.

I intend my agent to have the authority to consent to giving, withholding, or stopping my health care treatment, service or diagnostic procedure. All of this is to be in keeping with my instructions below or in my Directive to Physicians (Living Will).

Instructions:_____

_____

_____

By completing this document, I intend to create a durable power of attorney for health care. It shall take effect upon my incapacity to make my own health care decisions and shall continue during that incapacity to the extent permitted by law or until I revoke it.

By signing this document, I indicate that I understand the purpose and effect of this durable power of attorney for health care.

(You must sign this in the presence of a Notary Public for it to be valid.)

Dated this _____ day of _____, 19_____   Signed_____

State of _____ County of _____

On this day personally appeared before me, _____ to me known to be the individual described in and who executed the within and foregoing instrument, and acknowledged that he/she signed the same as his/her free and voluntary act and deed for the uses and purposes therein mentioned.

Given under my hand and official seal this _____day of _____, 19_____

_____   Notary Public in and for the State of _____

residing in_____   my appointment expires_____

Living Well—A Gay Man's Personal Health Checklist

I t's easy to be overwhelmed by a book full of health advice. I'd like to leave you with a summary of some of the more important ways a gay man can have a good, healthy life. Take an inventory and see where you stand. And remember: We all age. Accept this, and do it gracefully. Focus on living well each day of your life.

☐ Find yourself a primary health care provider, and keep your preventive care up to date.

☐ Don't smoke tobacco at all.

☐ Use moderation if you drink alcohol or if you use recreational drugs. If you cannot enjoy these in moderation, avoid them completely.

☐ Eat sensibly. Avoid too much fat, and consume plenty of fiber.

☐ Get regular vigorous physical activity. Exercise regularly, or incorporate strenuous activity into your daily routine.

☐ Appreciate that sex is a wonderful and powerful gift. Be careful with it. Protect yourself and your partner(s) from sexually transmitted diseases.

☐ Make sure you are immune to hepatitis A and B. Get vaccinated if need be.

☐ Get tested for HIV as often as appropriate, and seek medical care if your test is positive.

☐ Don't delay in checking out any worrisome symptoms.

☐ Be proud and grateful that you are a gay man. Work to get rid of internalized homophobia. Come out to your family and friends, and participate in your larger community.

Appendix

The information in this book is basic. It is intended to provide you with a foundation of knowledge about aspects of gay men's health. Your doctor can provide you with more information about any particular areas of concern. In addition, you may want to explore certain health topics on your own. On the following pages, I provide an eclectic assortment of information sources on some of the topics covered in this book. Phone numbers, postal addresses, World Wide Web sites, periodicals, and books are included.

This is a very selective list, and it is not meant to be an exhaustive bibliography. It is limited to those resources that I or my patients have found useful. Many of the resources are not specifically gay-oriented but can provide general information to complement the gay-oriented information in this book. I have included my unbiased comments where appropriate. Omission of a publication, organization, or Web site from this list does not mean it is not of value. If you know of another valuable resource on a particular topic, please inform me. Web sites are predominant on the list because they are so abundant and easy to explore free of charge once one has access to the Web.

Each entry has been checked for accuracy. Keep in mind, though, that organizations may move or fold. Phone numbers and Web addresses often change. Books go out of print. If you are unable to access a resource listed here, please let me know. I will correct the information in a future edition of the book.

When seeking further information, be critical, and consider the source. Every organization, author, or Web site sponsor has a particular bias and point of view. Just because something is written in a book or pamphlet or published on the Internet does not mean it is correct.

Some Tips on Gathering and Exchanging Information Via the Internet

The Internet is a unique and wonderful new way for people around the world to communicate. People with similar interests can meet electronically to have "real time" conversations or to post messages on bulletin boards for others to read and comment on. Many of my patients have found other kindred souls with similar interests this way.

The World Wide Web is a portion of the Internet that features not only text but graphics. Web sites, made up of one or more electronic "pages," can easily be accessed electronically from anywhere in the world, via a computer connected via a modem to a phone line.

Each Web site and each page has a unique address that is used to enable a computer to find it on the Internet. A valuable feature of the Web is called a "link." Links are words or phrases or icons on a Web site that, when chosen, will take the user to a related site. Moving from site to site via links can be great fun and is called "surfing the Web." All sorts of useful and useless information can be found this way, intentionally and serendipitously. The amount of information on the Web is already vast, and it is doubling every couple of months.

Be careful when looking for health-related information on the Web. You should keep in mind several things:

> **Anyone can post anything they want on the Web.** Just because you find something on the Web does not mean that the information is accurate or true. Find out who posted or sponsored the site you are looking at. Is it a drug company, a government agency, an advocacy organization, a person with a product or service to sell, or an individual with a particular ax to grind? All of these things will give a particular slant to the information. Be skeptical.
>
> **Web sites are ephemeral.** The content can be changed at any time. This is an advantage in that it is possible to keep them updated continuously. But a site or part of a site can disappear overnight. If you find some useful information on the Web, don't assume it'll be there the next time you look. Print out a copy, or at least save a copy on your computer.
>
> **Web sites can go stale.** Check out when the site was last updated. It may have been a few years ago, and health knowledge changes fast. There is much outdated information on the Web.
>
> **The Web is not a complete resource.** You will only find information on a subject

there if someone has made an effort to post it. Some topics have legions of devotees. You will find thousands of pages devoted to popular areas such as body piercing, HIV, or foreskins. On the other hand, good luck trying to find anything useful on the subject of diarrhea in gay men. That is not a particularly sexy topic, and it does not have an advocacy group. There are many other "orphan" topics.

The Web can be a magical way to get information or find kindred souls. But surfing the Web is not always an efficient way to spend time. A person can spend hours and not find the answer to his question. Sometimes it is just easier to ask your doctor.

Resources by Topic

Aging

☐ **National Institute on Aging:** (800) 222-2225; Information Office, National Institutes of Health, Building 31, Room 5C27, 9000 Rockville Pike, Bethesda, MD 20892; brochures available on many aging-related health topics; http://www.nih.gov/nia/health/health.htm brochures available for downloading, apparently no specifically gay-related materials

☐ **American Society on Aging:** (415) 974-9600; www.asaging.org: general advocacy organization with a constituent unit for gay and lesbian issues that is accessible via their home page

Coming Out

☐ *Outing Yourself:* by Michelangelo Signorile, Fireside, 1995; helpful, commonsense advice or those who are in the coming out process

☐ **Parents, Families, and Friends of Lesbians and Gays:** (202) 638-4200; 1101 14th Street, NW, Suite 1030, Washington, DC 20005; http://pflag.org/; supportive organization for those coming out, dealing with family issues

Dealing With Illness

☐ *Eighty-Sixed; Spontaneous Combustion; Queer and Loathing:* all by David B. Feinberg; Penguin Books, 1989, 1991, and 1994; Funny, bitter, and angry series of autobiographical novels by a man who died of AIDS at age 37. Feinberg is my personal favorite AIDS author, though there are many, many other good books by and about gay men dealing with AIDS.

☐ *It's Always Something*: by Gilda Radner; Avon Books, New York; if you are dealing with HIV/AIDS, it's a refreshing change of pace to read about people's struggles with other illnesses. This is another funny book about facing death, by the Saturday Night Live comedian who died of ovarian cancer. Easily found for a dollar or two at your local thrift shop, and worth picking up.

☐ *God Said "Ha!"*: by Julia Sweeney; Bantam Books, New York, 1997; Julia, who played the androgynous Pat on Saturday Night Live and is a great friend and ally of gay people, writes about "laughing through the worst year of my life," dealing with her brother's illness with cancer and then her own cancer diagnosis.

Death and Dying

☐ **National Hospice Organization Referral Line:** (800) 658-8898
☐ **Hospice Web:** http://www.teleport.com/~hospice/
☐ **The Hemlock Society:** (800) 247-7421; PO Box 101810, Denver, CO 80250-1810; http://www.hemlock.org/hemlock; organization advocating right to die for terminally ill individuals
☐ **Compassion In Dying:** http://www.compassionindying.org; nonprofit organization supporting the right of terminally ill patients to choose to die without pain, without suffering, and with personal assistance, if necessary, to intentionally hasten death

Depression

☐ **National Depression and Manic-depressive Association:** (800) 826-3632; http://ndmda.org/ excellent information and links to support groups and other resources

Domestic Violence

☐ **National Domestic Violence Hotline:** (800) 799-7233; staffed 24 hours

☐ ***Men Who Beat The Men Who Love Them:*** by David Island, Ph.D. and Patrick Letellier, M.A.; Harrington Press, 1991; explores the phenomenon of gay male domestic violence, its causes, and who the batterers and victims are

Finding a Health Care Provider: Sources of Physician Referrals

☐ **National Gay and Lesbian Health Association:** (202) 939-7880; nonprofit organization dedicated to improving the health of lesbians and gay men

☐ **The Gay and Lesbian National Hotline:** (888) THE-GLNH (843-4564); nonprofit organization providing nationwide toll-free peer counseling, information, and referrals

☐ **Gay and Lesbian Medical Association:** (415) 255-4547; an organization of gay and lesbian physicians and their supporters; referrals available

Foreskin Advocacy and Restoration

☐ ***The Joy of Uncircumcising: Restore your Birthright and Maximize Sexual Pleasure:*** by Jim Bigelow, Ph.D., Hourglass Book Publishing, PO Box 171, Aptos, CA 95001; wonderful, thorough book on foreskins, circumcision, and foreskin restoration, with many first-person stories

☐ **http://www.nocirc.org/** home page for anti-circumcision organization, links re: circumcision)

☐ **http://www.foreskin.denver.co.us/** "Derrick Townsend's Foreskin Restoration Site;" much very useful information, stories, links to personal home pages with illustrated diaries of foreskin restoration)

HIV

☐ **National Association of People with AIDS Hotline:** (202) 898-0414

☐ **National HIV/AIDS Hotline:** (800) 342-2437, English; (800) 344-7432, Spanish;

(800) 243-7889, deaf; information and referrals. In addition, each state has a toll-free hot-line that can be identified via calling the national number.

☐ **Project Inform:** treatment hotline (800) 822-7422 or (415) 558-9051; 1965 Market Street, Suite 220, San Francisco, CA 94103; San Francisco–based treatment advocacy organization

☐ **http://projinf.org/** huge site, much useful treatment information

☐ *The HIV Drug Book:* Pocket Books, Second Edition, 1998

☐ **http://www.thebody.com/cgi-bin/body.cgi** "A Multimedia AIDS and HIV Resource"; compilation of information from various sources

☐ **http://aids.miningco.com/** similar, rich Web site

☐ **http://healthcg.com/hiv/links.html#patient** a site by the Healthcare Communications Group, made up solely of links to many HIV-oriented web sites

Insomnia

☐ **American Sleep Disorders Association:** (507) 287-6006; 1610 14th Street NW, Suite 300, Rochester, MN 55901; http://www.asda.org; with links and booklets available

Male Sexual Health

☐ **http://www.testosteronesource.com/support/other.html** drug company–sponsored Web site with good links on many aspects of male sexual health

☐ **American Foundation for Urologic Disease:** (800) 242-2383; 1128 North Charles Street, Baltimore, MD 21201; http://www.access.digex.net/~afud

Medical-Legal Issues

☐ **Lambda Legal Defense and Education:** (212) 809-8585; 120 Wall Street, Suite 1500, New York, NY 10005; http://www.lambdalegal.org/; general legal advocacy organization for the rights of all sexual-minority people, as well as those with HIV/AIDS

☐ **Partners Task Force for Gay & Lesbian Couples:** (206) 935-1206; Box 9685, Seattle, WA

98109-0685; http://www.buddybuddy.com/toc.html; advocacy and information regarding marriage rights, immigration, etc.

Parenthood

☐ **Gay and Lesbian Parents Coalition International:** (202) 583-8029; http://glpci.org/ excellent home page with many links

☐ **http://studio8prod.com/familyq/** "Family Q: The Internet Resource for Lesbian Moms and Gay Dads"

☐ **http://www.adopting.org/gaychild.html** Child Welfare League of America's policy regarding adoption by gay or lesbian individuals

☐ **http://www.adopting.org/ar.html** general adoption resources

Piercing, Tattooing, Branding, Scarification

☐ **Association of Professional Piercers:** 519 Castro Street, Box 120, San Francisco, CA 94114; http://www.sfo.com/~app/; Web site does not have referrals but has useful information about the ethics and safety of piercing, to help inform consumers

☐ ***Modern Primitives (Issue of Re/Search):*** edited by V. Vale and Andrea Juno, Re/Search Publications, 1989; illustrated interviews with people who have been tattooed and/or pierced

☐ **The Total Tattoo Book:** Amy Krakow, Warner Books, 1994; detailed and down-to-earth; list of tattooists included

☐ **http://www.mayohealth.org/ivi/mayo/9605/htm/tattoos.htm** "You Get Under My Skin—The Risks of Getting—and Getting Rid of—A Tattoo"; medical advice on tattooing

☐ **http://www.medaccess.com/consumer_rep/hc0044.htm** another page of medical advice

☐ **http://www.cybercondo.com/PUB/BODYART/scarfaq.html** Web site devoted to information on branding, cutting, and scarification as a form of body art

Plastic Surgery

☐ **Plastic Surgery Information Service:** (800) 635-0635; provides a list of five board-certified plastic surgeons in your area)

Preventive Care, Fitness, Grooming, Nutrition

☐ *Men's Health:* Rodale Press, 33 Minor Street, Emmaus, PA, 18098; http://www.menshealth.com; excellent magazine packed with articles about health, fitness, and grooming, and lots of photos of vigorous, fit men of all ages—my waiting-room copy usually disappears in a few days; generally ignores the existence of gay men except when discussing HIV/AIDS

☐ *The Zone:* by Barry Sears, Ph.D.; HarperCollins, 1995; an eating approach that can increase energy and normalize weight; a little complicated to understand at first, but it works well for those who can follow it.

Prostate Cancer

☐ **National Cancer Institute Cancer Information Service:** (800)-4-CANCER; http://rex.nci.nih.gov; current cancer information from the NCI and patient-education resources

Sexual Dysfunction

☐ **Impotence Institute of America:** (800) 669-1603; 8201 Corporate Drive, Suite 320, Landover, MD 20715

☐ **Sexual Function Health Council, c/o American Foundation for Urologic Disease:** (800) 242-2383; 1128 North Charles Street, Baltimore, MD 21201; http://www.access.digex.net/~afud/takes2.html

Sexuality

☐ *The New Joy of Gay Sex:* by Charles Silverstein and Felice Picano; HarperPerennial, Revised Edition, 1993; enjoyable to read but presented as numerous short essays arranged alphabetically rather than logically

☐ *Anal Pleasure and Health: A Guide for Men and Women:* by Jack Morin, Ph.D.; Down There Press, 3rd Revised Edition, 1998; a unique and valuable book for those interested in enjoying their anus

Sexually Transmitted Diseases

☐ **National STD Hotline:** (800) 227-8922; referrals, STD and prevention info, written info

☐ **CDC STD home page:** http://www.cdc.gov/nchstp/dstd/dstdp.htm; much info, fact sheets on individual STDs

☐ **National Herpes Hotline:** (919) 361-8488

☐ **Hepatitis B Coalition:** (612) 647-900; 91573 Selby Avenue, St. Paul, MN 55104

☐ **http://www.immunize.org/** info and links regarding hepatitis A and B

☐ **The Hepatitis Information Network:** http://hepnet.com/

☐ **http://www.boymeetsboy.com** cute site advertising hepatitis A vaccine to gay men

☐ **American Liver Foundation:** (800) 233-0179; information and referrals regarding hepatitis

Substance Use and Addiction

☐ **National Clearinghouse on Alcohol and Drug Information:** (800) 729-6686; PO Box 2345, Rockville, MD 20847; http://www.health.org

☐ **National Council on Alcoholism and Drug Dependence:** (800) 622-2255; http://www.ncadd.org links, publications, referrals

☐ **Resource Guide for Lesbians, Gays, and Bisexuals:** http://www.drugs.indiana.edu/publications/ncadi/radar/rguides/lgb.html

☐ **Alcoholics Anonymous:** check local phone directory for AA or Al-Anon orNA; gay or gay-friendly meetings exist in most areas; on-line Intergroup of AA at http://aa-intergroup.org/

☐ **American Lung Association:** (800) LUNG-USA; routed automatically to local state association; information on smoking cessation); http://www.lungusa.org/

Travel

☐ **International Gay Travel Association:** (800) 448-8550; provides information on gay tours, cruises, etc.

☐ ***Out & About:*** (800) 929-2260; PO Box 1792, New York, NY 10114-0831; home page at http://www.outandabout.com/index.html; *Out & About* is "the gay and lesbian travel newsletter;" the Web site is packed with good information and has lots of useful links.

☐ **Centers for Disease Control and Prevention:**
Travel Information Web page: http://www.cdc.gov/travel/travel.html
CDC Immunization Hotline (automated, 24-hours): (404) 332-4559

☐ **U.S. Public Health Service Information for Travelers:**

City	Phone Number
Chicago	(312) 894-2960
Honolulu	(808) 861-8530
Los Angeles	(310) 215-2365
Miami	(305) 526-2910
New York	(718) 553-1685
San Francisco	(415) 876-2872
Seattle	(206) 553-4519

Index